Qìgōng
Meditation
Embryonic Breathing

Don’t be afraid!
不用害怕！

Dare to challenge.....
敢於挑戰.....

Dare to accept.....
敢於接受.....

Dare to dream.....
敢於夢想.....

- Dare to emerge from the traditional matrix -
- be free from spiritual bondage -

“The philosopher should be a man willing to listen to every suggestion, but determined to judge for himself. He should not be biased by appearances, have no favorite hypothesis, be of no school, and in doctrine have no master. He should not be a respecter of persons, but of things. Truth should be his primary object. If to these qualities be added industry, he may indeed hope to walk within the veil of the temple of Nature.”

—Michael Faraday (1791–1867)

Qìgōng Meditation

Embryonic Breathing

Second Edition

The Foundation of Internal Elixir Cultivation

Dr. Yáng, Jwìng-Mǐng

YMAA Publication Center
Wolfeboro, NH. USA

YMAA Publication Center
PO Box 480
Wolfeboro, NH 03894
1-800-669-8892 www.ymaa.com info@ymaa.com

Second Edition Copyright ©2003, 2022

ISBN 9781594399145 (print)
ISBN 9781594399152 (ebook)
ISBN 9781594399169 (hardcover)

This book set in EB Garamond and Avenir.

First edition edited by Keith Brown and James O'Leary
Second edition copyedited by Doran Hunter
Cover design by Axie Breen
Photos by YMAA Publication Center unless otherwise noted.

20220831

Publisher's Cataloging in Publication

Names: Yang, Jwing-Ming, 1946- author.

Title: Qìgōng meditation embryonic breathing : the foundation of internal elixir cultivation / Dr. Yáng, Jwìng-Mǐng.

Description: Second edition. | Wolfeboro, NH USA : YMAA Publication Center, [2022] | Revises the 2003 first edition. | Includes bibliographical references, translation and glossary of Chinese terms, and index.

Identifiers: ISBN: 9781594399145 (paperback) | 978194399169 (hardcover) | 9781594399152 (ebook) | LCCN: 2022944129

Subjects: LCSH: Qi gong. | Qi gong--Therapeutic use. | Breathing exercises--Therapeutic use. | Mind and body. | Well-being. | Meditation. | Longevity. | Spirituality. | Medicine, Chinese. | BISAC: HEALTH & FITNESS / Longevity. | HEALTH & FITNESS / Tai Chi. | BODY, MIND & SPIRIT / Healing / Energy (Qigong, Reiki, Polarity) | SELF-HELP / Meditations.

Classification: LCC: RA781.8 .Y36 2022 | DDC: 613.7/148--dc22

Figures 1-23, 1-24, 1-25, 1-26, 1-27, 1-35, 1-38, 2-16, 3-3, and 3-5 are used by permission from the LifeART Collection of Images © 1989-1997 by Techpool Studios, Cleveland, OH.

Printed in Canada.

MIX
Paper from responsible sources
FSC® C103567
FSC www.fsc.org

Contents

ROMANIZATION OF CHINESE TERMS VIII
DEDICATION IX
FOREWORD BY DR. THOMAS G. GUTHEIL, M.D. XVII
PREFACE XIX
PUBLISHER'S NOTE ON THE 2ND EDITION XV

PART I FOUNDATIONS

CHAPTER 1 GENERAL CONCEPTS

1.1 Introduction (Jièshào, 介紹) 3
1.2 General Qìgōng Concepts (Yībān Qìgōng Gàiniàn, 一般氣功概念) 6
1.3 The Network of Qì Vessels and Channels (Qìmài Yǔ Jīngluò Wǎnglù, 氣脈與經絡網路) 31
1.4 Buddhist and Daoist Qìgōng Concepts (Fójiā Yǔ Dàojiā Zhī Qìgōng Gàiniàn, 佛家與道家之氣功概念) 38
1.5 Four Refinements (Sìhuà, 四化) 43
1.6 Five Regulatings (Wǔtiáo, 五調) 63
1.7 Muscle/Tendon Changing and Marrow/Brain Washing Qìgōng (Yìjīnjīng Yǔ Xǐsuǐjīng Qìgōng, 易筋經與洗髓經氣功) 85
1.8 Small Circulation, Grand Circulation, and Enlightenment Meditation (Xiǎozhōutiān, Dàzhōutiān, Yǔ Xiāndào Wùzhēn Jìngzuò, 小周天、大周天、與仙道悟真靜坐) 88
1.9 Definition of Embryonic Breathing (Tāixí Zhī Dìngyì, 胎息之定義) 94
1.10 Embryonic Breathing and Cultivation of the Dào (Tāixí Yǔ Xiūdào, 胎息與修道) 97
1.11 About This Book (Guānyú Zhèběnshū, 關於這本書) 102

CHAPTER 2 THEORETICAL FOUNDATION OF EMBRYONIC BREATHING

2.1 Introduction (Jièshào, 介紹) 107
2.2 Human Qìgōng Science (Rénlèi Qìgōng Kēxué, 人類氣功科學) 113
2.3 Theoretical Foundations of Embryonic Breathing (Tāixí Zhī Lǐlùn Jīchǔ, 胎息之理論基礎) 134
2.4 Meanings and Purposes of Meditation (Jìngzuò Zhī Yìyì Yǔ Mùdì, 靜坐之意義與目的) ... 144

PART II TRANSLATIONS AND COMMENTARIES OF ANCIENT DOCUMENTS RELATED TO EMBRYONIC BREATHING

CHAPTER 3 TRANSLATIONS AND COMMENTARIES OF ANCIENT DOCUMENTS

3.1 Introduction (Jièshào, 介紹) 155
3.2 General Concepts (Yībān Gàiniàn, 一般概念) 157
3.3 About the Dāntián (Guānyú Dāntián, 關於丹田) 220
3.4 Regulating the Breathing (Tiáoxí, 調息) 229
3.5 Regulating the Mind (Tiáoxīn, 調心) 241
3.6 Regulating the Spirit (Tiáoshén, 調神) 267
3.7 Methods of Embryonic Breathing (Tāixífǎ, 胎息法) 287
3.8 Other Related Documents (Qítā Yǒuguān Wénxiàn, 其他有關文獻) 306

Chapter 4 Summaries from Ancient Documents
4.1 Introduction (Jièshào, 介紹) 313
4.2 Summaries of Important Points (Yàodiǎn Zǒngjié, 要點總結) 314

Part III Practice of Embryonic Breathing
Chapter 5 Practice of Embryonic Breathing
5.1 Introduction (Jièshào, 介紹) 323
5.2 Preparation for Embryonic Breathing (Tāixí Liànxí Zhī Zhǔnbèi, 胎息練習之準備) 324
5.3 Practice of Embryonic Breathing (Tāixí Zhī Liànxí, 胎息之練習) 329
5.4 Recovery from the Meditative State (Jìngzuòhòu Zhī Huīfù, 靜坐後之恢復) 343

Chapter 6 Conclusion (Jiélùn, 結論) 347

ACKNOWLEDGMENTS 349
APPENDIX A TRANSLATION AND GLOSSARY OF CHINESE TERMS 351
INDEX 385
ABOUT THE AUTHOR 390

Dedication

To my friend whom I can't forget, Mr. Wolfgang Pastore

Dear Wolfgang:

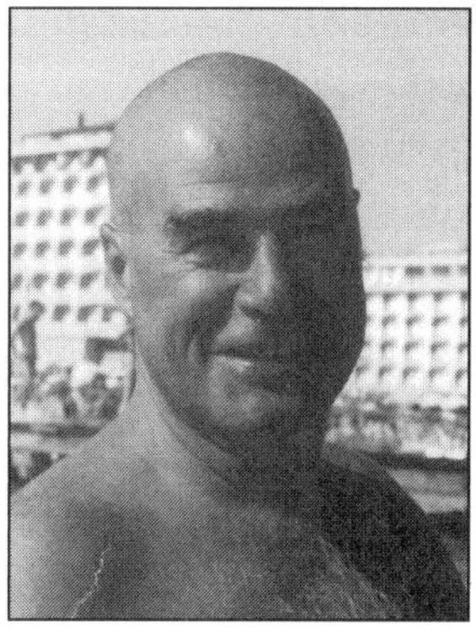

Less than three months ago we practiced Chén Style Tàijíquan together in Boston. We went to Cape Cod with others and had a great time. I remember when the other four were swimming; only you, Siu Hung, and I sat on the beach and talked. We had such a good time, and it reminded me that you took me everywhere in Italy for sightseeing. You told me that someday, you would take me to see the Tower of Pisa. Now, I don't think my dream will come true. Even if I have a chance to see it someday, the feeling will not be the same simply because you will not be there.

I was so shocked and lost when Franco called me on the 18th of July and told me the bad news. Even now, I still believe that I am dreaming and still wait to wake up. You were not just a student, but a good friend. It has not been easy to find people like you in my lifetime. However, you have passed and gone on. I promised you that I would complete the book *Small Circulation* in a couple of years. Now, I am so disappointed that you will not be able to see it. In fact, my motivation was to write a good book about Small Circulation and Grand Circulation to surprise and please you. Since I promised you, I have started to compile and research the documents, study them, ponder them, and blend them with my thirty years of experience. I was just ready to put down what I had planned for this book and was waiting to tell you when I came to Venice this September. Now, I am so sad. I wish time could return to before the 18th of this month. However, days have passed and my sorrow has grown deeper.

I looked at some of the pictures we took. I remember you took Master Liáng and me to Florence. I remember you walked with me in Venice and explained its history. I remember your expression when you saw me rowing the gondola and could not wait to take a picture of me. I also remember your depression when you could not learn the Chén Style Tàijíquan as fast as the others. I promised you that we would go over it together when I came to Venice this September. Now when I practice Chén Style Tàijíquan, I am unable to continue and finish. It reminds me of you. Only now, I start to realize how much your friendship has influenced me.

Though we were born in the same year, you always treated me as a teacher and more than a friend. We were so close that we could share philosophies and feelings without hesitation. I don't know how I could not miss you whenever I visit Venice again. It seems that you will still be there waiting for me, waiting to tell me things at which we can laugh together.

One thing that both of us agreed upon was that there was another dimension coexisting with ours, and that we will enter that dimension when we die. I hope you will be waiting for me there to tell me we were right. The end of life is not an end but the beginning of another life. That is the nature of this universe, isn't it?

I will complete the book which I promised. Your death has made me understand that I should value the rest of my life more, and try my best to share what I know with others. Knowledge is an accumulation of many lifetimes from countless ages. We should not let this knowledge die with us. If we let this happen, then we really die; otherwise, we can continue to live forever.

Whenever I am discouraged, I will remember you. Whenever I am sad, I will recall your smile and laughter. Whenever I am calm and spiritual, I will try to communicate with you. I hope you will try the same on the other side until we meet again. Good bye, dear friend.

Most sincerely yours,
Dr. Yáng, Jwìng-Mǐng
July 24, 1995

Foreword

Thomas G. Gutheil, M.D.

> *"And the Lord God formed man of the dust of the ground and breathed into his nostrils the breath of life; and man became a living soul."*
>
> —Genesis 2:7

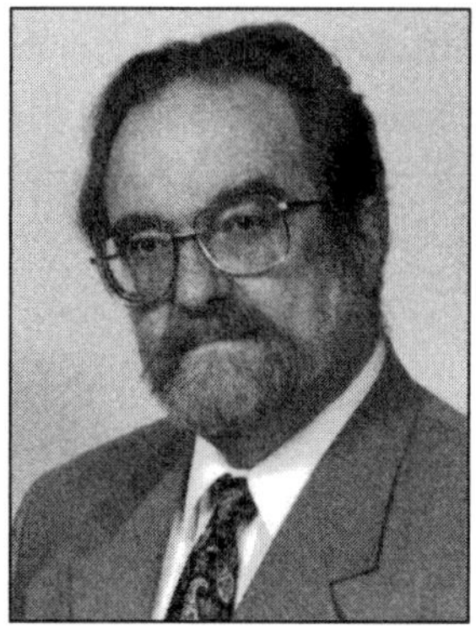

The Bible in the above quote gives to breath the ultimate creative force, not only giving life, but creating all human life. For the ancient Greeks, "psyche" meant "breath-soul," capturing how closely identified the breath of life is with life itself. For the ancient Romans, the term "inspired" literally meant "breathed into by a god or muse."

The essential role of proper breathing is recognized in vocal and instrumental music, rhetoric, public speaking, athletics, meditation, yoga and all the martial arts. This central subject receives clarification in depth by Dr. Yáng, Jwìng-Mǐng, one of the most lauded and successful translators and interpreters of ancient Chinese documents: lost works, ancient writings, mistranslated or never-translated archives and forgotten teachings that are as relevant and true today as in the remote past, when they were set down, often in secret. Bringing light to such dark corners has been a long-standing goal, even an obsession, of Dr. Yáng, a master and master teacher of martial arts with schools all over the world. His bibliography records a number of previous presentations of ancient Chinese classics now made available in English to the general reader. The present volume joins this distinguished list.

The effort to translate these arcane documents from the ancient Chinese faces formidable obstacles, each Chinese character—nay, each sound—can have multiple meanings and nuances, many totally dependent on context and many of those contexts lost. Further complicating the task are the often metaphoric and poetic imagery used instead of literal meanings and the fact that some expressions have specific meanings in Qì (energy) theory and nowhere else. Many of the writings make use of paradoxes familiar from Zen teaching: "doing without doing," for example. It is only Dr. Yáng's intimate familiarity with Qì Gōng (Qìgōng) theory and its extensive writing (many translated by himself) that permits his effort to succeed in bringing these old teachings to our present use.

One further point must be made. Few areas like the present topic so vividly demonstrate the separateness and compartmentalization of Western approaches to the mind-body synergy and the contrast with Eastern unity. We Westerners take our philosophy in school, our spiritual needs in houses of worship, our physical exercise in the gymnasium and our mental or meditative needs in holistic classes. In this text, the mental, physical and spiritual aspects of a human being are combined, not separated, integrated, not divided.

Why "embryonic" breathing? As this volume describes breathing methods in relation to Qì theory aimed at longevity and health, imagery is invoked that is related to the effortless breathless breathing of the baby in the womb; but the essential idea of an embryo captures the vision of potential mental, physical and spiritual growth towards ultimate enlightenment. After a review of Qì and Qì Gōng theory, Dr. Yáng translates and then provides detailed and essential commentary on these writings to aid the modern reader to appreciate the valuable concepts therein. As future readers, you are invited to breathe in this rare opportunity.

(Dr. Gutheil is Professor of Psychiatry at Harvard Medical School and a student at Yáng's Martial Arts Association)

Thomas G. Gutheil, M.D.
Harvard Medical School

Preface

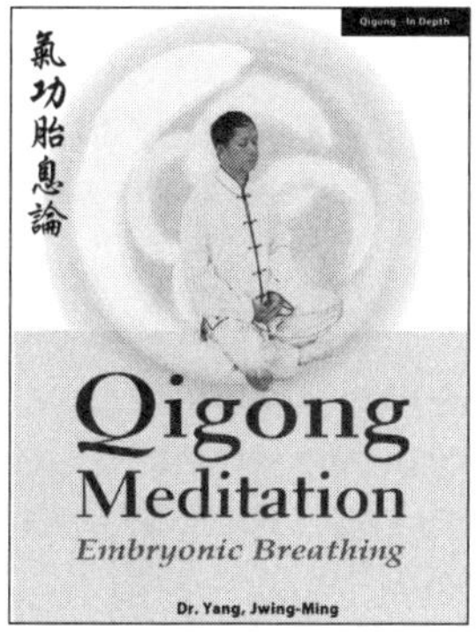

First edition, as published in 2003.

Chinese Qìgōng can generally be categorized into External Elixir (Wàidān, 外丹) and Internal Elixir (Nèidān, 內丹) Qìgōng. From External Elixir Qìgōng practice, a student learns how to build up the Qì to a higher level in the limbs and at the surface of the body. He then allows it to flow inward to the center of the body and the internal organs to nourish them. Through this practice, Qì circulation in the body can be improved and enhanced to achieve the goal of maintaining health.

In Internal Elixir Qìgōng practice, a practitioner will build up the Qì internally through correct breathing and meditation methods. When the Qì has been built up to an abundant level, this Qì will then be distributed outward to nourish the entire body and enhance its vital functions.

Experience teaches that, compared to Internal Elixir Qìgōng, External Elixir Qìgōng practice is simpler, easier, and also safer. However, the benefits that can be obtained from External Elixir practice are limited to enhancing the health of the physical body. If one wishes to reach the goal of longevity and spiritual enlightenment, Internal Elixir Qìgōng practice is essential.

The first step in practicing Internal Elixir Qìgōng is called "Small Cyclic Heaven Meditation" (Xiǎozhōutiān Jìngzuò, 小周天靜坐) or "Small Circulation Meditation." This is also commonly known as "Microcosmic Meditation" in Indian Yoga (Yújiā, 瑜珈). Although many people have heard of it, not many practice this kind of meditation, due to the difficulties and dangers involved. The reasons for this are simple: 1. There are very few experienced and qualified teachers in Qìgōng society today who are willing to take the risk of being sued due to the dangers involved in the practice. 2. It is much harder to find a sincere and committed student given today's lifestyle who will listen and last till the end of practice. The relationship between a teacher and a student is much shallower nowadays than before. This has downgraded the mutual trust between teacher and student. 3. To create a desirable environment for a profound level of meditation, such as "Small Circulation," "Grand Circulation" (Dàzhōutiān, 大周天), and "Enlightenment Meditation" (Xiāndào Jìngzuò, 仙道靜坐), is very difficult in today's society. So there are very few books or documents written and revealed to the general public. It is even harder to find any experienced teacher who is able to interpret the entire practice from a scientific point of view.

Through practicing Small Circulation Meditation, one can circulate the Qì (i.e., bioelectricity) smoothly in the Conception (Rènmài, 任脈) and Governing Vessels (Dūmài, 督脈), the two major Qì vessels which regulate the Qì circulating in the Twelve Primary

Qì Channels (Shíèrjīng, 十二經). In addition, a practitioner will also learn how to build up the Qì and store it to an abundant level in his Real Lower Dāntián (Zhēn Xiàdāntián, 真下丹田) (bio-battery). This enables the storage of a higher level of vital energy (i.e., Qì) in the body in order to strengthen the immune system and increase the lifespan. Furthermore, through practicing Small Circulation Meditation, a practitioner can find his peaceful mind and the spiritual center.

Success in Internal Elixir Qìgōng practice depends on whether a practitioner knows how to build up the Qì (i.e., Elixir) to a higher level and then store it inside his body. In order to store the Qì to an abundant level, a practitioner must locate the Dāntiáns (丹田) (i.e., Elixir Fields), and know how to build up and store the Qì. To reach this goal, a practitioner must first know the theory and techniques of Embryonic Breathing (Tāixí, 胎息). Usually, these theories and techniques were kept top secret in ancient Qìgōng society. It was not until the second half of the last century that documents on Embryonic Breathing were gradually revealed to the general public. This book covers most of the available documents. These documents have been translated and commented on from my personal point of view. I sincerely believe, for those who wish to study and practice Embryonic Breathing, that this book will provide them with an important guideline and crucial key to reach this goal. In "Grand Circulation Meditation" and "Spiritual Enlightenment Meditation," Embryonic Breathing is a vital practice for those who wish to reach their final goal of spiritual cultivation.

Originally, this book was only one part of the book entitled, *Small Circulation Meditation*. However, after five years of writing, I began to realize that it was impossible to include Embryonic Breathing with thorough and detailed discussion and analysis in that book. Translations of the available ancient documents about Embryonic Breathing, together with a scientific commentary, took more than 150 pages. Therefore, I decided that Embryonic Breathing merited a book of its own. In this way, the subject of Embryonic Breathing can be treated independently. I believe that I have tried my best to convey the information with a thorough and scientific discussion of the subject.

In order to help those interested Qìgōng practitioners without general Qìgōng knowledge, the first part of this book will review and summarize important Qìgōng concepts. This is followed by the theoretical discussion of Embryonic Breathing.

In the second, core part of this book, the available documents are translated with commentary. However, before you read them, you need to understand a few important points. It is very difficult to translate these ancient Chinese writings. Because of cultural differences, many expressions would not make sense to the Westerner if translated literally. Often, knowledge of the historical context is necessary. Furthermore, since in Chinese every sound has several possible meanings, when anyone tried to understand a poem or write it down, he had to choose from among these meanings. For this reason, many of the poems have several variations. The same problem occurs when the poems are read. Many

Chinese characters have several possible meanings, so reading involves interpretation of the text even for the Chinese. Also, the meaning of many words has changed over the course of time. When you add to this the grammatical differences (generally no tenses, articles, singular or plural, or differentiation between parts of speech), you find that it is almost impossible to translate Chinese literally into English completely. In addition to all this, the translator must have had much the same experience and understanding, as well as similar intuitive feelings as the original author, in order to convey the same meaning.

With these difficulties in mind, I have attempted to convey as much of the original meaning of the Chinese as possible, based on my own Qìgōng experience and understanding. Although it is impossible to fully translate the original meaning, I feel I have managed to express the majority of the important points. The translation has been made as close to the original Chinese as possible, including such things as double negatives and, sometimes, idiosyncratic sentence structure. Words that are understood but not actually written in the Chinese text have been included in parentheses. Also, some Chinese words are followed by the English in parentheses, e.g., Shén (Spirit). To further assist the reader, I have included my personal commentary with each document.

Finally, in the third part of this book, I will summarize the methods of practice from translated documents and also from my personal practical experience. From this part, you will know how to practice correctly without too much danger.

After you practice Embryonic Breathing for a period of time, you will soon discover that it seems there is another world (i.e., spiritual world) which other regular people cannot reach. This world has not yet been understood by today's science. If you are able to step in and practice, you will become a pioneer of the study and practice of spiritual science. Compared to material science which has been well developed, spiritual science is still far behind. This is why we have encountered the biggest crises and challenges today. On one hand we have developed the material science which is able to destroy the entire world; on the other, we still don't know how to control human desires and temperament.

Compared with the Western spiritual science and understanding, in my personal opinion, the East has developed far beyond the West. The reason for this is simply because of the involvement of politics in Western religion. Glory, dignity, power, and wealth have become the major concerns in Western religious societies. Although, of course, there have been examples of the same thing in Eastern religions, this has been more of an exception. For this reason, in Europe and the Americas, it was more common for those people who had natural inborn spiritual capabilities to be accused as witches and burned to death. In China, the situation was very different. Those spiritual people would usually hide themselves in the mountains for spiritual cultivation. Many of them would write their experiences down and these were passed down to us. In China, it was very common that when those spiritually talented people were found, they were said to have affinity for Buddhahood (Fóyuán, 佛緣) or the Dào (Dàoyuán, 道緣). These people were usually sent to the monasteries for further training.

I sincerely believe that in order to promote human spiritual science to a higher level, the first priority is to translate these existing ancient documents written by those experienced spiritual practitioners. However, there are now too many documents available to society. In the last few years, I have realized that even having spent my last forty years collecting the ancient documents, studying and interpreting them, all my effort has only contributed probably less than 0.1 percent to the entire study. To expedite the spiritual study, we will need a well-funded non-profit organization to translate these documents which can thus allow the Western general public to study and practice them.

Before I finish this preface, I would like to point out an important fact. It does not matter how long a person has studied and practiced Qìgōng, still his knowledge, experience, and understanding of Qìgōng will be limited and shallow, compared with the vast and profound nature of Qìgōng itself. Therefore, there is no single person who is able to understand all of the practices and share them with you. If you are wise, you should remain humble and search for other sources of knowledge and experience. Only if you can keep an open mind, can you accept the nature of truth.

Publisher's Note on the 2nd Edition

This 2nd edition includes pinyin with tonal marks, a new Chinese character font (Biau-Kai), and selected illustration enhancements.

An important contribution to this new edition is the use of tonal marks on the pinyin. Pinyin is the current standard for Romanizing Chinese characters so they can be read by non-Chinese speaking readers. By adding tonal marks to the Romanized Chinese words (pinyin), we can have a guide for properly pronouncing these words.

Before we can begin learning how to pronounce pinyin words, we must recognize some common differences in how some letters sound.[1]

ü Start pronouncing "ee" in English and then round your lips to pronounce "oo".
q Pronounced like "ch" in chin.
x Pronounced like a blend of "she" and "he".
z Pronounced like "ds" in kids.
c Pronounced like "ts" in bats.
zh Pronounced like "ger" in germ.
ch Pronounced like "chur" in church.
sh Pronounced like "sur" in sure.
er Pronounced like "ar" in are.
i When i follows z, c, s, it sounds like "zz": zzz, czz, szz.
When i follows zh, ch, sh, r, it sounds like "rr": zhrr, chrr, shrr, rrr.

There are primarily four tonal categories written in pinyin.[2]

1. mā 媽 (mom). Begins high and stays high.
2. má 麻 (hemp). Begins at mid-range and ends high.
3. mǎ 馬 (horse). Begins mid-range, dips low, ends mid-range.
4. mà 罵 (scold). Begins high and ends low.

There are many websites offering guides for the pronunciation of Chinese words and how to interpret and pronounce pinyin words with the tonal marks. We encourage readers to explore these valuable online tools. Some are provided below for your reference.

https://dictionary.hantrainerpro.com/
https://en.wikipedia.org/wiki/Pinyin
https://ymaa.com/publishing/spoken-chinese-glossary

1 https://www.mandarintutor.com/resources/pinyinintro
2 https://www.duchinese.net/blog/learn-to-read-chinese-tones/

PART I
Foundations

CHAPTER 1

General Concepts

1.1 INTRODUCTION (JIÈSHÀO, 介紹)

Throughout human history, we have been wondering at the how and why of our existence. What kind of role are we playing in this universe? What is the meaning of our lives? What will happen after our death? Countless questions and confusions have always been in our mind. Therefore, since ancient times, we have continued to search for ourselves and tried to understand our inner original natural being. Externally, we have sought ways to survive physically and satisfy ourselves through material enjoyment. In order to understand ourselves and our surrounding environment better, through our five sense organs—eyes (seeing), ears (hearing), skin (touching), tongue (tasting), and nose (smelling)—we constantly collect information from all around us. As this information has been compiled, analyzed, recorded, and slowly understood, we have gradually untied the knots of the questions and increased our knowledge. From this learning process we have made our lives better, and also enabled the evolution of our spirit to advance one more tiny step.

Humanity's process of learning the truth, about ourselves and about Great Nature, has been very long and painful, as we have been subject to the bondage of our own emotional mind. In the course of human history, in order to satisfy our emotional desire for power or glory, our pride and jealousy, our selfishness and greed, we have learned how to kill each other—but also how to love one another.

In the past, when we encountered difficult problems and unanswered questions, we turned to wise and long-lived humans, hoping that from their wisdom and experience the confusion of our lives could be answered. Therefore, philosophers and holy men were respected and worshipped. This led us to the path of religion. We hoped, through the guidance of these philosophers and holy men, to alleviate the inner pain and doubt in our lives, and also for a better understanding of this universe and ourselves. Through their wisdom, the rules of how to live peacefully and harmoniously with each other—and with nature—were interpreted and codified. Through their teachings, we have understood something about the relationship between nature and humanity. Our spirit has been gradually raised to a higher level. We have learned to be more civilized spiritually.

However, if we reflect sincerely on our past, we realize that, very unfortunately, we have also been seriously abused by many religions which have misled us to continue killing each other. I deeply believe that this was not the original intention of the teachings passed down to us from those wise holy men. For thousands of years, religions have been used as an excuse for killing and conquering. If you step into any European historical museum, you can see that the majority of the art created in the past is related to religion and war. Our spirit has been channeled and misused by religion to fulfill the wishes of those in power. Glory, wealth, and power have been the symbols of religion. I believe that this was a wrong turn.

Many of the spiritual people in the past could see the tragedy of this spiritual abuse and retired to the mountains, far from the bondage of the human emotional mind. They meditated and pondered, hoping to find their spirit and connect it to nature. However, this is not an easy task. After all, since birth we have been brainwashed into wrong thought patterns created in the past, and taught to place a mask on our face in order to survive in this masked society. It will take a great effort for us to open our minds and remove this mask, and face the truth of nature. Naturally, most of this mask is generated from our emotional bondage and desires. Through the years this mask has become thicker and heavier and, without realizing it, we have forgotten our true face hidden behind the mask. In this way we have isolated ourselves from the true, pure nature to which we originally belonged.

To unify with the natural spirit, the spiritual people both in the East and the West realized that they must first learn to calm down their emotional disturbances, filter them through the brain, and finally bring their spirit to a more purified, neutral, and peaceful state. From this spiritual purification, they found that the natural spirit can be reached. From continued pondering, they also discovered that many of our questions could be answered. Therefore, meditation methods which were able to lead us into this spiritual and peaceful state were developed and passed down through writing and instruction. Through meditation, a stronger intuition and psychic feeling (extrasensory perception, or ESP) was developed. Even today, this kind of special talent or training cannot yet be explained by modern science; it is still in its infant stage. The reason for this is simply that humans have been paying more attention to material science than to spiritual science in the last several centuries. Spiritual science remains mysterious and confused, and the human spirit has continued to be abused.

It is amazing that the experiences of both Eastern and Western meditating traditions agree that meditation is the best way to better understand the human spirit and to further unify it with the spirit of nature. Both Eastern and Western meditators believe that our spirit resides in our brain and that, through opening the Third Eye (center of the forehead), we are capable of communicating and unifying with the nature spirit. The Third Eye is called "Tiānyǎn" (Heaven Eye, 天眼), or "Shàng Dāntián" (Upper Elixir Field, 上丹田) in the tradition of Chinese Qìgōng spiritual cultivation.

Naturally, the final goal of this spiritual cultivation is continuing to search for the meaning of our lives and hopefully to build a connection with the natural spirit. In order to reach the natural spirit, natural Qì such as heaven Qì (energy which flows down to us from the heavens) and earth Qì are studied. You should understand that this natural Qì has not only been studied by the Chinese spiritual Qìgōng practitioners but also by other human cultures. For example, this natural energy is called "prana" in India, "pneuma" in Greece, and "ki" in Japan. Today, it is commonly called "cosmic energy," "orgone energy," or simply "natural energy/force."

This energy exists everywhere and takes many different forms. This energy manifests in a living body as heat, bioelectricity, or light. This energy supports the spirit when the physical body is alive and also after death. When this energy remains in dead objects without the spirit, though the object does not grow, it can also manifest in different energy forms.

Because the spiritual energy can only be felt but not perceived easily by humans, it has remained a mystery since ancient times. Since then, humans have tended to develop what they know best. While mystified by this spiritual energy, we have continued to develop, and have reached a very high level in the material sciences.

According to Chinese philosophy, the material world ("color world") is Yáng and is the manifestation of the spiritual world ("colorless world") which is Yīn. These two worlds coexist and are closely related to and mutually influenced by each other. If we can build a bridge or a connection between these two and harmonize them smoothly, we can better promote our understanding of our lives. Not only that, we can achieve better health and longevity each time we come back as a physical form. Consequently, this will provide us with a longer time for our spiritual cultivation.

After several hundred years of material development, though we have reached a high level of understanding about the material world, we are still in the dark about our spiritual being. It is now up to us to use what we have developed and learned in material and energy science to study the spiritual world. It is now time for us to step into the spiritual world and to understand it. The 21st century is the spiritual century.

To achieve this we should first study the traditional theory and methods of practice which have been passed down to us, both in the East and in the West. We must educate the next generation about what we have known about the spiritual world—the world without human emotional bondage. Then, we must teach our children how to meditate and find their inborn natural spiritual self. Through meditation, they can recognize their original spiritual being, and therefore be able to distinguish the pure spiritual world from the contaminated physical world. If we are able to teach them how to meditate from childhood, we will have provided them with a firm foundation for their spiritual development and growth. Only then can we expect, after a few more generations, to achieve progress in cultivating our spiritual being.

In order to help those interested Qìgōng practitioners who have not had a clear idea of general Qìgōng knowledge, the first part of this book will review and summarize those important Qìgōng concepts. This will be followed by the theoretical discussion of Embryonic Breathing. Readers of my other Qìgōng books may find many of the contents in the first chapter to be similar to those of other books. The reason for this is simply that the basic general concepts of Qìgōng remain the same. To those who have never read my other Qìgōng books, this part is very important. Without the first chapter, the fundamental structure of the entire practice would be incomplete. To those already familiar with these basic concepts, this chapter will serve the purpose of reviewing. From these basic concepts, the theoretical discussion of Embryonic Breathing in Chapter 2 will make sense.

In Part II, the core of this book, the available documents will be translated and then commented on. Finally, in Part III I will summarize the methods of practice, from translated documents and also from my personal practical experience. From this part, you will know how to practice correctly without encountering too much danger.

1.2 General Qìgōng Concepts (Yībān Qìgōng Gàiniàn, 一般氣功概念)

In this section, we will first review the traditional concept of Qì and Qìgōng. Next, we will discuss the scope of Qìgōng practice, the differences between External Elixir (Wàidān, 外丹) and Internal Elixir (Nèidān, 內丹) Qìgōng practice, and differences between Qìgōng schools in Chinese history. Then, in order to understand the practice concepts, the theories of Yīn-Yáng (陰陽) and Kǎn-Lí (坎離) will be explained. Finally, we will summarize the relationship of Qìgōng practice to health, longevity, and spiritual enlightenment.

1.2.1 Traditional Definition of Qì (Qì Zhī Chuántǒng Gàiniàn, 氣之傳統概念)

In this subsection, we will first define the general concept of Qì, followed by the narrow concept of Qì. In order to understand the meaning of Qìgōng practice, you must first have a clear idea of how Qì is defined. After you have understood these traditional concepts, we will, from a scientific point of view, discuss and define the modern concept of Qì in Chapter 2.

A General Definition of Qì. Qì is the energy or natural force that fills the universe. The Chinese have traditionally believed that there are three major powers in the universe. These Three Powers (Sāncái, 三才) are Heaven (Tiān, 天), Earth (Dì, 地), and Man (Rén, 人). Heaven (the sky or universe) has Heaven Qì (Tiānqì, 天氣), the most important of the three, which is made up of the forces that the heavenly bodies exert on the earth, such as sunshine, moonlight, the moon's gravity, and the energy from the stars. In ancient times, the Chinese believed that weather, climate, and natural disasters were governed by Heaven Qì. Chinese people still refer to the weather as Heaven Qì (Tiānqì, 天氣). Every energy field strives to stay in balance, so whenever the Heaven Qì loses its balance, it tries to rebalance itself. Then the wind must blow, rain must fall, even tornadoes or hurricanes become necessary in order for the Heaven Qì to reach a new energy balance.

Under Heaven Qì, there is Earth Qì. It is influenced and controlled by Heaven Qì. For example, too much rain will force a river to flood or change its path. Without rain, the plants will die. The Chinese believe that Earth Qì is made up of lines and patterns of energy, as well as the earth's magnetic field and the heat concealed underground. These energies must also balance, otherwise disasters such as earthquakes will occur. When the Qì of the earth is balanced and harmonized, plants will grow and animals thrive.

Finally, within the Earth Qì, each individual person, animal, and plant has its own Qì field, which always seeks to be balanced. When any individual living thing loses its Qì balance, it will sicken, die, and decompose. All natural things, including mankind and our Human Qì, grow within and are influenced by the natural cycles of Heaven Qì and Earth Qì. Throughout the history of Qìgōng, people have been most interested in Human Qì and its relationship with Heaven Qì and Earth Qì.

In the Chinese tradition, Qì can also be defined as any type of energy which is able to demonstrate power and strength. This energy can be electricity, magnetism, heat, or light. For example, electric power is called "Electric Qì" (Diànqì, 電氣), and heat is called "Heat Qì" (Rèqì, 熱氣). When a person is alive, his body's energy is called "Human Qì" (Rénqì, 人氣).

Qì is also commonly used to express the energy state of something, especially living things. As mentioned before, the weather is called "Heaven Qì" (Tiānqì, 天氣) because it indicates the energy state of the heavens. When something is alive it has "Vital Qì" (Huóqì, 活氣), and when it is dead it has "Dead Qì" (Sǐqì, 死氣) or "Ghost Qì" (Guǐqì, 鬼氣). When a person is righteous and has the spiritual strength to do good, he is said to have "Normal Qì" or "Righteous Qì" (Zhèngqì, 正氣). The spiritual state or morale of an army is called "energy state" (Qìshì, 氣勢).

You can see that the word "Qì" has a wider and more general definition than most people think. It does not refer only to the energy circulating in the human body. Furthermore, the word "Qì" can represent the energy itself, but it can even be used to express the manner or state of the energy. It is important to understand this when you practice Qìgōng, so that your mind is not channeled into a narrow understanding of Qì, which would limit your future understanding and development.

A Narrow Definition of Qì. Now that you understand the general definition of Qì, let us look at how Qì is defined in Qìgōng society today. As mentioned before, among the Three Powers, the Chinese have been most concerned with the Qì that affects our health and longevity. Therefore, after four thousand years of emphasizing Human Qì, when people mention Qì they usually mean the Qì circulating in our bodies.

If we look at the Chinese medical and Qìgōng documents that were written in ancient times, the word "Qì" was written "炁." This character is constructed of two words, "旡" on the top, which means "nothing," and "灬" on the bottom, which means "fire." This means that the word Qì was actually written as "no fire" in ancient times. If we go back through Chinese medical and Qìgōng history, it is not hard to understand this expression.

In ancient times, Chinese physicians or Qìgōng practitioners were actually looking for the Yīn-Yáng balance of the Qì which was circulating in the body. When this goal was reached, there was "no fire" in the internal organs. This concept is very simple. According to Chinese medicine, each of our internal organs needs to receive a specific amount of Qì to function properly. If an organ receives an improper amount of Qì (usually too much, i.e., too Yáng or on fire), it will start to malfunction, and, in time, physical damage will occur. Therefore, the goal of the medical or Qìgōng practitioner was to attain a state of "no fire," which eventually became the word "Qì."

However, in more recent publications, the Qì of "no fire" has been replaced by the word "氣," which is again constructed of two words: "气" which means "air," and "米" which means "rice." This shows that later practitioners realized that, after each of us is born, the Qì circulating in our bodies is produced mainly by the inhalation of air (oxygen) and the consumption of food (rice). Air is called Kōngqì (空氣), which means literally "space energy."

For a long time, people were confused about just what type of energy was circulating in our bodies. Many people believed that it was heat, others considered it to be electricity, and many others assumed that it was a mixture of heat, electricity, and light.

This confusion lasted until the early 1980's, when the concept of Qì gradually became clear. If we think carefully about what we know from science today, we can see that (except possibly for gravity) there is actually only one type of energy in this universe, and that is electromagnetic energy (electromagnetic waves). This means that light and heat (infrared waves) are also defined as electromagnetic energy. This makes it very clear that the Qì circulating in our bodies is actually "bioelectricity," and that our body is a "living electromagnetic field."[1] This field is affected by our thoughts, feelings, activities, the food we eat, the quality of the air we breathe, our lifestyle, the natural energy that surrounds us, and also the unnatural energy which modern science inflicts upon us.

1.2.2 Traditional Definition of Qìgōng (Qìgōng Zhī Chuántǒng Gàiniàn, 氣功之傳統概念)

Now that you have a clear concept of Qì, let us discuss how Qìgōng is traditionally defined. Again, we can define it from a general and narrow point of view. In Chapter 2, after you have become familiar with the modern concept of Qì, we will define the meaning of Qìgōng based on the scientific understanding of today.

A General Definition of Qìgōng. We have explained that Qì is energy, and that it is found in the heavens, in the earth, and in every living thing. In China, the word "Gōng" (功) is often used instead of "Gōngfū" (or Kūng Fū, 功夫), which means energy and time. Any study or training which requires a lot of energy and time to learn or to accomplish is called Gōngfū. The term can be applied to any special skill or study as long as it requires time, energy, and patience. Therefore, the correct definition of Qìgōng is any training or study dealing with Qì which takes a long time and a lot of effort. You can see from this definition that Qìgōng is a science which studies the energy in nature. The main difference between this energy science and Western energy science is that Qìgōng focuses on the inner energy of human beings, while Western energy science pays more attention to the energy outside of the human body. When you study Qìgōng, it is worthwhile to also consider the modern, scientific point of view, and not restrict yourself to only the traditional beliefs.

The Chinese have studied Qì for thousands of years. Some of the information on the patterns and cycles of nature has been recorded in books, one of which is the *Yìjīng* (*Book of Changes*, 易經) (1122 BCE). When the *Yìjīng* was written, the Chinese people, as mentioned earlier, believed that natural power included Heaven (Tiān, 天), Earth (Dì, 地), and Man (Rén, 人). These are called "The Three Powers" (Sāncái, 三才) and are manifested by the three Qì's: Heaven Qì, Earth Qì, and Human Qì. These three facets of nature have their definite rules and cycles. The rules never change, and the cycles are repeated regularly. The Chinese people used an understanding of these natural principles and the "*Yìjīng*" to calculate the changes of natural Qì. This calculation is called the "Eight Trigrams" (Bāguà, 八卦). From the Eight Trigrams the Sixty-Four Hexagrams are derived. Therefore, the "*Yìjīng*" was probably the first book that taught the Chinese people about Qì and its variations in nature and man. The relationship of the Three Natural Powers to their Qì variations was later discussed extensively in the book *Theory of Qì's Variation* (*Qìhuàlùn*, 氣化論).

Understanding Heaven Qì is very difficult, and it was especially so in ancient times when the science was just developing. But since nature is always repeating itself, the experiences accumulated over the years have made it possible to trace the natural patterns. Understanding the rules and cycles of "heavenly timing" (Tiānshí, 天時) will help you to understand natural changes of the seasons, climate, weather, and all other natural occurrences. If you observe carefully, you can see many of these routine patterns and cycles are caused by the rebalancing of the Qì fields. Among the natural cycles are those which repeat every day, month, or year, as well as cycles of twelve years and sixty years.

Earth Qì is a part of Heaven Qì. If you can understand the rules and the structure of the earth, you can understand how mountains are formed, how rivers move, how plants grow, what part of the country is best for someone, where to build a house and which direction it should face so that it is a healthy place to live, and many other things related to the earth. In China there are people, called "geomancy teachers" (Dìlǐshī, 地理師) or "wind water teachers" (Fēngshuǐshī, 風水師), who make their living this way. The term "wind water" (Fēngshuǐ, 風水) is commonly used because the location and character of the wind and water in a landscape are the most important factors in evaluating a location. These experts use the accumulated body of geomantic knowledge and the "*Yìjīng*" to help people make important decisions such as where and how to build a house, where to bury their dead, and how to rearrange or redecorate homes and offices so that they are better places to live and work in. Many people even believe that setting up a store or business according to the guidance of Fēngshuǐ can make it more prosperous.

Among the three Qì's, Human Qì is probably the one studied most thoroughly. The study of Human Qì covers a large number of different subjects. The Chinese people believe that Human Qì is affected and controlled by Heaven Qì and Earth Qì, and that they in fact determine your destiny. Therefore, if you understand the relationship between nature and people, in addition to understanding "human relations" (Rénshì, 人事), you can predict wars, the destiny of a country, a person's desires and temperament, and even his future. The people who practice this profession are called "calculate life teachers" (Suànmìngshī, 算命師).

However, the greatest achievement in the study of Human Qì is in regard to health and longevity. Since Qì is the source of life, if you understand how Qì functions and know how to regulate it correctly, you should be able to live a long and healthy life. Remember that you are part of nature, and you are channeled into the cycles of nature. If you go against this natural cycle, you may become sick, so it is in your best interest to follow the way of nature. This is the meaning of "Dào" (道), which can be translated as "The Natural Way."

Many different aspects of Human Qì have been researched, including acupuncture, acupressure, massage, herbal treatment, meditation, and Qìgōng exercises. The use of acupuncture, acupressure, and herbal treatment to adjust Human Qì flow has become the root of Chinese medical science. Meditation and moving Qìgōng exercises are widely used by the Chinese people to improve their health or even to cure certain illnesses. In addition, Daoists and Buddhists use meditation and Qìgōng exercises in their pursuit of enlightenment.

In conclusion, the study of any of the aspects of Qì including Heaven Qì, Earth Qì, and Human Qì should be called Qìgōng. However, since the term is usually used today only in reference to the cultivation of Human Qì through meditation and exercise, we will only use it in this narrower sense to avoid confusion.

A Narrow Definition of Qìgōng. As mentioned earlier, the narrow definition of Qì is "the energy circulating in the human body." Therefore, the narrow definition of Qìgōng is "the study or the practice of circulating the Qì in the human body." Because our bodies are part of nature, the narrow definition of Qìgōng should also include the study of how our bodies relate to Heaven Qì and Earth Qì. Today, Chinese Qìgōng consists of several different fields: acupuncture, herbal treatment, martial arts Qìgōng, Qìgōng massage, Qìgōng exercises, Qìgōng healing, and religious enlightenment Qìgōng. Naturally, these fields are mutually related, and in many cases cannot be separated.

In ancient times, Qìgōng was also commonly called "Tǔ-Nà" (吐納). Tǔ-Nà means to "utter and admit" which implies uttering and admitting the air through the nose. The reason for this is simply that Qìgōng practice is closely related to the methods of how to inhale and exhale correctly. Zhuāngzi (莊子), during the Chinese Warring States Period (403–222 BCE) (戰國) said: "Blowing puffing to breathe, uttering the old and admitting the new, the bear's natural (action) and the bird's extending (the neck), are all for longevity. This is also favored by those people living as long as Péng, Zǔ (彭祖) who practice Dǎo-Yǐn (Direct-Lead, 導引) and nourishing the shapes (i.e., cultivating the physical body)."[2] Péng, Zǔ was a legendary Qìgōng practitioner during the period of Emperor Yáo (堯) (2356–2255 BCE), who was said to have lived for 800 years. From this saying, we can see that Qìgōng was also commonly called "Dǎo-Yǐn" (Direct-Lead, 導引) which means to use the mind and physical movements to direct and to lead the Qì's circulation in the correct way. The physical movements commonly imitate the natural instinctive movements of animals such as bears and birds. A famous medical Qìgōng set passed down at this time was "Five Animal Sports" (Wǔqínxì, 五禽戲) that imitates the movements of the tiger, deer, bear, ape, and bird.

The Chinese have discovered that the human body has twelve major Qì channels (Shíèrjīng, 十二經) which branch out with countless secondary channels (Luò, 絡). This is similar to the blood circulatory system in the body. The primary channels are like arteries and veins while the secondary channels are like capillaries. The twelve primary channels are like rivers and the secondary channels are like streams which branch out from rivers. From this network, the Qì is distributed throughout the entire body, connecting the extremities (fingers and toes) to the internal organs and also the skin to the bone marrow. Here you should understand that the "internal organs" of Chinese medicine do not necessarily correspond to the physical organs as understood in the West, but rather to a set of clinical functions similar to each other, and related to the organ system.

The human body also has eight vessels (Bāmài, 八脈). The eight vessels, which are often referred to as the extraordinary vessels, function like reservoirs and regulate the distribution and circulation of Qì in your body. The famous Chinese Daoist medical doctor, Lǐ, Shí-Zhēn (李時珍) in his book, *The Study of Strange Meridians and Eight Vessels* (*Qíjīng Bāmài Kǎo*, 奇經八脈考) said: "It is because the regular meridians (i.e., 12 Primary Qì Channels) are like rivers, while the strange meridians (i.e., eight vessels) are like lakes. (When) the regular meridians' (Qì) is abundant and flourishing, then overflow to the strange meridians."[3] We will discuss the Qì network more in the next section of this chapter.

When the Qì in the eight reservoirs is full and strong, the Qì in the rivers is strong and will be regulated efficiently. When there is stagnation in any of these twelve channels or rivers, the Qì which flows to the body's extremities and to the internal organs will be abnormal, and illness may develop. You should understand that every channel has its particular Qì flow strength, and every channel is different. All of these different levels of Qì strength are affected by your mind, the weather, the time of day, the food you have eaten, and even your mood. For example, when the weather is dry the Qì in the lungs will tend to be more positive (i.e., Yáng, 陽) than when it is moist. When you are angry, the Qì flow in your liver channel will be abnormal. The Qì strength in the different channels varies throughout the day in a regular cycle, and at any particular time one channel is strongest. For example, between 11:00 a.m. and 1:00 p.m. the Qì flow in the heart channel is the strongest. Furthermore, the Qì level of the same organ can be different from one person to another.

Whenever the Qì flow in the twelve rivers or channels is not normal, the eight reservoirs will regulate the Qì flow and bring it back into balance. For example, when you experience a sudden shock, the Qì flow in the bladder immediately becomes deficient. Normally, the reservoir will immediately regulate the Qì in this channel so that you recover from the shock. However, if the reservoir Qì is also deficient, or if the effect of the shock is too great and there is not enough time to regulate the Qì, the bladder will suddenly contract, causing unavoidable urination.

When a person is sick, his Qì level tends to be either too positive (excessive, Yáng, 陽) or too negative (deficient, Yīn, 陰). A Chinese physician would either use a prescription of herbs to adjust the Qì, or else he would insert acupuncture needles at various spots on the channels to inhibit the flow in some channels and stimulate the flow in others, so that balance could be restored. However, there is another alternative, and that is to use certain physical and mental exercises to adjust the Qì. In other words, to use Qìgōng exercises.

However, when Qìgōng is defined in scholarly society, it is somewhat different. The Qìgōng practice is focused on regulating the disturbed emotional mind. When the emotional mind is regulated into a peaceful and calm state, the body will be relaxed, which will assist the Qì to circulate smoothly in the body, and therefore regulate itself into a more harmonious state. From this, mental and physical health can be achieved.

When Qìgōng is defined in Daoist and Buddhist society, it refers to the method or training of leading the Qì from the Lower Dāntián (Lower Elixir Field) (Xiàdāntián, 下

丹田) to the brain for spiritual enlightenment or Buddhahood. The Lower Dāntián is the place at the abdominal area where one is able to store the Qì. It is considered a Qì storage area or bioelectric battery. Naturally, its training theory and methods will not be easy. In fact, religious Qìgōng is considered one of the highest levels of Qìgōng training in China.

Finally, when Qìgōng is defined in martial arts society, it refers to the theory and methods of using Qì to energize the physical body to its maximum efficiency for manifestation of power. However, since a great portion of martial arts Qìgōng was derived from religious Qìgōng, Muscle/Tendon Changing and Marrow/Brain Washing Qìgōng (Yìjīnjīng and Xǐsuǐjīng, 易筋經、洗髓經), it is not surprising that the profound level of training of martial arts Qìgōng remains the same as that of religious Qìgōng.

In order to make the above concepts clearer, we will discuss more about different Qìgōng categories later. If you wish to know more about medical Qìgōng, please refer to the books, *Qìgōng for Health and Martial Arts* and *The Root of Chinese Qìgōng*. If you wish to know more about religious Qìgōng, please refer to the book, *Qìgōng—The Secret of Youth*. However, if you are interested in martial Qìgōng, the book *The Essence of Shàolín White Crane*, is highly recommended. Please see the YMAA website (www.ymaa.com) for more information about these books.

1.2.3 Scope of Qìgōng Practice (Qìgōng Liànxí Zhī Guīfàn, 氣功練習之規範)

Often, people ask me the same question: is jogging, weightlifting, dancing, or even walking a kind of Qìgōng practice? To answer this question, let us trace back Qìgōng history to before the Chinese Qín and Hàn dynastic periods (秦、漢, 255 BCE–220 CE). Then you can see that the origins of many Qìgōng practices were actually in dancing. Through dancing, the physical body was exercised and its healthy condition was maintained. Also, through dancing and matching movements with music, the mind was regulated into a harmonious state. From this harmonious mind, the spirit was raised to a more energized state, or calmed down to a peaceful level. This Qìgōng dancing later passed to Japan during the Chinese Hàn Dynasty (206 BCE–220 CE) (漢朝) and became a very elegant, slow, and high class of dance in the Japanese royal court. This Tàijíquán-like court dancing is still practiced in Japan today as "Bugaku".

The ways of African or Native American dancing, in which the body is bounced up and down, also assists in loosening the joints and improving Qì circulation. Naturally, jogging, weightlifting, or even walking are kinds of Qìgōng practices. Therefore, we can say that any activity which is able to regulate the Qì circulation in the body is a Qìgōng practice. This can also include the food we eat, the air we breathe, and even emotions and thoughts.

Let us define it more clearly. In Figure 1-1, if the left vertical line represents the amount of usage of the physical body (Yáng), and the right vertical line the usage of the mind (Yīn), then we can see that the more you practice toward the left, the more physical effort and less mental effort are needed. This can be applied to aerobic dancing, walking, or jogging in which the use of the mind is relatively small compared to physical action. In this kind of Qìgōng practice, normally you do not need special training, and it is classified as layman Qìgōng. At the middle point, the mind and the physical activity are almost equally important. This kind of Qìgōng will be the slow-moving Qìgōng commonly practiced, in which the mind is used to lead the Qì in coordination with the movements. Theoretically speaking, when the body is in its state of slow and relaxed movements, the Qì led by the mind can reach the deeper places of the body such as ligaments, marrow, and internal organs. Consequently, the internal self-feeling can also be deep and the Qì can be led there significantly. For example, Tàijí Qìgōng, White Crane Qìgōng, Snake Qìgōng, Dragon Qìgōng, and many others are very typical body-mind Qìgōng exercises. These are specifically practiced in Chinese medical and martial arts societies.

However, when you reach a profound level of Qìgōng practice, the mind becomes more critical and important. When you reach this high level, you are dealing with your mind while you are sitting or standing still and are extremely relaxed. Most of this mental Qìgōng training was practiced by scholars and religious Qìgōng practitioners. In this practice, you may have a little physical movement in the lower abdomen area. However, the main focus of this Qìgōng practice is to cultivate the peaceful and neutral mind and

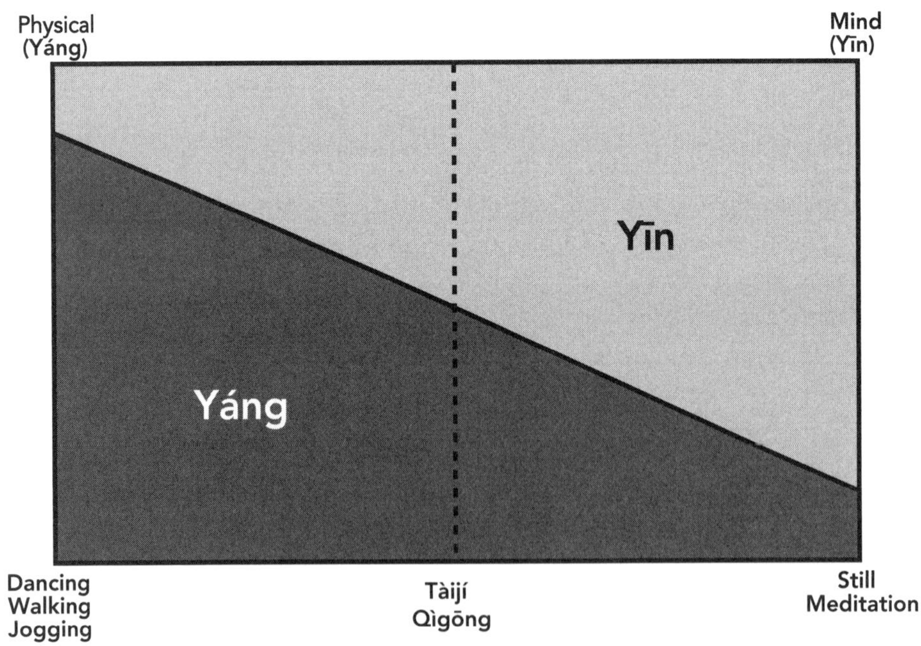

Figure 1-1. The Range of Defined Qìgōng

further pursue the final goal of spiritual enlightenment. This kind of Qìgōng practice includes Sitting Chán (Rěn) (坐禪，忍), Small Circulation Meditation (Xiǎozhōutiān, 小周天), Grand Circulation Meditation (Dàzhōutiān, 大周天), or Brain Washing Enlightenment Meditation (Xǐsuǐgōng, 洗髓功).

From this, you can see that different Qìgōng practices aim for different goals. Theoretically speaking, in order to have a good healthy, long, and happy life, both your physical body and your mind must be healthy. The best Qìgōng for health is actually located in the middle of our model, where you learn how to regulate your physical body and also your mind. Naturally, you may practice the Yīn side through still meditation and the Yáng side from physical action separately. From this Yīn and Yáng balancing practice, your Qì can be built up to a more abundant level and the Qì can also be circulated smoothly in the body.

From this, we can conclude:

1. Any activity which is able to improve the Qì circulation in our body is called Qìgōng.
2. Those Qìgōng forms which emphasize the physical body will improve the physical strength and Qì circulation of those areas being exercised. Normally, the muscles, tendons, ligaments, and bones are conditioned.
3. Through those Qìgōng forms using both body and mind, one can achieve a deeper level of physical strength and Qì circulation. Normally, with the coordination of the relaxed physical body and concentrated mind, the Qì circulation is able to reach to the internal organs, deep places of the joints, and even the marrow.
4. Through those Qìgōng forms using mostly the mind, one may reach a deep and profound meditative state. However, due to the lack of physical movements, physical strength will tend to degenerate, unless the physical body is also exercised.

1.2.4 Definition of External and Internal Elixirs (Wàidān Yǔ Nèidān Zhī Dìngyì, 外丹與內丹之定義)

Let us now review the traditional classifications of Qìgōng. Generally speaking, all Qìgōng practices can be divided, according to their training theory and methods, into two general categories: Wàidān (External Elixir, 外丹) and Nèidān (Internal Elixir, 內丹). Understanding the differences between them will give you an overview of most Chinese Qìgōng practice.

Wàidān (External Elixir, 外丹)

"Wài" (外) means "external" or "outside," and "Dān" (丹) means "elixir." External here means the skin surface of the body, or the limbs, as opposed to the torso or the center of the body, which includes all of the vital organs. Elixir is a hypothetical, life-prolonging substance for which Chinese Daoists have been searching for several millennia. They originally thought that the elixir was something physical which could be prepared from herbs or chemicals purified in a furnace. After thousands of years of study and experimentation, they found that the elixir is in the body. In other words, if you want to prolong your life, you must find the elixir in your body, and then learn to cultivate, protect, and nourish it. Actually, the elixir is the essence of the inner energy or Qì circulating in the body.

There are many ways of producing elixir or Qì in the body. In Wàidān Qìgōng practice, you may exercise your limbs through dancing or even walking. As you exercise, the Qì builds up in your arms and legs. When the Qì potential in your limbs builds to a high enough level, the Qì will flow through the twelve primary Qì channels, clearing any obstructions and flowing into the center of the body to nourish the organs. This is the main reason that a person who works out, or has a physical job, is generally healthier than someone who sits around all day.

Naturally, you may simply massage your body to produce the Qì. Through massage, you may stimulate the cells of your body to a highly energized state and therefore the Qì concentration will be raised and the circulation enhanced. After massage, when you relax, the higher levels of Qì on the skin surface and in the muscles will flow into the center of the body and thereby improve the Qì circulatory conditions in your internal organs. This is the theoretical foundation of the Tuīná (推拿) (i.e., pushing and grabbing) Qìgōng massage.

Through acupuncture, you may also bring the Qì level near the skin surface to a higher level and from this stimulation, the Qì condition of the internal organs can be regulated through Qì channels. Therefore, acupressure (Diǎnxuè, 點穴) (i.e., cavity press) can also be classified as Wàidān Qìgōng practice. Naturally, the herbal treatments are a way of Wàidān practice as well.

From this, we can briefly conclude that any possible stimulation or exercise which accumulates a high level of Qì in the limbs or at the surface of the body, and then flows inward toward the center of the body, can be classified as Wàidān (External Elixir) (Figure 1-2).

Nèidān (Internal Elixir, 內丹)

"Nèi" (內) means "internal" and "Dān" (丹) again means "elixir." Thus, Nèidān means to build the elixir internally. Here, "internally" means inside the body instead of in the limbs. Normally, the Qì is accumulated in the Qì vessels instead of the primary

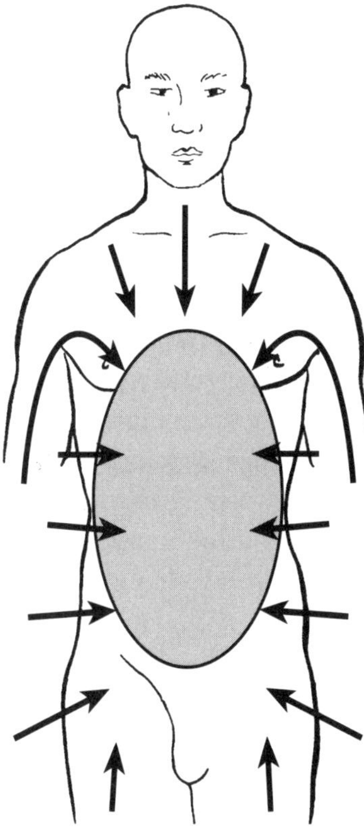

Figure 1-2. External Elixir (Wàidān)

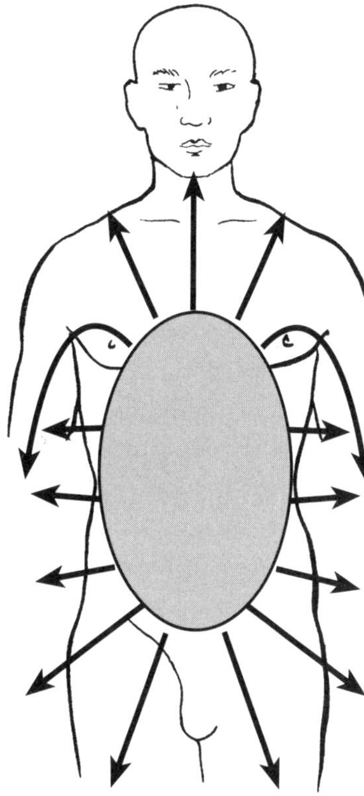

Figure 1-3. Internal Elixir (Nèidān)

Qì channels. Whereas in Wàidān the Qì is built up in the limbs or skin surface and then moved into the body through primary Qì channels, Nèidān exercises build up Qì in the body and lead it out to the limbs (Figure 1-3). Normally, Nèidān Qìgōng is accomplished by special breathing techniques during the meditation process. The first step of Nèidān practice is to build up abundant Qì in the Lower Dāntián (i.e., human bioelectric battery). This abundant Qì can then be distributed to the eight vessels to increase the store of Qì. Only then can the Qì circulating in the twelve primary Qì channels be regulated smoothly and efficiently.

In order to build up the Qì and store it internally, you must first have a deep and profound feeling which allows your mind to reach the deep places of your body. You should know that feeling is the language by which your mind and body communicate. Therefore, to improve the communication ability, your feeling of your physical body and Qì body must reach a high level. The training to increase this sensitivity of feeling is called "Nèishì Gōngfū" (內視功夫), which means the "Gōngfū of internal vision or observation." In fact, to see or to observe inside your body means to feel it. It is called Gōngfū (功夫) simply because it will take a great deal of time and practice to reach a high level of accurate feeling.

Generally speaking, Nèidān theory is deeper than Wàidān theory, and is more difficult to understand and practice. Traditionally, most of the Nèidān Qìgōng practices have been passed down more secretly than those of the Wàidān. This is especially true for the highest levels of Nèidān, such as Marrow/Brain Washing, which were passed down to only a few trusted disciples.

Normally, the first step of practicing Internal Elixir Qìgōng has been known by Daoists as "Small Cyclic Heaven" (Xiǎozhōutiān, 小周天) or "Small Circulation Meditation." This is also commonly known as "Microcosmic Meditation" in Yoga (Yújiā, 瑜珈) or as "Turning the Wheel of Natural Law" (Zhuǎnfǎlún, 轉法輪) by Buddhist society.

Small Circulation can be considered as the foundation of the Internal Elixir Qìgōng. Through practicing Small Circulation Meditation, a practitioner can circulate the Qì smoothly in the Conception and Governing Vessels (Rènmài, Dūmài; 任脈・督脈), the two major Qì vessels which regulate the Qì circulating in the Twelve Primary Qì Channels (Shíèrjīng, 十二經). After completing Small Circulation, a practitioner will learn "Grand Cyclic Heaven" (Dàzhōutiān, 大周天) or "Grand Circulation." This is also commonly called "Macrocosmic Meditation" in Indian Yoga. Through Grand Circulation meditation practice, a practitioner will learn how to circulate the Qì throughout his body, and then learn to exchange the Qì with partners or surrounding environments. The purpose of Grand Circulation meditation is to reopen the "Heaven Eye" (Tiānyǎn, 天眼) (i.e., The Third Eye) so as to unify the natural spirit and human spirit (Tiānrén Héyī, 天人合一). This is the ultimate goal of spiritual enlightenment in both Daoism and Buddhism.

In order to reach the goal of Internal Elixir Qìgōng practice, a practitioner must first know how to store the Qì to an abundant level in the Real Lower Dāntián (Zhēn Xiàdāntián, 真下丹田) (i.e., human bio-battery), using the theory and the techniques of Embryonic Breathing (Tāixí, 胎息). These were kept top-secret in ancient Qìgōng society. It was not until the second half of the last century that documents expounding on Embryonic Breathing were gradually revealed to the general public.

1.2.5 Schools of Qìgōng Practice (Qìgōng Liànxí Zhī Ménpài, 氣功練習之門派)

We can also classify Qìgōng into four major categories according to the purpose or final goal of the training: A. curing sickness; B. maintaining health; C. enlightenment or Buddhahood; D. martial arts. These are only general guidelines, however, since almost every style of Qìgōng serves more than one of the above purposes. For example, although martial Qìgōng focuses on increasing fighting effectiveness, it can also improve your health. Daoist Qìgōng aims for longevity and enlightenment, but to reach this goal you need to be in good health and know how to cure sickness. Because of this multi-purpose aspect of the categories, it will be simpler to discuss their backgrounds rather than the goals of their training. Knowing the history and basic principles of each category will help you to understand their Qìgōng more clearly.

Medical Qìgōng—for Healing. In ancient Chinese society, most emperors respected the scholars and were affected by their philosophy. Doctors were not regarded highly because they made their diagnosis by touching the patient's body, which was considered characteristic of the lower classes in society. Although the doctors developed a profound and successful medical science, they were commonly looked down on by society. However, they continued to work hard and study, and quietly passed down the results of their research to succeeding generations.

Of all the groups studying Qìgōng in China, the doctors pursued it the longest. Since the discovery of Qì circulation in the human body about four thousand years ago, Chinese doctors have devoted a major portion of their efforts to studying the behavior of Qì. Their efforts resulted in acupuncture, acupressure or cavity press massage, and herbal treatment.

In addition, many Chinese doctors used their medical knowledge to create different sets of Qìgōng exercises, either for maintaining health or for curing specific illnesses. Chinese medical doctors believed that doing only sitting or still meditation to regulate the body, mind, and breathing, as the scholars' Qìgōng or Buddhist Chán (禪) (i.e., Zen) meditation did, was not enough to cure sickness. They believed that in order to increase Qì circulation, you must move. Although a calm and peaceful mind was important for health, exercising the body was more important. They learned through their medical practice that people who exercised properly became sick less often, and their bodies degenerated less quickly, than was the case with people who just sat around. They also realized that specific body movements could increase the Qì circulation in specific organs. From this, they reasoned that these exercises could also be used to treat specific illnesses and to restore the normal functioning of the organs.

Some of these movements are similar to the ways certain animals move. For an animal to survive in the wild, it must instinctively know how to protect its body. Part of this instinct is concerned with how to build up its Qì and how to keep its Qì from being lost. We humans have lost many of these instincts over the years that we have been separating ourselves from nature.

Many doctors developed Qìgōng exercises which were modeled after animal movements to maintain health and cure sickness. A typical, well-known set of such exercises is "Wǔqínxì" (五禽戲) (Five Animal Sports) created by Dr. Huátuó (華佗) nearly two thousand years ago. (Others say Wǔqínxì was created by Jūnqiàn (君倩) and was publicized by Huátuó.) Another famous set based on similar principles is called "Bāduànjǐn" (八段錦) (The Eight Pieces of Brocade). It was created by Marshal Yuè, Fēi (岳飛) during the Southern Sòng Dynasty (南宋) (1127–1280 CE). Yuè, Fēi, interestingly enough, was a soldier and scholar rather than a doctor.

In addition, using their medical knowledge of Qì circulation, Chinese doctors researched until they found which movements could help cure particular illnesses and health problems. Not surprisingly, many of these movements were not unlike the ones used to maintain health, since many illnesses are caused by unbalanced Qì. When an imbalance continues for a long period of time, the organs will be affected, and may be physically damaged. It is just like running a machine without supplying the proper electrical current—over time, the machine will be damaged. Chinese doctors believe that before physical damage to an organ shows up in a patient's body, there is first an abnormality in the Qì balance and circulation. Abnormal Qì circulation is the very beginning of illness and organ damage. When Qì is too positive (Yáng) or too negative (Yīn) in a specific organ's Qì channel, your physical organ begins to suffer damage. If you do not correct the Qì circulation, that organ will malfunction or degenerate. The best way to heal someone is to adjust and balance the Qì even before there is any physical problem. Therefore, correcting or increasing the normal Qì circulation is the major goal of acupuncture or acupressure treatments. Herbs and special diets are also considered important treatments in regulating the Qì in the body.

As long as the illness is limited to the level of Qì stagnation and there is no physical organ damage, the Qìgōng exercises used for maintaining health can be used to readjust the Qì circulation and treat the problem. However, if the sickness is already so serious that the physical organs have started to fail, then the situation has become critical and a specific treatment is necessary. The treatment can include acupuncture, herbs, or even an operation, as well as specific Qìgōng exercises designed to accelerate healing. For example, ulcers and asthma can often be cured or helped by some simple exercises. Recently in both mainland China and Táiwān, certain Qìgōng exercises have been shown to be effective in treating certain kinds of cancer.

Over thousands of years of observing nature and themselves, some Qìgōng practitioners went even deeper. They realized that the body's Qì circulation changes with the seasons, and that it is a good idea to help the body out during these periodic adjustments. They noticed also that in each season different organs have characteristic problems. For example, in the beginning of autumn the lungs must adapt to the colder air that you are breathing. While this adjustment is going on, the lungs are susceptible to disturbance, so your lungs may feel uncomfortable and you may catch colds easily. Your digestive system is also affected during seasonal changes. Your appetite may increase, or you may have diarrhea. When your temperature drops, your kidneys and bladder will start to give you trouble. For example, if the kidneys are stressed, you may feel pain in the back. Focusing on these seasonal Qì disorders, the meditators created a set of movements which can be used to speed up the body's adjustment.

In addition to Marshal Yuè, Fēi, many people who were not doctors also created sets of medical Qìgōng. These sets were probably originally created to maintain health, and were also later used for curing sickness.

Scholar Qìgōng—for Maintaining Health. In China before the Hàn Dynasty, there were two major schools of scholarship. One of them was created by Confucius (Kǒngzǐ, 孔子) (551–479 BCE) during the Spring and Autumn Period (722–484 BCE) (Chūnqiū, 春秋). Later, his philosophy was popularized and enlarged by Mencius (Mèngzǐ, 孟子) (372–289 BCE) in the Warring States Period (403–222 BCE) (Zhànguó, 戰國). The scholars who practice his philosophy are commonly called Confucians or Confucianists (Rújiā, 儒家). The key words to their basic philosophy are Loyalty (Zhōng, 忠), Filial Piety (Xiào, 孝), Humanity (Rén, 仁), Kindness (Ài, 愛), Trust (Xìn, 信), Justice (Yì, 義), Harmony (Hé, 和), and Peace (Píng, 平). Humanity and human feelings are the main subjects of study. Confucius' philosophy has become the center of much of Chinese culture.

The second major school of scholarship was called Daoism (Dàojiā, 道家) and was created by Lǎozi (老子) (604–531 BCE). Lǎozi is considered to be the author of a book called the *Dào Dé Jīng* (*Classic on the Virtue of the Dào*) (道德經) which describes the "virtue of the Dào such as human moralities." Later, in the Warring States Period (403–222 BCE), his follower Zhuāngzhōu (莊周) wrote a book called *Zhuāngzi* (莊子) which led to the formation of another strong branch of Daoism. Before the Hàn Dynasty, Daoism was considered a branch of scholarship. However, in the East Hàn Dynasty (25–168 CE), traditional Daoism was combined with the Buddhism imported from India by Zhāng, Dào-Líng (張道陵); it gradually began to be treated as a religion. Therefore, the Daoism before the Hàn Dynasty should be considered scholarly Daoism rather than religious.

With regard to their contribution to Qìgōng, both schools emphasized maintaining health and preventing disease. They believed that many illnesses are caused by mental and emotional excesses. When a person's mind is not calm, balanced, and peaceful, the organs will not function normally. For example, depression can cause stomach ulcers and indigestion. Anger will cause the liver to malfunction. Sadness will cause stagnation and tightness in the lungs, and fear can disturb the normal functioning of the kidneys and bladder. They realized that if you want to avoid illness, you must learn to balance and relax your thoughts and emotions. This is called "regulating the mind" (Tiáoxīn, 調心).

Therefore, the scholars emphasize gaining a peaceful mind through meditation. In their still meditation, the main part of the training is getting rid of thoughts so that the mind is clear and calm. When you become calm, the flow of thoughts and emotions slows down, and you feel mentally and emotionally neutral. This kind of meditation can be thought of as practicing emotional self-control. When you are in this "no thought" state, you become very relaxed, and can even relax deep down into your internal organs. When your body is this relaxed, your Qì will naturally flow smoothly and strongly. This kind of still meditation was very common in ancient Chinese scholar society.

In order to reach the goal of a calm and peaceful mind, their training focused on regulating the mind, body, and breath. They believed that as long as these three things were regulated, the Qì flow would be smooth and sickness would not occur. This is why the Qì training of the scholars is called "Xiūqì" (修氣), which means "cultivating Qì." "Xiū" (修) in Chinese means to regulate, to cultivate, to repair, or to maintain in good condition. This is very different from the religious Daoist Qì training after the East Hàn Dynasty which was called "Liànqì" (煉氣), and is translated "train Qì." "Liàn" (煉) means to drill or to practice to make stronger. They believed that it is possible to train your Qì to make it stronger; and to extend your life. It is said in scholarly society: "in human life, seventy is rare."[4] You should understand that few of the common people in ancient times lived past seventy because of the lack of good food and modern medical technology. It is also said: "peace with Heaven and delight in your destiny" (Āntiān Lèmìng, 安天樂命); and "cultivate the body and await destiny" (Xiūshēn Qímìng, 修身俟命). Compare this with the philosophy of the later Daoists, who said: "one hundred and twenty means dying young."[5] They believed and have proven that human life can be lengthened and destiny can be resisted and overcome.

Confucianism and Daoism were the two major scholarly schools in China, but there were many other schools which were also more or less involved in Qìgōng practices. We will not discuss them here because there are only a very limited number of Qìgōng documents from these schools.

Religious Qìgōng—for Enlightenment or Buddhahood. Religious Qìgōng, though not as popular as other categories in China, is recognized as having achieved the highest accomplishments of all the Qìgōng categories. It used to be kept secret in monastic society, and only in the 20th century was it revealed to laymen.

In China, religious Qìgōng includes mainly Daoist and Buddhist Qìgōng. The main purpose of their training is striving for enlightenment (Shéntōng, 神通), or what the Buddhists refer to as Buddhahood (Chéngfó, 成佛). They are looking for a way to lift themselves above normal human suffering, and to escape from the cycle of continual reincarnation. They believe that all human suffering is caused by the seven passions and six desires (Qīqíng Liùyù, 七情六慾). The seven passions are happiness (Xǐ, 喜), anger (Nù, 怒), sorrow (Āi, 哀), joy (Lè, 樂), love (Ài, 愛), hate (Hèn, 恨), and desire (Yù, 慾). The six desires are the six sensory pleasures derived from the eyes, ears, nose, tongue, body, and mind. If you are still bound to these emotions and desires, you will reincarnate after your death. To avoid reincarnation, you must train your spirit to reach a very high stage where it is strong enough to be independent after your death. This spirit will enter the heavenly kingdom and gain eternal peace. This final stage of training is called "unification of heaven and man" (Tiānrén Héyī, 天人合一). This training is hard to do in the everyday world, so practitioners frequently flee society and move into the solitude of the mountains, where they can concentrate all of their energies on self-cultivation.

Religious Qìgōng practitioners train to strengthen their internal Qì to nourish their Shén (神) (i.e., spirit) until the Shén is able to survive the death of the physical body. Marrow/Brain Washing Qìgōng (Xǐsuǐgōng, 洗髓功) training is necessary to reach this stage. It enables them to lead Qì to the brain, where the Shén resides, and raise the brain cells to a higher energy state. This training used to be restricted to only a few priests who had reached an advanced level. Tibetan Buddhists were also heavily involved in this training. Over the last two thousand years the Tibetan Buddhists, the Chinese Buddhists, and the religious Daoists have followed the same principles to become the three major religious schools of Qìgōng training.

This religious striving toward enlightenment or Buddhahood is recognized as the highest and most difficult level of Qìgōng. Many Qìgōng practitioners reject the rigors of this religious striving, and practice Marrow/Brain Washing Qìgōng solely for the purpose of longevity. It was these people who eventually revealed the secrets of Marrow/Brain Washing to the outside world. If you are interested in knowing more about this training, you may refer to: *Qìgōng—The Secret of Youth*, by Dr. Yáng.

Martial Qìgōng—for Fighting. Chinese martial Qìgōng was probably not developed until Dámó (達磨) wrote the *Muscle/Tendon Changing* and *Marrow/Brain Washing Qìgōng Classic* (*Yìjīnjīng*, *Xǐsuǐjīng*; 易筋經，洗髓經) in the Shàolín Temple (少林寺) during the Liáng Dynasty (梁朝) (502–557 CE). When Shàolín monks trained Dámó's Muscle/Tendon Changing Qìgōng, they found they could not only improve their health, but also greatly increase the power of their martial techniques. Since then, many martial styles have developed Qìgōng sets to increase their fighting effectiveness. In addition, many martial styles have been created based on Qìgōng theory. Martial artists have played a major role in Chinese Qìgōng society.

When Qìgōng theory was first applied to the martial arts, it was used to increase the power and efficiency of the muscles. The theory is very simple—the mind (Yì) is used to lead Qì to the muscles to energize them so that they function more efficiently. The average person generally uses his muscles at about 65–75 percent of maximum efficiency. If one can train his concentration and use his strong Yì (意) (i.e., the mind generated from clear thinking) to lead Qì to the muscles effectively, he can energize the muscles to a higher level and, therefore, increase his fighting effectiveness.

As acupuncture theory became better understood, fighting techniques were able to reach even more advanced levels. Martial artists learned to attack specific areas, such as vital acupuncture cavities, to disturb the enemy's Qì flow, and create imbalances which caused injury or even death. In order to do this, the practitioner must understand the route and timing of the Qì circulation in the human body. He also has to train so that he can strike the cavities accurately and to the correct depth. These cavity strike techniques are called "Diǎnxuè" (點穴) (Pointing Cavities) or "Diǎnmài" (點脈) (Pointing Vessels).

Most of the martial Qìgōng practices help to improve the practitioner's health. However, there are other martial Qìgōng practices which, although they build up some special skill which is useful for fighting, also damage the practitioner's health. An example of this is Iron Sand Palm (Tiěshāzhǎng, 鐵砂掌). Although this training can build up amazing destructive power, it can also harm your hands and affect the Qì circulation in the hands and internal organs.

Since the 6th century, many martial styles have been created that were based on Dámó's Qìgōng theory and methods. They can be roughly divided into external and internal styles.

The external styles emphasize building Qì in the limbs to coordinate with the physical martial techniques. They follow the theory of Wàidān (External Elixir) Qìgōng, which usually generates Qì in the limbs through special exercises. The concentrated mind is used during the exercises to energize the Qì. This increases muscular strength significantly, and therefore increases the effectiveness of the martial techniques. Qìgōng can also be used to train the body to resist punches and kicks. In this training, Qì is led to energize the skin and the muscles, enabling them to resist a blow without injury. This training is commonly called "Iron Shirt" (Tiěbùshān, 鐵布衫) or "Golden Bell Cover" (Jīnzhōngzhào, 金鐘罩). The martial styles which use Wàidān Qìgōng training are normally called external styles (Wàijiā, 外家). Hard Qìgōng training is called Hard Gōng (Yìnggōng, 硬功). Shàolín Gōngfū is a typical example of a style which uses Wàidān martial Qìgōng.

Although Wàidān Qìgōng can help the martial artist increase his power, there is a disadvantage. Because Wàidān Qìgōng emphasizes training the external muscles, it can cause over-development. This can cause a problem called "energy dispersion" (Sàngōng, 散功) when the practitioner gets older. In order to remedy this, when an external martial artist reaches a high level of external Qìgōng training he will start training internal Qìgōng, which specializes in curing the energy dispersion problem. That is why it is said: "External Gōngfū is from external to internal."

Internal Martial Qìgōng is based on the theory of Nèidān (Internal Elixir). In this method, Qì is generated in the body instead of the limbs, and this Qì is then led to the limbs to increase power. In order to lead Qì to the limbs, the techniques must be soft and muscle usage must be kept to a minimum. The training and theory of Nèidān martial Qìgōng is much more difficult than those of Wàidān martial Qìgōng. Interested readers should refer to the author's book *Tài Chí Theory and Martial Power,* published by YMAA Publication Center.

Several internal martial styles were created in the Wǔdāng (武當山) and Éméi (峨嵋山) Mountains. Popular styles are Tàijíquán (太極拳), Bāguàzhǎng (八卦掌), Liùhé Bāfǎ (六合八法), and Xíngyìquán (形意拳). However, you should understand that even the internal martial styles, which are commonly called Soft Styles (Ruǎnquán, 軟

拳), must on some occasions use muscular strength while fighting. In order to have strong power in the fight, the Qì must be led to the muscular body and manifested externally. Therefore, once an internal martial artist has achieved a degree of competence in internal Qìgōng, he or she should also learn how to use harder, more external techniques. That is why it is said: "The internal styles are from internal to external and from soft to hard."

You can see that, although Qìgōng is widely studied in Chinese martial society, the main focus of training was originally on increasing fighting ability rather than health. Good health was considered a by-product of training. It was not until this century that the health aspect of martial Qìgōng started receiving greater attention. This is especially true in the internal martial arts. If you would like to know more about Martial Qìgōng, please refer to the book *The Essence of Shàolín White Crane*, published by YMAA Publication Center.

From the above brief summary, you may obtain a general concept of how Chinese Qìgōng can be categorized, and should not have further doubt about any Qìgōng you are training.

1.2.6 Theory of Yīn-Yáng and Kǎn-Lí (Yīn-Yáng, Kǎn-Lí Zhī Lǐlùn, 陰陽、坎離之理論)

To practice Qìgōng accurately, you must not only understand the theory but also the correct methods of practice. Knowing the theory correctly places a clear and accurate map in your hands leading you to your goal in the shortest time. Without this map, you may take many years to find the correct path.

Two of the most important concepts in Qìgōng practice are the theory of Yīn and Yáng, and of Kǎn and Lí. These two concepts have been commonly confused in Qìgōng society, even in China. If you are able to understand them clearly, you will have grasped an important key to the practice of Qìgōng.

What are Kǎn and Lí? (Shénme Shì Kǎn-Lí?, 什麼是坎離？)

Kǎn and Lí training has long been of major importance to Qìgōng practitioners. In order to understand why, you must understand these two words, and the theory behind them. The terms Kǎn (坎) and Lí (離) occur frequently in Qìgōng documents. In the Eight Trigrams Kǎn represents "Water," while Lí represents "Fire." However, the everyday terms for water and fire are also often used.

First you should understand that though Kǎn-Lí and Yīn-Yáng are related, Kǎn and Lí are not Yīn and Yáng. Kǎn is Water, which is able to cool your body down and make it more Yīn, while Lí is Fire, which warms your body and makes it more Yáng. Kǎn and Lí are the methods or causes, while Yīn and Yáng are the results. When Kǎn and Lí are adjusted or regulated correctly, Yīn and Yáng will be balanced and interact harmoniously.

Qìgōng practitioners believe that your body is always too Yáng, unless you are sick or have not eaten for a long time, in which case your body may be more Yīn. When your body is always Yáng, it is degenerating and burning out. It is believed that this is the cause of aging. If you are able to use Water to cool down your body, you can slow down the process of degeneration, and thereby lengthen your life. This is the main reason why Qìgōng practitioners have been studying ways of improving the quality of Water in their bodies, and of reducing the quantity of Fire. I believe that as a Qìgōng practitioner, you should always keep this subject at the top of your list for study and research. If you earnestly ponder and experiment, you can grasp the trick of adjusting them.

If you want to learn how to adjust them, you must understand that Water and Fire mean many things in your body. The first concern is your Qì. Qì is classified as Fire or Water. When your Qì is not pure, and causes your physical body to heat up and your mental/spiritual body to become unstable (Yáng), it is classified as Fire Qì. The Qì which is pure and is able to cool both your physical and spiritual bodies (make them more Yīn) is considered Water Qì. However, your body can never be purely Water. Water can cool down the Fire, but it must never totally quench it, because then you would be dead. It is also said that Fire Qì is able to agitate and stimulate the emotions, and from these emotions generate a "mind." This mind is called Xīn (心), and is considered the Fire mind, Yáng mind, or emotional mind. On the other hand, the mind that Water Qì generates is calm, steady, and wise. This mind is called Yì (意), and is considered to be the Water mind or Wisdom Mind. If your Shén is nourished by Fire Qì, although your Shén may be high, it will be scattered and confused (a Yángshén). Naturally, if the Shén is nourished and raised up by Water Qì, it will be firm and steady (a Yīn mind). When your Yì is able to govern your emotional Xīn effectively, your will (strong emotional intention) can be firm.

You can see from this discussion that your Qì is the main cause of the Yīn and Yáng of your physical body, your mind, and your Shén. To regulate your body's Yīn and Yáng, you must learn how to regulate your body's Water and Fire Qì, and to do this efficiently you must know their sources.

In order to understand Kǎn and Lí clearly and to adjust them efficiently, you are urged to use the modern scientific, medical point of view to analyze the concepts. This will allow you to marry the past and present, and give birth to the future.

Kǎn and Lí in Breathing, Mind, and Shén (Hūxī, Xīnyì, Hé Shén De Kǎn-Lí, 呼吸、心意、和神的坎離)

Here we introduce the general concepts of how Kǎn and Lí relate to your breathing, mind, and Shén. Then, we will combine them together and construct a secret key which will lead you to the Qìgōng treasure.

Breathing's Kǎn and Lí. In Qìgōng, breathing is considered a "strategy" which enables you to lead the Qì effectively. For example, you can use your breath to lead the Qì to your skin or marrow. Slow or fast breathing can make the flow of Qì calm or vigorous. When you are excited your body is Yáng, and you exhale more than you inhale. This leads the Qì to the skin so that you sweat, and the excess dissipates in the surrounding air. When you are sad your body is Yīn, and you inhale more than you exhale to lead the Qì inward to conserve it, and you feel cold. You can see that breathing can be the main cause of changing the body's Yīn and Yáng. Therefore, breathing has Kǎn and Lí.

Generally speaking, in the normal state of your body, inhaling is considered to be a Water activity (Kǎn) because you lead the Qì inward to the bone marrow where it is stored. This reduces the Qì in the muscles and tendons, which calms down the body's Yáng. Exhaling is considered a Fire activity (Lí) because it brings Qì outward to the muscles, tendons, and skin to energize them, making the body more Yáng. When the body is more Yáng than its surroundings, the Qì in the body is automatically dissipated outward.

Normally, Yīn and Yáng should be balanced so that your body will function harmoniously. The trick to maintaining this balance is using breathing strategy. Usually your inhalations and exhalations should be equal. However, when you are excited your body is too Yáng, so you may inhale longer and deeper to calm down your mind and lead the Qì inside your body to make it more Yīn.

In Qìgōng practice, it is very important to grasp the trick of correct breathing. It is the exhalation which leads Qì to the five centers (head, two Láogōng cavities at the center of the palms, and two Yǒngquán cavities near the center of the soles) and the skin to exchange Qì with the surroundings. Inhalation leads Qì deep inside your body to reach the internal organs and marrow. Table 1–1 summarizes how different breathing strategies affect the body's Yīn and Yáng in their various manifestations.

The Mind's Kǎn and Lí. According to Chinese tradition, a human has two minds: Xīn (心) and Yì (意). Xīn is translated literally as "heart" and is considered as the mind generated from emotional disturbance. Therefore, Xīn can be translated as "emotional mind." The Chinese word for Yì is constructed of three characters. The top one means "establish" (立), the middle one means "speaking" (曰), and the bottom one is "heart" (心). That means the emotional mind is under control when you speak. Therefore, Yì can be translated as "Wisdom Mind" or "Rational Mind." Because the emotional mind makes you excited and emotionally disturbed, which results in the excitement of your body (Yáng), it is considered as Lí. The Wisdom Mind which makes you calm, peaceful, and able to think clearly (Yīn) is considered to be Kǎn.

In Qìgōng training, the mind is considered the "general" who directs the entire battle. It is the general who decides the fighting strategy (breathing) and controls the movement of the soldiers (Qì). Therefore, as a general, you must control your Xīn (emotional

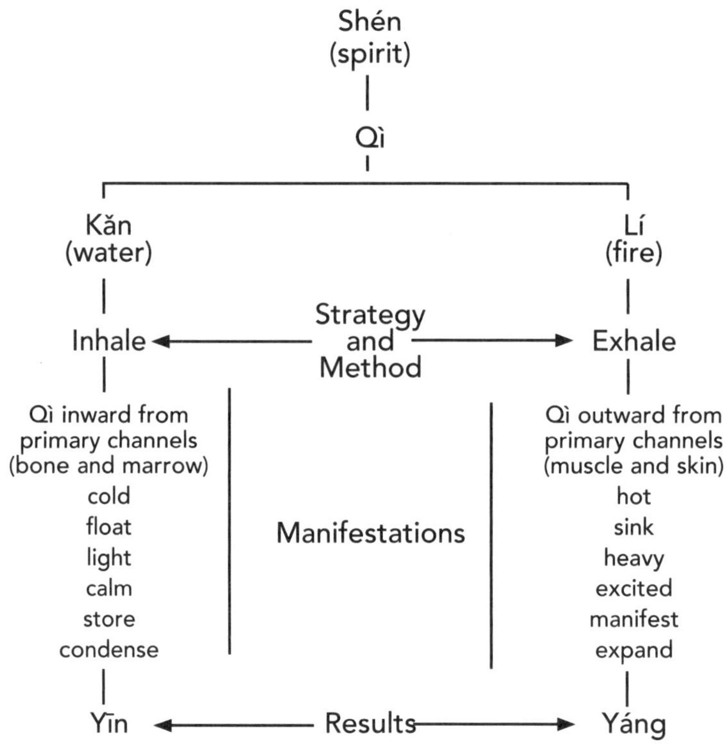

Table 1-1. The Effects of Breathing on the Body's Yīn and Yáng in their Various Manifestations

mind) and use your Yì (Wisdom Mind) to judge and understand the situation and finally decide on the proper strategy.

In Qìgōng, your Wisdom Mind must first dominate the situation and generate an idea. This idea generates and executes the strategy (breathing) and is also the force that moves the Qì. Generally speaking, when your mind is excited, aggressive, and energized, the strategy (breathing) is more offensive (emphasizing exhalation) and the Qì circulation is more vigorous and expansive. This aggressive mind is then considered a Fire mind, since it is able to make your body more Yáng. However, when the strategy is more defensive (i.e., emphasizing inhalation), the Qì circulation will be more calm and condensed. Therefore, a calm or depressed mind is considered a Water mind, since it can make your body more Yīn.

You can see that the Kǎn and Lí of the mind are more important than those of breathing. After all, it is the mind which makes the strategy. Regulating the mind and the breathing are two of the basic techniques for controlling your body's Yīn and Yáng. Regulating the mind cannot be separated from regulating the breathing. When the mind is regulated, the breathing can be regulated. When the breathing is regulated, the mind is able to enter a deeper state of calm.

The Shén's Kǎn and Lí. Now it is time to consider the final and most decisive element in winning a battle—the Shén (神). Shén is compared to the morale of the general's officers and soldiers. There are many cases throughout history of armies winning battles against great odds because the morale of their soldiers was high. If a soldier's morale is high enough, he can defeat ten enemies.

It is the same in Qìgōng training. It is the Shén which determines how successful your Qìgōng practice will be. Your Yì (Wisdom Mind), which is the general who makes the strategy, must also be concerned with raising up the fighting morale (Shén) of the soldiers (Qì). When their morale is raised the soldiers can be led more efficiently, and consequently the strategy can be executed more effectively.

You can see that knowing how to use the Yì to raise the Shén is the major key to successful Qìgōng training. In Qìgōng, Shén is considered the headquarters which governs the Qì. In fact, both Yì and Shén govern the Qì. They are closely related and cannot be separated.

Generally speaking, when the Wisdom Mind (Yì) is energized, the Shén is also raised. You should understand that in Qìgōng training, you want to raise your Shén but not let it get excited. When the Shén is raised, the strategy can be carried out effectively. However, if the Shén is excited, the body will become too Yáng, and that is not desirable in Qìgōng practice. When you are practicing Qìgōng, you want to keep your Shén high all the time and use it to govern the strategy and the Qì. This will enable you to readjust or regulate your Kǎn and Lí efficiently.

Shén is the control tower which is able to adjust the Kǎn and Lí, but it does not have Kǎn and Lí itself. However, some Qìgōng practitioners consider the raised Shén to be Lí (Fire) and the calm Shén to be Kǎn (Water).

Now, let us draw a few important conclusions from the above discussion:

A. Kǎn (Water) and Lí (Fire) are not Yīn and Yáng. Kǎn and Lí are methods which can cause Yīn or Yáng.

B. Qì itself is only a form of energy and does not have Kǎn and Lí. When Qì is excessive or deficient, it can cause the body to be too Yáng or too Yīn.

C. When you adjust Kǎn and Lí in the body, the mind is the first concern. The mind can be Kǎn or Lí. It determines the strategy (breathing) for withdrawing the Qì (Kǎn) or expanding it (Lí).

D. Breathing has Kǎn and Lí. Usually inhaling, which makes the body more Yīn, is Kǎn. Exhaling, which makes the body more Yáng, is Lí.

E. The Shén does not have Kǎn and Lí. Shén is the key to making the Kǎn and Lí adjustment effective and efficient.

The Key Secrets of Adjusting Kǎn and Lí (Tiáozhěng Kǎn-Lí De Guānjiàn Mìjué, 調整坎離的關鍵秘訣)

In light of these conclusions, let us discuss the keys of Kǎn and Lí adjustment. These keys are repeatedly mentioned in the ancient documents. The first key is that Shén and Breathing mutually rely on each other. The second key is that Shén and Qì mutually combine and harmonize with each other.

Shén and Breathing Mutually Dependent (Shénxí Xiāngyī, 神息相依). We know that breathing is the strategy which directs the Qì in various ways and therefore controls and adjusts the Kǎn and Lí, which in turn control the body's Yīn and Yáng. We also know that the Shén is the control tower which is able to make the strategy work in the most efficient way. Therefore, Shén governs the strategy directly, and controls Kǎn and Lí and the body's Yīn and Yáng indirectly. You can see that the success of your Kǎn and Lí adjustment depends upon your Shén.

When the Shén matches your inhaling and exhaling, it can lead the Qì to condense and expand directly in the most efficient way. Your Shén must match with the breathing to be raised up or calmed down, and the breathing must rely on the Shén to make the strategy work efficiently. In this case, it seems that the Shén and breathing are dependent on each other and cannot be separated. In Qìgōng practice, this training is called "Shénxí Xiāngyī" (神息相依) which means "Shén and Breathing Mutually Dependent." When your Shén and Breathing match each other, it is called "Shénxí" (神息) (Shén Breathing), because it seems that your Shén is actually doing the breathing.

You can see that "Shénxí Xiāngyī" is a technique or method in which, when the Shén and breathing are united, the Shén is able to control the Qì more directly.

Shén and Qì Mutually Combined (Shénqì Xiànghé, 神氣相合). When your Shén and Breathing are able to match with each other as one, the Qì can be led directly, and thus Shén and Qì also become one. In Qìgōng practice it is called "Shénqì Xiànghé" (神氣相合), which means "Shén and Qì mutually combined or harmonized." When this happens, the Shén can govern the Qì directly and more efficiently. You can see from this that the Shén and Qì combining is the result of the Shén and breathing being mutually dependent.

Dámó (達磨) believed that in order to have a long and peaceful life, Shén and Qì must be coordinated and harmonized with each other. He said: "If (one) does not know how to keep the mother (Qì) and son (Shén) together, though the Qì (is directed) by breathing internally, (nevertheless) the Shén is labored and craves external (objects), resulting in the Shén being always debauched and dirty; the Shén is thus not clear. (If) the Shén is not clear, the original harmonious Qì will disperse gradually, (Shén and Qì) cannot be kept together."[6] From this, you can see that Shén is very important. To regulate the Shén is one of the highest levels of Qìgōng practice. The reason for this is simply that in order to reach a high degree of harmony, you must first regulate your emotional mind. This is hard to achieve in lay society.

1.3 The Network of Qì Vessels and Channels (Qìmài Yǔ Jīngluò Wǎnglù, 氣脈與經絡網路)

As explained earlier, we have two bodies: the physical body and the Qì body (or bio-electric body). The physical body can be seen, but Qì can only be felt. The Qì body is the vital source of the physical body (i.e., all living cells) and the foundation of our lives. The Qì body is not only related to our cells, but also to our thinking and Shén, since it is the energy source which maintains the brain's functioning. Therefore, any Qì imbalance or stagnation will be the root and cause of any physical sickness or mental disorder.

Western medical science has long studied the physical body, but ignored the Qì body for the most part. This has begun to change since the late 20th century. The scientific understanding of the Qì body, and how it affects our health and longevity, is still in its infancy. Under these circumstances, we may still accept the ancient Chinese understanding of our body's Qì network.

1.3.1 Twelve Primary Qì Channels and the Eight Vessels (Shíèrjīng, Luò Yǔ Bāmài, 十二經、絡與八脈)

From the understanding of Chinese medicine, the Qì circulatory system in a human body includes eight vessels (Bāmài, 八脈), twelve primary Qì channels (Shíèrjīng, 十二經), and thousands of secondary channels branching out from the primary channels (Luò, 絡). On two of the vessels (Conception and Governing Vessels) (Rènmài and Dūmài, 任脈・督脈) and the twelve primary Qì channels, there are more than seven hundred acupuncture cavities, through which the Qì level in the channels can be adjusted and regulated. From this Qì adjustment, the Qì circulation in the body, especially in the internal organs, can be regulated to a harmonious state, and the body's sickness can be cured and health maintained. Here, we will briefly review these three circulatory networks. If you are interested in learning more about this Qì network, you may refer to Chinese acupuncture books or to the book: *The Root of Chinese Qìgōng*, published by YMAA Publication Center.

1. **Eight Vessels** (Bāmài) (Bāmài, 八脈)

   a. The eight vessels include four Yáng vessels and four Yīn vessels. They therefore balance each other.

   b. The Four Yáng Vessels are:

      Governing Vessel (Dūmài, 督脈) (Figure 1–4)

      Girdle (or Belt) Vessel (Dàimài, 帶脈) (Figure 1–5)

      Yáng Heel Vessel (Yángqiāomài, 陽蹻脈) (Figure 1–6)

      Yáng Linking Vessel (Yángwéimài, 陽維脈) (Figure 1–7)

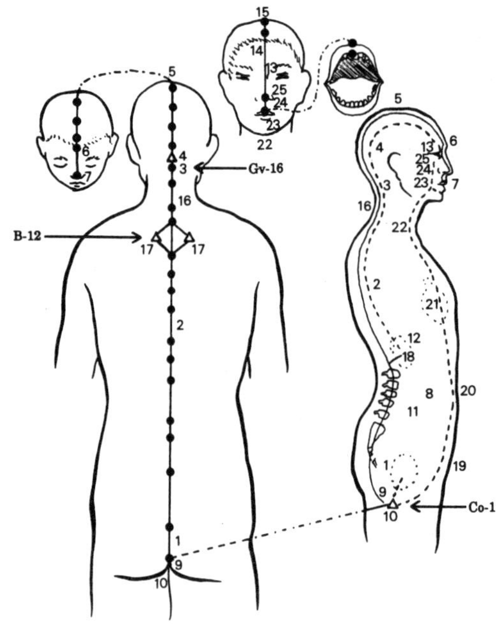

Figure 1-4. The Governing Vessel (Dūmài)

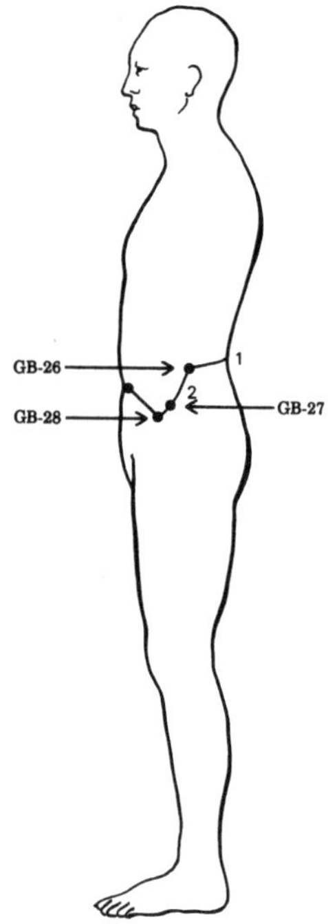

Figure 1-5. The Girdle Vessel (Dàimài)

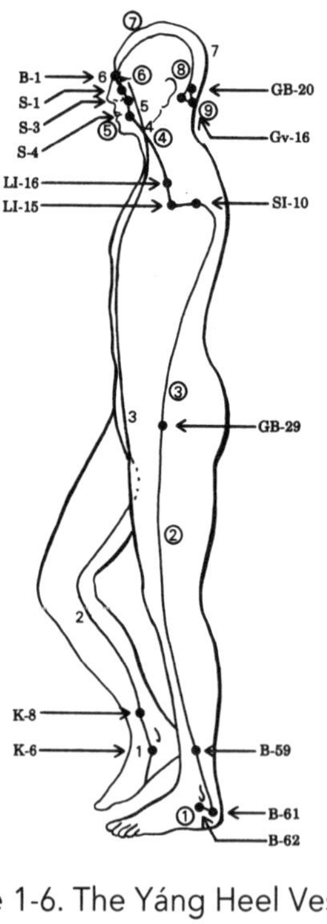

Figure 1-6. The Yáng Heel Vessel (Yángqiāomài) and the Yīn Heel Vessel (Yīnqiāomài)

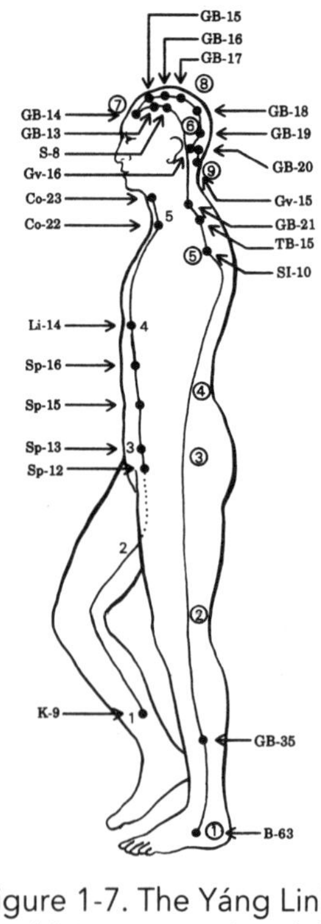

Figure 1-7. The Yáng Linking Vessel (Yángwéimài) and the Yīn Linking Vessel (Yīnwéimài)

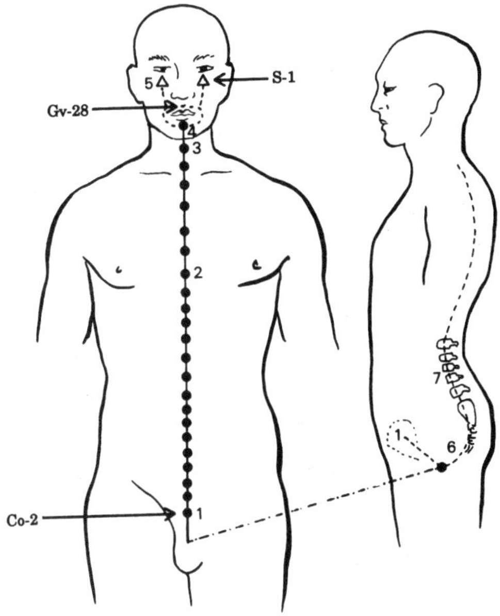

Figure 1-8. The Conception Vessel (Rènmài)

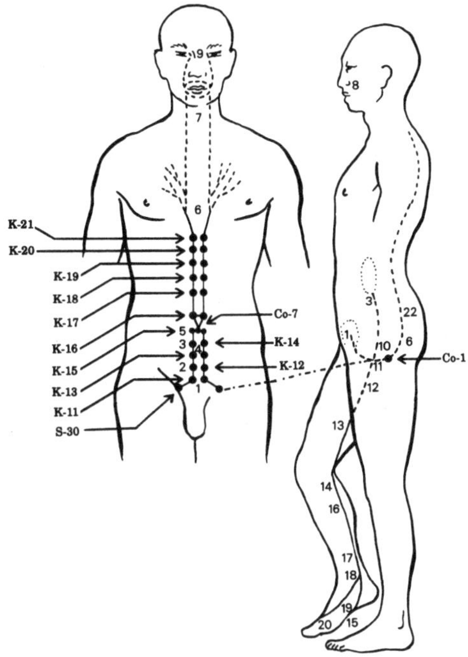

Figure 1-9. The Thrusting Vessel (Chōngmài)

The Four Yīn Vessels are:

Conception Vessel (Rènmài, 任脈) (Figure 1–8)

Thrusting Vessel (Chōngmài, 衝脈) (Figure 1–9)

Yīn Heel Vessel (Yīnqiāomài, 陰蹻脈) (Figure 1–6)

Yīn Linking Vessel (Yīnwéimài, 陰維脈) (Figure 1–7).

c. According to Chinese medicine, vessels function as reservoirs, connected to the twelve primary Qì channels and regulating the Qì level circulating in these channels. When the Qì level in some specific channel is too high, one or more of the reservoirs will absorb the excess Qì, and if the Qì is too low, the shortfall will be supplied from these vessels. This enables a harmonious level to be maintained.

d. The two Yáng vessels (Governing and Girdle Vessels), and the two Yīn vessels (Conception and Thrusting Vessels), are individual and located in the torso. The other four vessels exist in pairs, and are located in the legs. There are no vessels in the arms.

e. Among the eight vessels, according to Chinese medicine, the Governing and Conception Vessels are the most important, since they are the main vessels that regulate the twelve primary Qì channels. The Governing Vessel regulates the Qì in the six primary Yáng Qì channels, while the Conception Vessel regulates the Qì in the six primary Yīn Qì Channels. There are acupuncture cavities on these two vessels, and none on the other six vessels. However, there are many cavities on these six vessels that belong to the twelve primary Qì channels. These cavities are considered to be gates that allow the Qì to pass between the vessels and channels.

f. According to Chinese Qìgōng practice for health and longevity, the methods of learning how to expand the Qì in the vessels are very important. The reason for this is that these eight vessels are the reservoirs for the Qì. When the Qì in these reservoirs is abundant, the Qì-regulating potential of the primary Qì channels will be high and efficient. Among these eight vessels, the Governing and Conception Vessels are the most important, since they regulate the twelve primary Qì channels. The Qì circulates in these two vessels and distributes to the twelve primary Qì channels throughout the day.

g. In religious Qìgōng meditation practice for enlightenment, the Thrusting Vessel (i.e., spinal cord) is very important. The Thrusting Vessel connects the brain and the perineum, and the Qì is abundant in this vessel at midnight. Typically, during the midnight hours, we are sleeping and the physical body is extremely relaxed. In this situation, the physical body does not need a great amount of Qì to support its activities, and the Qì circulates abundantly in the spinal cord to nourish the brain and sexual organs. Hormone production from the pineal, pituitary, and adrenal glands, as well as the testicles or ovaries, is therefore increased at night. When the brain is nourished and its functioning is raised to a high level, the Shén can be raised and enlightenment can be achieved. If you are interested in more on this subject, please refer to the book: *Qìgōng—The Secret of Youth*, published by YMAA Publication Center.

h. The Governing Vessel, which is located at the center of the back, is the main vessel supplying Qì to the nervous system branching out from the spinal cord. The nervous system is constructed of physical cells which need to be nourished with Qì (bioelectricity) to function and stay alive. This tells us that Qì is ultimately the root of the nerves' functioning. To maintain abundant Qì circulation in this vessel, your physical condition is extremely important. If there is any physical injury or damage along the course of this vessel, the Qì supply to the nervous system will be stagnant and irregular. Moreover, in order to have healthy and abundant Qì circulation in this vessel, you must learn how to increase Qì storage in the Real Lower Dāntián (Zhēn Xiàdāntián, 真下丹田), which is the main Qì reservoir or bioelectric battery in our body.

i. The Yáng Girdle Vessel is the only vessel in which the Qì circulates horizontally. To Qìgōng practitioners, this vessel is very important. Since the Qì status in this vessel is Yáng, the Qì is expanding outward. It is from this vessel that we feel our balance. It is just like an airplane or a tight-rope walker: the longer the wings or the balancing pole, the easier it will be to find and maintain balance. A Qìgōng practitioner or a Chinese martial artist will train this vessel and make the Qì expand outward farther, therefore increasing the balance and stability of both the physical and mental bodies. When you have more balance and stability, you can find your center. *When you find your physical and mental center, then you will be rooted. Once you are rooted, your Shén can be raised to a higher level.*

1.3.2 The Twelve Primary Qì Channels and Their Branches (Shíèr Jīngluò, 十二經絡)

a. The Twelve Primary Qì Channels include six Yáng channels and six Yīn channels. They therefore balance each other.

b. The Six Yáng channels are:
Arm Yáng Brightness Large Intestine Channel (Shǒu Yángmíng Dàchángjīng, 手陽明大腸經) (Figure 1–10)
Leg Yáng Brightness Stomach Channel (Zú Yángmíng Wèijīng, 足陽明胃經) (Figure 1–11)

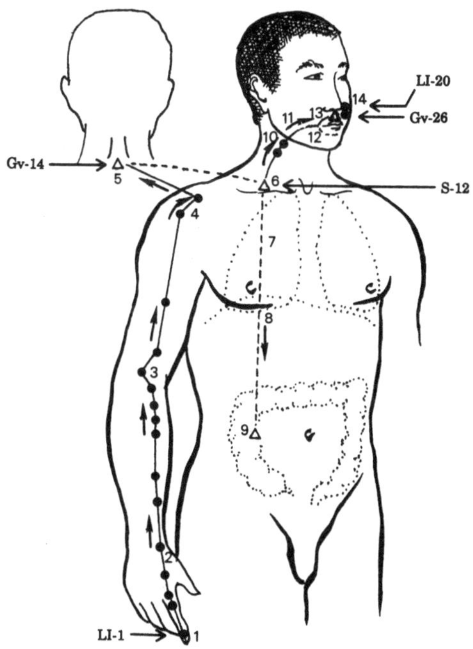

Figure 1-10. Arm Yáng Brightness Large Intestine Channel

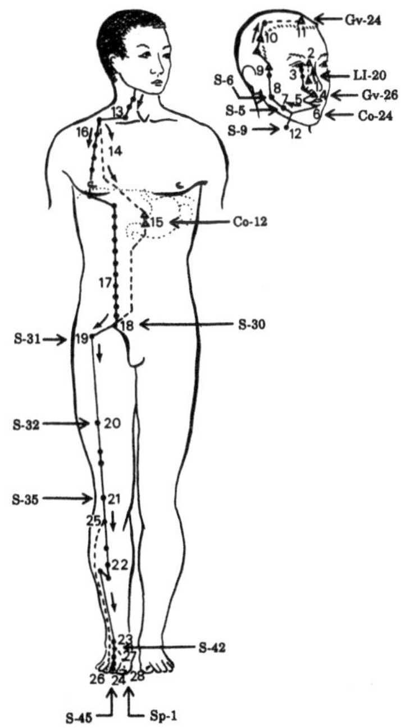

Figure 1-11. Leg Yáng Brightness Stomach Channel

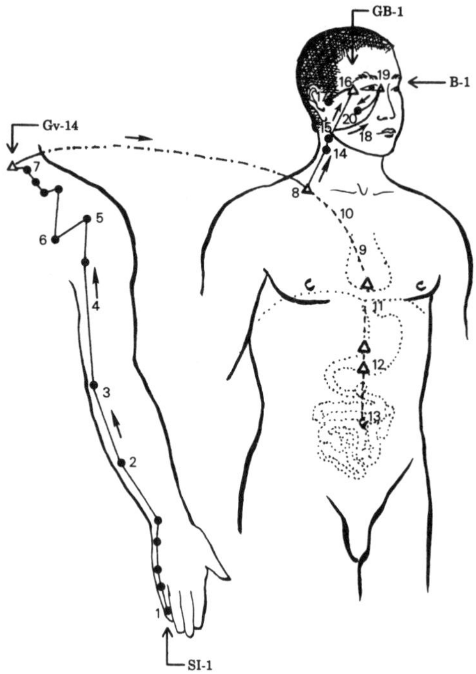

Figure 1-12. Arm Greater Yáng Small Intestine Channel

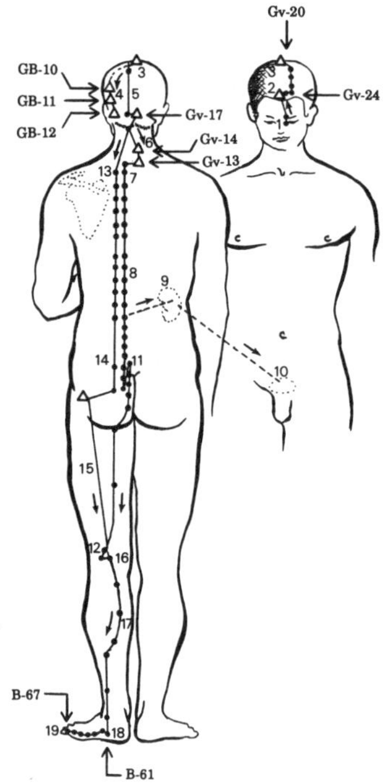

Figure 1-13. Leg Greater Yáng Bladder Channel

Arm Greater Yáng Small Intestine Channel (Shǒu Tàiyáng Xiǎochángjīng, 手太陽小腸經) (Figure 1–12)
Leg Greater Yáng Bladder Channel (Zú Tàiyáng Pángguāngjīng, 足太陽膀胱經) (Figure 1–13)
Arm Lesser Yáng Triple Burner Channel (Shǒu Shǎoyáng Sānjiāojīng, 手少陽三焦經) (Figure 1–14)
Leg Lesser Yáng Gall Bladder Channel (Zú Shǎoyáng Dǎnjīng, 足少陽膽經) (Figure 1–15)

The Six Yīn channels are:
Arm Greater Yīn Lung Channel (Shǒu Tàiyīn Fèijīng, 手太陰肺經) (Figure 1–16)
Leg Greater Yīn Spleen Channel (Zú Tàiyīn Píjīng, 足太陰脾經) (Figure 1–17)
Arm Lesser Yīn Heart Channel (Shǒu Shǎoyīn Xīnjīng, 手少陰心經) (Figure 1–18)
Leg Lesser Yīn Kidney Channel (Zú Shǎoyīn Shènjīng, 足少陰腎經) (Figure 1–19)

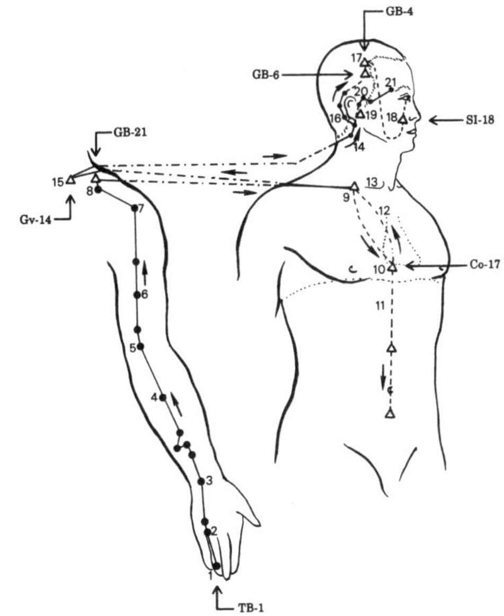

Figure 1-14. Arm Lesser Yáng
Triple Burner Channel

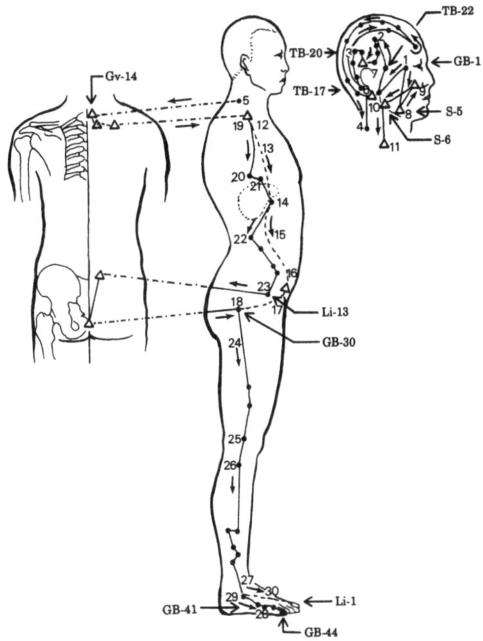

Figure 1-15. Leg Lesser Yáng
Gall Bladder Channel

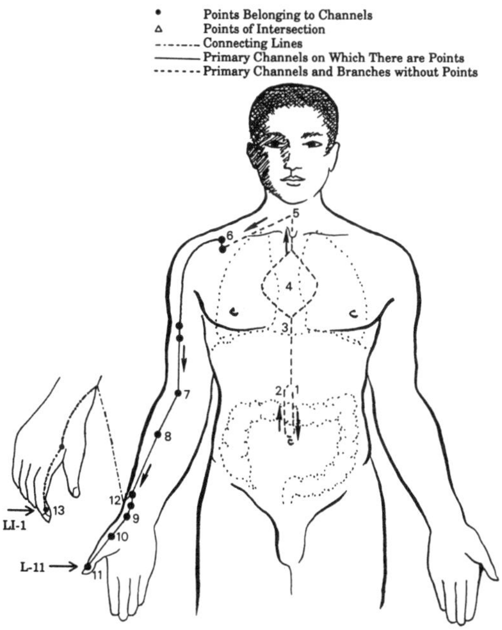

Figure 1-16. Arm Greater Yīn
Lung Channel

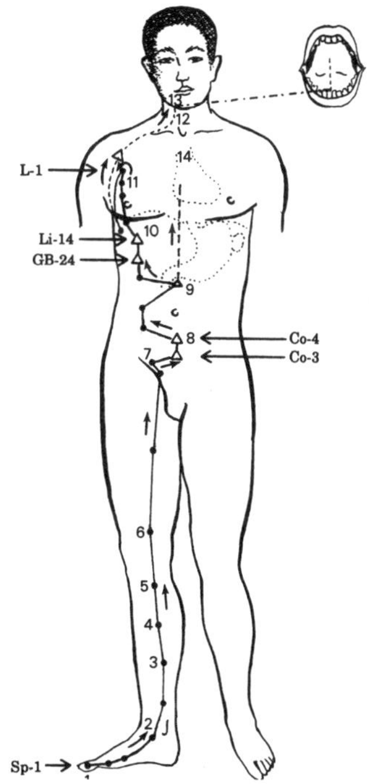

Figure 1-17. Leg Greater Yīn
Spleen Channel

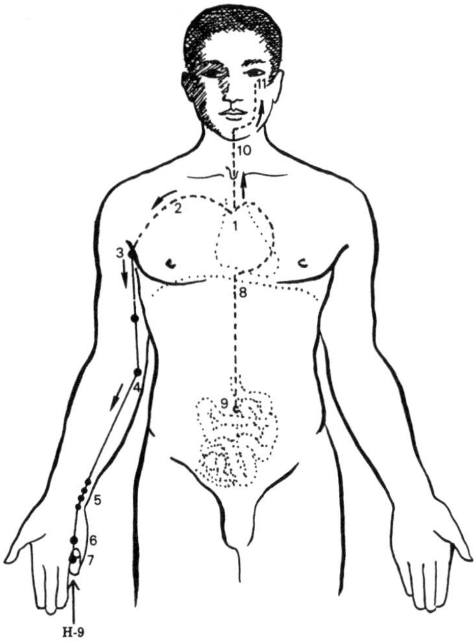

Figure 1-18. Arm Lesser Yīn Heart Channel

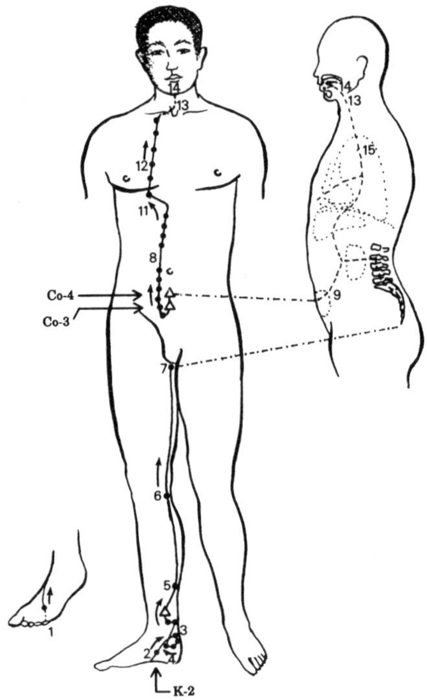

Figure 1-19. Leg Lesser Yīn Kidney Channel

Arm Absolute Yīn Pericardium Channel (Shǒu Juéyīn Xīnbāoluòjīng, 手厥陰心包絡經) (Figure 1–20)
Leg Absolute Yīn Liver Channel (Zú Juéyīn Gānjīng, 足厥陰肝經) (Figure 1–21)

c. From the above, you can see that one end of each channel connects to an extremity, and the other end connects with a different internal organ. In each channel, there are many acupuncture cavities through which the Qì condition in each channel can be regulated. This is the basic theory of acupuncture.

d. There are thousands of secondary channels (Luò, 絡) branching out from each primary; these lead the Qì to the surface of the skin and to the bone marrow. It is very similar to the artery and capillary system. Instead of blood, Qì is being distributed.

1.4 Buddhist and Daoist Qìgōng Concepts (Fójiā Yǔ Dàojiā Zhī Qìgōng Gàiniàn, 佛家與道家之氣功概念)

Because it was kept so secret, religious Qìgōng did not become as popular as the other categories in China before the Qīng Dynasty (清朝) (1644–1912 CE). It was not until the 20th century, when the secrets were gradually released to the public, that religious

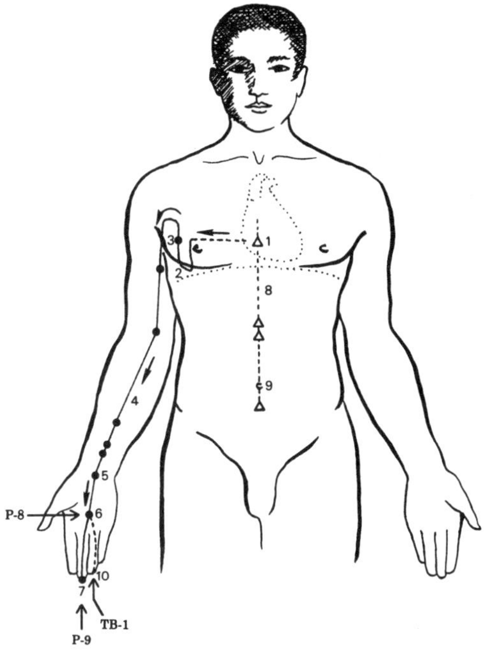

Figure 1-20. Arm Absolute Yīn Pericardium Channel

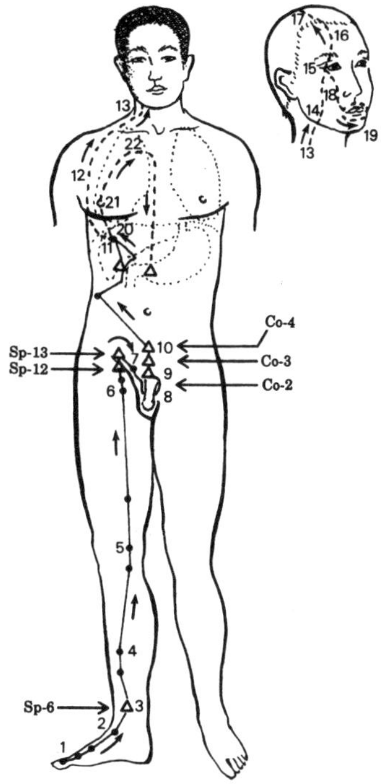

Figure 1-21. Leg Absolute Yīn Liver Channel

Qìgōng became popular in China. Religious Qìgōng is mostly Daoist and Buddhist, and its main purpose is to aid in one's striving for enlightenment, or what the Buddhists refer to as Buddhahood.

In order to help you understand both the training theory and methods studied in Buddhist and Daoist societies, I would like to give a brief introduction to Buddhist and Daoist Qìgōng, followed by a comparison of their training.

Buddhist Qìgōng (Fójiā Qìgōng, 佛家氣功). Three main schools of Buddhist Qìgōng developed in Asia during the last two thousand years: Indian, Chinese, and Tibetan. Because Buddhism was created in India by an Indian prince named Gautama between 558 BCE and 478 BCE, Indian Buddhist Qìgōng has the longest history. Buddhism was imported into China during the Eastern Hàn Dynasty (Dōnghàn, 東漢) (58 CE), and the Chinese Buddhists gradually learned its methods of spiritual cultivation. Their practice was influenced by traditional Chinese Scholar and Medical Qìgōng, which had been developing for about two thousand years. What resulted was a unique system of training which was different from its ancestors.

According to the available document fragments, it is believed that, at least in the first few hundred years after Buddhism's importation, only the philosophy and doctrines were passed down to the Chinese. The actual methods of cultivation and Qìgōng training were not known. There are several reasons for this:

1. Because of the difficulty of transportation and communication at that time, the transferral of Buddhist documents from India to China was limited. Although a few Indian priests were invited to China to preach, the problems remained.
2. Even if the documents had been transferred, because of the profound theory and philosophy of Buddhism, very few people were qualified to translate the documents accurately from the Indian languages to Chinese. This problem was exacerbated by the different cultural backgrounds. Even today, cultural differences are always the main problem in translating accurately.
3. The main reason was probably that most of the actual training methods need to be taught and guided personally by an experienced master. Only a limited amount can be learned from the documents. This problem was exacerbated by the tradition of passing information secretly from master to disciple.

You can see that the transferral process was very slow and painful, especially with regard to the actual training methods. For several hundred years it was believed that as long as you were able to purify your mind and sincerely strive for Buddhahood, sooner or later you would succeed. This situation was not improved until Dámó (達磨) wrote the *Muscle/Tendon Changing Classic* and the *Marrow/Brain Washing Classic* (*Yìjīnjīng, Xǐsuǐjīng*; 易筋經、洗髓經). Then, finally, there was a firm direction for the training to reach the goal of Buddhahood.

Before Dámó, Chinese Buddhist Qìgōng training was very similar to Chinese Scholar Qìgōng. The main difference was that while Scholar Qìgōng aimed at maintaining health, Buddhist Qìgōng aimed at becoming a Buddha. Meditation is a necessary process in training a priest to stay emotionally neutral. Buddhism believes that all human spiritual suffering is caused by the seven passions and six desires (Qīqíng Liùyù, 七情六慾). As mentioned earlier, the seven passions are happiness (Xǐ, 喜), anger (Nù, 怒), sorrow (Āi, 哀), joy (Lè, 樂), love (Ài, 愛), hate (Hèn, 恨), and desire (Yù, 慾). The six desires are the six sensory pleasures derived from the eyes, ears, nose, tongue, body, and mind. Buddhists also cultivate within themselves a neutral state, separated from the four emptinesses of earth, water, fire, and wind (Sìdà Jiēkōng, 四大皆空). They believe that this training enables them to keep their spirits independent so they can escape from the cycle of repeated reincarnation.

Tibetan Buddhism has always been kept secret and isolated from the outside world. Because of this, it is very difficult to determine exactly when Tibetan Buddhism was established. Because Tibet is near India, it is reasonable to assume that Tibetan Qìgōng training has had more influence from India than Chinese Qìgōng has. However, over thousands of years of study and research, the Tibetans established their own unique style of Qìgōng meditation. The Tibetan priests are called Lamas (Lǎma, 喇嘛), and many of them also learned martial arts. Because of the different cultural background, not only are the Lamas' meditation techniques different from those of the Chinese or Indian Buddhists, but their martial techniques are also different. Tibetan Qìgōng meditation and martial arts were kept secret from the outside world, and were therefore called "Mìzōng" (秘宗), which means "secret style." Generally speaking, Tibetan Qìgōng and martial arts did not spread into Chinese society until almost the Qīng Dynasty (清朝) (1644–1912 CE). Since then, however, they have become more popular.

Daoist Qìgōng (Dàojiā Qìgōng, 道家氣功). Like the Buddhists, Daoists believe that if they can build up their Shén (神) so that it is independent and strong, they can escape from the cycle of repeated reincarnation. When a Daoist has reached this stage, he has reached the goal of enlightenment, and it is said that he has attained eternal life. However, if he cannot build his Shén quite strong enough before he dies, his soul or Shén will not go to hell, and he can control his own destiny, either remaining a spirit or being reborn as a human. They believe that it is only possible to develop the human spirit while in a body, so that the continual cycle of rebirth is necessary to attain enlightenment.

Daoist monks, in the past, found that in order to enhance their Shén, they had to cultivate the Qì which was converted from their Essence (Jīng, 精). The normal Daoist Qìgōng training process is: 1. To convert the Essence (Jīng) into Qì (Liànjīng Huàqì, 煉精化氣); 2. To nourish the Shén with Qì (Liànqì Huàshén, 煉氣化神); 3. To refine the Shén and return into nothingness (Liànshén Fǎnxū, 煉神返虛); and 4. To crush the nothingness (Fěnsuì Xūkōng, 粉碎虛空).

The first step involved firming and strengthening the Jīng, then converting this Jīng into Qì through meditation or other methods. This Qì is then led to the top of the head to nourish the brain and raise the Shén. When a Daoist has reached this stage, it is called "the three flowers meet at the top" (Sānhuā Jùdǐng, 三花聚頂). The three flowers mean essence (Jīng), Qì, and Shén. This stage is necessary to gain health and longevity. Finally, the Daoist can start training to reach the goal of enlightenment. However, the biggest obstacle to achieving this goal is the emotions, which affect the thinking and upset the balance of the Shén. This is the reason why Daoists hid themselves in the mountains, away from other people and their distractions. Usually they also abstained from eating meat, feeling that it muddied thinking and increased the emotions, leading the Shén away from self-cultivation.

An important part of this training to prolong life is Yìjīnjīng (易筋經) (Muscle/Tendon Changing) and Xǐsuǐjīng (洗髓經) (Marrow/Brain Washing) Qìgōng. While the Yìjīnjīng Qìgōng is able to build up an abundant Qì in the Lower Dāntián and strengthen the physical body, the basic idea of Xǐsuǐjīng Qìgōng is to lead the Qì to the brain to raise up the Shén and keep the Qì circulating in the marrow so that the marrow stays clean and healthy. Your bone marrow manufactures most of your blood cells. The blood cells bring nourishment to the organs and all the other cells of the body, and also take waste products away. When your blood is healthy and functions properly, your whole body is well-nourished and healthy, and can resist disease effectively. When the marrow is clean and fresh, it manufactures a plentiful quantity of healthy blood cells which will do their job properly. Your whole body will stay healthy, and the degeneration of your physical body will be significantly slowed.

For longevity, although the theory is simple, the training is very difficult. You must first learn how to build up your Qì at the Lower Dāntián (human bio-battery) and fill up your eight Qì vessels, and then you must know how to lead this Qì into the bone marrow to "wash" the marrow. Except for some Daoist monks, there are very few people who have lived longer than 150 years. The reason for this is that the training process is long and hard. You must have a pure mind and a simple lifestyle so that you can concentrate entirely on the training. Without a peaceful life, your training will not be effective.

Many Daoist Qìgōng styles are based on the theory of cultivating both the Shén and the physical body. It is said: "Talking about human temperament (i.e., Shén) and life (i.e., physical life), (one) must cultivate both of them. (One must) place the lead (Pb, i.e., Yīn) and mercury (Hg, i.e., Yáng) together (i.e., they interact harmoniously). This message (secret) is hard to comprehend. Cultivating human temperament is to refine self-being, while cultivating life is to return the essence (i.e., convert the essence into Qì). The Xīn (i.e., mind) is the house of the Shén while the body is the residence of the Qì. Life is the Qì. Those who cultivate human temperament, must blend the body and the Xīn as a family, Jīng (essence), Qì, and Shén must be combined into one unit. Then the cultivation of life can be approached."[7] This paragraph emphasizes that in order to reach enlightenment, you must cultivate both human temperament and physical life. The key is to harmonize the Yīn and Yáng. Yīn is the spiritual body related to human temperament, while Yáng is the physical life related to physical condition. Only when these Yīn and Yáng are harmonious and the three treasures (Jīng, Qì, and Shén) have reached the top (brain) are you able to achieve the goal of enlightenment.

In Daoism, there are generally three ways of training: Golden Elixir Large Way (Jīndān Dàdào, 金丹大道), Dual Cultivation (Shuāngxiū, 雙修), and Herb Picking Outside of the Dào (Dàowài Cǎiyào, 道外採藥). Generally, there are two meanings to "Dual Cultivation;" one is to cultivate the Qì with a partner, while the other implies the cultivation of both the human temperament and the physical body.

Golden Elixir Large Way teaches the ways of Qìgōng training within yourself. This approach believes that you can find the elixir of longevity or even enlightenment within your own body.

In the second approach, Dual Cultivation, a partner is used to balance one's Qì more quickly. Most people's Qì is not entirely balanced. Some people are a bit too positive, others too negative, and individual channels are also positive or negative. If you know how to exchange Qì with your partner, you can help each other out and speed your training. Your partner can be either the same sex or the opposite.

The third way, Herb Picking Outside of the Dào, uses herbs to speed and control the cultivation. "Herbs" can be plants such as ginseng, or animal products such as musk from the musk-deer. To many Daoists, "herbs" can also mean the Qì which can be obtained from sexual practices.

According to the training methods used, Daoist Qìgōng can again be divided into two major schools: Peaceful Cultivation Division (Qīngxiūpài, 清修派) and Plant and Graft Division (Zāijiēpài, 栽接派). This division was especially clear after the Sòng and Yuán dynasties (960–1367 CE, 宋、元). The meditation, training theory and methods of the Peaceful Cultivation Division are close to those of the Buddhists. They believe that the only way to reach enlightenment is Golden Elixir Large Way, according to which you build up the elixir within your body. Using a partner for the cultivation is immoral and will cause emotional problems which may significantly affect the cultivation.

However, the Plant and Graft Division claims that their approach of using Dual Cultivation and Herb Picking Outside of the Dào in addition to Golden Elixir Large Way makes the cultivation faster and more practical. For this reason, Daoist Qìgōng training is also commonly called "Dāndǐng Dàogōng" (丹鼎道功) which means "the Dào Training in the Elixir Crucible." The Daoists originally believed that they would be able to find and purify the elixir from herbs. Later, they realized that the only real elixir was in your body.

1.5 Four Refinements (Sìhuà, 四化)

Before you start to read this section, you should first clearly understand the concepts of Jīng (精) (essence), Qì (氣) (inner energy or bioelectricity), and Shén (神).

Understanding Jīng (精) (Essence), Qì (氣) (internal energy), and Shén (神) spirit) is one of the most important requirements for effective Qìgōng training. They are the root of your life and therefore also the root of Qìgōng practice. Jīng, Qì, and Shén are called "Sānbǎo" (三寶), which means "The Three Treasures," "Sānyuán" (三元), which means "The Three Origins," or "Sānběn" (三本), which means "The Three Foundations." In Qìgōng training, a practitioner learns how to "firm his Jīng" (Gùjīng, 固精; Gù means to firm, solidify, retain, and conserve) and how to convert it into Qì. This is called "Liànjīng Huàqì" (煉精化氣), which means "to refine the Jīng and convert it into Qì." Then he learns how to lead the Qì to the head to convert it into Shén (also called nourishing Shén). This is called "Liànqì Huàshén" (煉氣化神), which means "to refine the Qì and convert it into (nourish) the Shén." Finally, the practitioner learns to use his energized Shén to govern the emotional part of his personality. This is called "Liànshén Liǎoxìng" (煉神了性), or "to refine the Shén to end human (emotional) nature."

These conversion processes are what enable you to gain health and longevity. As a Qìgōng practitioner, you must pay a great deal of attention to these three elements during the course of your training. If you keep these three elements strong and healthy, you will live a long and healthy life. If you neglect or abuse them, you will frequently be sick and will age fast. Each one of these three elements or treasures has its own root. You must know the roots so that you can strengthen and protect your three treasures.

Jīng (Essence) 精. The Chinese word Jīng means a number of things depending on where, when, and how it is used. Jīng can be used as a verb, an adjective, or a noun. When it is used as a verb, it means "to refine." For example, to refine or purify a liquid to a high quality is called "Jīngliàn" (精煉). When it is used as an adjective, it is used to describe or signify something which is "refined," "polished" and "pure without mixture." For example, when a piece of art work is well done, people say "Jīngxì" (精細), which means "delicate and painstaking" (literally, "pure and fine"), or "Jīngliáng" (精良), which means "excellent quality" (literally "pure and good"). When Jīng is used to apply to personal wisdom or personality, it means "keen" and "sharp." For example, when someone is smart or wise, they are called "Jīngmíng" (精明), which means "keen and clever." When Jīng is applied to a thought, it means "profound" or "astute," and indicates that the idea or plan was well and carefully considered. When used as a noun for an object, Jīng means "the essence" or "the essentials." When it is used for the energy side of a being, it means "spirit" or "ghost." Since Chinese tradition believes that the male sperm or semen is the refined and the most essential product of a man, Jīng also means sperm or semen.

When Jīng is used as "essence," it exists in everything. Jīng may be considered the primal substance or original source from which a thing is made, and which exhibits the true nature of that thing. When Jīng refers to animals or humans, it means the very original and essential source of life and growth. This Jīng is the origin of the Shén which makes an animal different from a tree. In humans, Jīng is passed down from the parents. Sperm is called "Jīngzǐ" (精子), which means "the sons of essence." When this essence is mixed with the mother's Jīng (egg), a new life is generated which, in certain fundamental respects, is an intertwinement of the Jīngs of both parents. The child is formed, the Qì circulates, and the Shén grows. The Jīng which has been carried over from the parents is called "Yuánjīng" (元精), which means "Original Essence."

Once you are born, Original Jīng is the fountainhead and root of your life. It is what enables you to grow stronger and bigger. After birth you start to absorb the Jīng of food and air, converting these Jīngs into the Qì which supplies your body's needs. You should understand that when Jīng is mentioned in Qìgōng society, it usually refers to Yuánjīng (元精) (Original Jīng). Qìgōng practitioners believe that Original Jīng is the most important part of you, because it is the root of your body's Qì and Shén. The quantity and quality of Original Jīng is different from person to person, and it is affected significantly by your parents' health and living habits while they were creating you. Generally speaking, it does not matter how much Original Jīng you have carried over from your parents. If you know how to conserve it, you will have more than enough for your lifetime. According to Chinese medicine, you probably cannot increase the amount of Jīng you have. However, it is believed that Qìgōng training can improve its quality.

In Qìgōng training, knowing how to conserve and firm your Original Jīng is of primary importance. To conserve means to refrain from abusing your Original Jīng through overuse. For example, if you overindulge in sexual activity, you will lose Original Jīng faster than other people and your body will degenerate faster. To firm your Jīng means to keep and protect it. For example, you should know how to keep your kidneys strong. Kidneys are thought of as the residence of Original Jīng. When your kidneys are strong, the Original Jīng will be kept firm and will not be lost without reason. The firming of your Original Jīng is called "Gùjīng" (固精), which is translated "to make solid, to firm the essence." Only after you know how to retain (meaning to conserve and firm) your Original Jīng can you start seeking ways to improve its quality. Therefore, conserving and firming your Jīng is the first step in training. You need to know the root of your Jīng, where the Original Jīng resides, and how Original Jīng is converted into Qì.

The root of your Original Jīng before your birth is in your parents. After birth, this Original Jīng stays in its residence, the kidneys, which are now also its root. When you keep this root strong, you will have plenty of Original Jīng to supply your body.

Qì (Inner Energy) 氣. Since we have already discussed Qì at the beginning of this chapter in general terms, we will now discuss Qì in the human body and in Qìgōng training. We must note that as of yet, there is no clear explanation of the relationship between all of the circulatory systems and the Qì circulatory system. The Western world knows of the blood system, nervous system, and lymphatic system. Now, there is the Qì circulation system from China. How are, for example, the Qì and the nervous system related? If the nervous system does not match the Qì system, where does the sensing energy in the nervous system come from? How is the lymphatic system related to the Qì system? All of these questions are still waiting for study by modern scientific methods and technology. Here, we can only offer you some theoretical assumptions based on the research conducted up to now.

Chinese medical society believes that Qì and blood are closely related. Where Qì goes, blood follows. That is why the term "Qìxuě" (氣血) (Qì Blood) is commonly used in Chinese medical texts. It is believed that Qì provides the energy for the blood cells to keep them alive. In fact, it is believed that blood is able to store Qì, and that it helps to transport air Qì to every cell of the body.

If you look carefully, you can see that the elements of your physical body such as the organs, nerves, blood, and even every tiny cell are all like separate machines, each with their own unique function. Just like electric motors, if there is no current in them, they are dead. If you compare the routes of the blood circulatory system, the nervous system, and the lymphatic system with the course of the Qì channels, you will see that there is a great deal of correspondence. This is simply because Qì is the energy needed to keep them all alive and functioning.

Now, let us look at your body as an entire system. Your body is composed of two major parts. The first is your physical body, and the second is the energy supply which your body needs to function. Your body is like a factory. Inside your body are many organs, which correspond to the machines required to process raw materials into the finished product. Some of the raw materials brought into a factory are used to create the energy with which other raw materials will be converted into finished goods. The raw materials for your body are food and air, and the finished product is life.

The Qì in your body is analogous to the electric current which the factory power plant obtains from coal or oil. The factory has many wires connecting the power plant to the machines, and other wires connecting telephones, intercoms, and computers. There are also many conveyer belts, elevators, wagons, and trucks to move material from one place to another. It is no different in your body, where there are systems of intestines, blood vessels, complex networks of nerves and Qì channels to facilitate the supply of blood, sensory information and energy to the entire body. However, unlike the digestive, circulatory, and central nervous systems — all of whose supportive vessels can be observed as material structures in the body — Qì channels cannot be observed as physical objects. The circulatory, nervous, and Qì systems all possess similar configurations within the body, and are distributed rather equally throughout the body.

In a factory, different machines require different levels of electrical current. It is the same for your organs, which require different levels of Qì. If a machine is supplied with an improper level of power, it will not function normally and may even be damaged. In the same way, when the Qì level supplied to your organs is either too positive or too negative, they will be damaged and will degenerate more rapidly.

In order for a factory to function smoothly and productively, it will not only need high quality machines, but also a reliable power supply. The same goes for your body. The quality of your organs is largely dependent upon what you inherited from your parents. To maintain your organs in a healthy state and to ensure that they function well for a long time, you must have an appropriate Qì supply. If you don't have it, you will become sick.

Qì is affected by the quality of air you inhale, the kind of food you eat, your lifestyle, and even your personality and emotional make-up. Food and air are like the fuel or power supply, and their quality affects you. Your lifestyle is like the way you run the machine, and your personality is like the management of the factory.

The above discussion clarifies the role that Qì plays in your body. However, it should be noted that the above metaphor is an oversimplification, and that the behavior and function of Qì is much more complex and difficult to handle than the power supply in a factory. You are neither a factory nor a robot; you are a human being with feelings and emotions. These feelings also have a major influence on your Qì circulation. For example, when you pinch yourself, the Qì in that area will be disturbed. This Qì disturbance will be sensed through the nervous system and interpreted by your brain as pain. No machine can do this. Moreover, after you have felt the pain, unlike a machine, you will react either as a result either of instinct or of conscious thought. Human feelings and thoughts affect Qì circulation in the body, whereas a machine cannot influence its power supply. In order to understand your Qì, you must use your feelings, rather than just the intellect, to sense its flow and make judgments about it.

Now a few words as to the source of human Qì. As mentioned, Chinese doctors and Qìgōng practitioners believe that the body contains two general types of Qì. The first type is called Pre-Birth Qì or Original Qì (Yuánqì, 元氣). Original Qì is also called "Xiāntiānqì" (先天氣) which, translated literally, means "Pre-Heaven Qì." "Heaven" here means the sky, so "Pre-Heaven" means before the baby sees the sky. In other words, before birth. Original Qì comes from converted Original Jīng (Yuánjīng, 元精) which you received before your birth. This is why Original Qì is also called Pre-Birth Qì. Once the Qì is converted, it will stay at its residence, the Lower Dāntián.

The second type is called Post-Birth Qì or "Hòutiānqì" (後天氣), which means "Post-Heaven Qì." This Qì is drawn from the Jīng (essence) of the food and air we take in. As mentioned, the residence of the Post-Birth Qì is the Middle Dāntián. This Qì then circulates and mixes with the Pre-Birth or Dāntián Qì (Original Qì; Yuánqì, 元氣). Together, they circulate down, passing into the Governing Vessel (Dūmài, 督脈), from where they are distributed to the entire body.

Pre-Birth Qì is commonly called "Water Qì" (Shuǐqì, 水氣) because it is able to cool down the Post-Birth Qì, which is called "Fire Qì" (Huǒqì, 火氣). Fire Qì usually brings the body to a positive (Yáng) state, which stimulates the emotions and scatters and confuses the mind. When the Water Qì cools your body down, the mind will become clear, neutral and centered. It is believed in Qìgōng society that Fire Qì supports the emotional part of the body, while Water Qì supports the wisdom part.

After the Fire Qì and Water Qì mix, this Qì will not only circulate to the Governing Vessel, but will also supply the "Thrusting Vessel" (Chōngmài, 衝脈) which will lead the Qì directly up through the spinal cord to nourish the brain and energize the Shén and soul. As will be discussed later, energizing the brain and raising the Shén are very important in Qìgōng practice.

Qì can be divided into two major categories, according to its function. The first is called "Yíngqì" (營氣) (Managing Qì), because it manages or controls the functioning of the body. This includes the functioning of the brain and the organs, and even body movement. Yíngqì is again divided into two major types. The first type circulates in the channels and is responsible for the functioning of the organs. The circulation of Qì to the organs and the extremities continues automatically as long as you have enough Qì in your reservoirs and you maintain your body in good condition. The second type of

Yíngqì is linked to your Yì (mind, intention). When your Yì decides to do something, for example to lift a box, this type of Yíngqì will automatically flow to the muscles needed to do the job. This type of Qì is directed by your thoughts, and is therefore closely related to your feelings and emotions.

The second major category of Qì is "Wèiqì" (衛氣) (Guardian Qì). Wèiqì forms a shield on the surface of the body to protect you from negative outside influences. Wèiqì is also involved in the growth of hair, the repair of skin injuries, and many other functions on the surface of the skin. Wèiqì comes from the Qì channels, and is led through millions of tiny channels to the surface of the skin. This Qì can even extend beyond the body. When your body is positive (Yáng), this Qì is strong, and your pores will be open. When your body is negative (Yīn), this Qì is weak, and your pores will close up to preserve Qì.

In the summertime, your body is Yáng and your Qì is strong, so your Qì shield will be bigger and extend beyond your physical body, and the pores will be wide open. In the wintertime, your body is relatively Yīn, and you must conserve your Qì in order to stay warm and keep pathogens out. The Qì shield is smaller and doesn't extend out much beyond your skin.

Wèiqì functions automatically in response to changes in the environment, but it is also influenced significantly by your feelings and emotions. For example, when you feel happy or angry, the Qì shield will be more expansive than when you are sad.

In order to keep your body healthy and functioning properly, you must keep the Yíngqì functioning smoothly and, at the same time, keep the Wèiqì strong to protect you from negative outside influences such as the cold. Chinese doctors and Qìgōng practitioners believe that the key to doing this is through Shén. Shén is considered to be the headquarters which directs and controls the Qì. Therefore, when you practice Qìgōng you must understand what your Shén is and know how to raise it. When people are ill and facing death, very often the ones with a strong Shén, which is indicative of a strong will to live, will survive. The people who are apathetic or depressed will generally not last long. A strong will to live raises the Shén, which energizes the body's Qì and keeps you alive and healthy.

In order to raise your Shén, you must first nourish your brain with Qì. This Qì energizes the brain so that you can concentrate more effectively. Your mind will then be steady, your will strong, and your Shén raised.

As a Qìgōng practitioner, in addition to paying attention to the food and air you take in, it is important for you to learn how to generate Water Qì and how to use it more effectively. Water Qì can cool down Fire Qì and, therefore, slow down the degeneration of the body. Water Qì also helps to calm your mind and keep it centered. This allows you to judge things objectively. During Qìgōng practice, you can sense your Qì and direct it effectively.

In order to generate Water Qì and use it efficiently, you must know how and where it is generated. Since Water Qì comes from the conversion of Original Jīng, they both have the kidneys for their root. Once Water Qì is generated, it resides in the Lower Dāntián below your navel. In order to conserve your Water Qì, you must keep your kidneys firm and strong.

Shén (Spirit) 神. It is very difficult to find an English word to exactly express Shén. As in so many other cases, the context determines the translation. Shén can be translated as spirit, god, immortal, soul, mind, divine, and supernatural.

When you are alive, Shén is the spirit which is directed by your mind. When your mind is not steady it is said "Xīnshén Bùníng" (心神不寧), which means "the (emotional) mind and spirit are not at peace." The average person can use his emotional mind to energize and stimulate his Shén to a higher state, but at the same time he must restrain his emotional mind with his Wisdom Mind (Yì). If his Yì can control the Xīn, the mind as a whole will be concentrated and the Yì can influence the Shén. When someone's Shén is excited, however, it is not being guided by his Yì, so we say, "Shénzhì Bùqīng" (神志不清), which means "the spirit and the will (generated from Yì) are not clear." In Qìgōng it is very important for you to train your wisdom Yì to control your emotional Xīn effectively. In order to reach this goal, Buddhists and Daoists train themselves to be free of emotions. Only in this way are they able to build a strong Shén which is completely under their control.

When you are healthy you are able to use your Yì to protect your Shén and keep it at its residence: the Upper Dāntián. Even when your Shén is energized, it is still controlled. However, when you are very sick or near death, your Yì becomes weak and your Shén will leave its residence and wander around. When you are dead, your Shén separates completely from the physical body. It is then called a "Hún" (魂) (soul). Often the term "Shénhún" (神魂) is used, since the Hún originated with the Shén. Sometimes "Shénhún" is also used to refer to the spirit of a dying person, since his spirit is between "Shén" and "Hún."

The Chinese believe that when your Shén reaches a higher and stronger state, you are able to sense and feel more sharply, and your mind is more clever and inspired. The world of living human beings is usually considered a Yáng world (Yángjiān, 陽間), and the spirit world after death is considered a Yīn world (Yīnjiān, 陰間). When your Shén has reached its higher, more sensitive state, you can transcend your mind's normal capacity. Ideas beyond your usual grasp can be understood and controlled, and you may develop the ability to sense or even communicate with the Yīn world. This supernatural Shén is called "Líng" (靈). "Líng" describes someone who is sharp, clever, nimble, and able to quickly empathize with people and things. It is believed that when you die this supernatural Shén will not die with your body right away. It is this supernatural Shén (Língshén, 靈神) which still holds your energy together as a "ghost" or "Guǐ" (鬼).

Therefore, a ghost is also called "Língguǐ" (靈鬼) meaning "spiritual ghost" or ""Línghún"" (靈魂) meaning "spiritual soul."

From this you can see that Líng is the supernatural part of the spirit. It is believed that if this supernatural spiritual soul is strong enough, it will live for a long time after the physical body is dead and have plenty of opportunity to reincarnate. Chinese people believe that if a person has reached the stage of enlightenment or Buddhahood when he is alive, after he dies this supernatural spirit will leave the cycle of reincarnation and live forever. These spirits are called "Shénmíng" (神明), which means "spiritually enlightened beings," or simply "Shén" (神), which here implies that this spirit has become divine. Normally, if you die and your supernatural spiritual soul is not strong, your spirit has only a short time to search for a new residence in which to be reborn before its energy disperses. In this case, the spirit is called "Guǐ" (鬼), which means "ghost."

Buddhists and Daoists believe that when you are alive you may use your Jīng and Qì to nourish the Shén (Yǎngshén, 養神) and make your Líng strong. When this "Língshén" (靈神) is built up to a high level, your will is able to lead it to separate from the physical body even while you are alive. When you have reached this stage, your physical body is able to live for many hundreds of years. People who can do this are called "Xiān" (仙), which means "immortal," "god," or "fairy." Since "Xiān" originated with the Shén, the "Xian" is sometimes called "Shénxiān" (神仙), which means "immortal spirit." The "Xiān" is a living person whose Shén has reached the stage of enlightenment or Buddhahood. After his death, his spirit will be called "Shénmíng" (神明).

The foundation of Buddhist and Daoist Qìgōng training is to firm your Shén, nourish it, and grow it until it is mature enough to separate from your physical body. In order to do this, the Qìgōng practitioner must know where the Shén resides and how to keep, protect, nourish, and train it. It is also essential for you to know the root or origin of your Shén.

Your Shén resides in the Upper Dāntián (i.e., the brain). When you concentrate on The Third Eye, the Shén can be firmed. "Firm" here means "to keep and protect." When someone's mind is scattered and confused, his Shén wanders. This is called "Shénbù Shǒushè" (神不守舍), which means "the spirit is not kept at its residence."

According to Qìgōng theory, though your Xīn (emotional mind, 心) is able to raise your spirit, this mind can also make your Shén confused, so that it leaves its residence. You must constantly engage your Yì (Wisdom Mind) to restrain and control your Shén at its residence.

In Qìgōng, when your Qì can reach and nourish your Shén efficiently, your Shén will be energized to a higher level and, in turn, conduct the Qì in its circulation. Shén is the force which keeps you alive, and it is also the control tower for the Qì. When your Shén is strong, your Qì is strong and you can lead it efficiently. When your Shén is weak, your Qì is weak and the body will degenerate rapidly. Likewise, Qì supports the Shén, energizing it and keeping it sharp, clear, and strong. If the Qì in your body is weak, your Shén will also be weak.

Once you know the residence of your Shén, you must understand the root of your Shén, and learn how to nourish it and make it grow. We have already discussed Original Essence (Yuánjīng, 元精), which is the essential life inherited from your parents. After your birth, this Original Essence is your most important energy source. Your Original Qì (Yuánqì, 元氣) is created from this Original Essence, and it mixes with the Qì generated from the food you eat and the air you breathe to supply the energy for your growth and activity. Naturally, this mixed Qì nourishes your Shén as well. While the Fire Qì will energize your Shén, Water Qì will strengthen the Wisdom Mind to control the energized Shén. The Shén which is kept in its residence by the Yì (which is nourished by the Original Qì) is called Original Shén (Yuánshén, 元神). Therefore, the root of your Original Shén is traced back to your Original Essence. When your Shén is energized but restrained by your Yì it is called "Jīngshén" (精神), literally "Essence Shén," which is commonly translated "Spirit of Vitality."

Original Shén is thought of as the center of your being. It is able to make you calm, clear your mind, and firm your will. When you concentrate your mind on doing something, it is called "Jùjīng Huìshén" (聚精會神), which means "gathering Jīng to meet Shén." This implies that when you concentrate, you must use your Original Jīng to meet and lift up your Original Shén, so that your mind will be calm, steady, and concentrated. Since this Shén is nourished by your Original Qì, which is considered Water Qì, Original Shén is considered Water Shén.

For those who have reached a higher level of Qìgōng practice, cultivating the Shén becomes the most important subject. For Buddhists and Daoists, the final goal of cultivating the Shén is to generate a Holy Embryo (Xiāntāi, 仙胎) from their Shén, and nourish it until the spiritual baby is born and can be independent. For the average Qìgōng practitioner however, the final goal of cultivating Shén is to raise the Shén through Qì nourishment while maintaining control with the Yì. This raised-up Shén can direct and govern the Qì efficiently to achieve health and longevity.

In conclusion, we would like to point out that your Shén and brain cannot be separated. Shén is the spiritual part of your being and is generated and controlled by your mind. The mind generates the will, which keeps the Shén firm. The Chinese commonly use Shén (spirit) and Zhì (will) together as "Shénzhì" (神志) because they are so related. In addition, you should understand that when your Shén is raised and firm, this raised spirit will firm your will. They are mutually related, and assist each other. From this you can see that the material foundation of the spirit is your brain. When it is said "nourish your Shén," it means "nourish your brain." As we discussed previously, the original nourishing source is your Jīng. This Jīng is then converted into Qì, which is led to the brain to nourish and energize it. In Qìgōng practice, this process is called "Fǎnjīng Bǔnǎo" (返精補腦), which means "to return the Jīng to nourish the brain."

Now you have grasped a clearer idea of Jīng, Qì, and Shén, you can understand how these three treasures interact in Buddhist and Daoist Qìgōng practice. Next, we will explain the Daoist and Buddhist training procedures of how to use these treasures to reach the final Dào of spiritual enlightenment.

After more than fourteen hundred years of meditation training and accumulation of experience, both Chinese Buddhist and Daoist societies agree that in order to reach the final goal of enlightenment or Buddhahood, you must follow four necessary steps of training:

A. **Refine the Essence and Convert it into Qì** (Liànjīng Huàqì)煉精化氣
—One Hundred Days of Building the Foundation (Bǎirì Zhújī, 百日築基)

B. **Purify Qì and Convert it into Shén** (Liànqì Huàshén) 煉氣化神
—Ten Months of Pregnancy (Shíyuè Huáitāi, 十月懷胎)

C. **Refine Shén and Return it to Nothingness** (Liànshén Fǎnxū) 煉神返虛
—Three Years of Nursing (Sānnián Bǔrǔ, 三年哺乳)

D. **Crush the Nothingness (Fěnsuì Xūkōng)** 粉碎虛空
—Nine Years of Facing the Wall (Jiǔnián Miànbì, 九年面壁)

You can see that the Dào of reaching enlightenment or becoming a Buddha requires years of training. It covers four stages of conversion training, first of which is the formation of a "spiritual baby embryo" (one hundred days of building the foundation) which is commonly called "Shèngtāi" (Holy Embryo, 聖胎) or "Língtāi" (Spiritual Embryo, 靈胎). This is followed by ten months of nourishing and growing, three years of nursing, and finally nine years of educating this baby Shén until it matures and becomes independent. In Daoist and Buddhist Qìgōng training, it is believed that in order to reach the final goal of enlightenment and Buddhahood, you must first build up an independent spiritual energy body. After your physical body is dead, this spiritual body will continue to live eternally and will not re-enter the path of reincarnation.

After the Xǐsuǐjīng training secret was revealed to laymen, a change took place in the training. Because the final goal of enlightenment or Buddhahood was not the main reason laymen practiced, and because the final step of training was hard to understand and to reach, many Xǐsuǐjīng practitioners who were looking only for longevity considered that there were only the first three steps of training, ignoring the final step. For this reason, there are very few documents which can lead you to this final step. We will now discuss these four training stages in the next four sections.

Refine the Essence and Convert it into Qì (Liànjīng Huàqì, 煉精化氣). This first step is also called: "One Hundred Days of Building the Foundation" (Bǎirì Zhújī, 百日

築基). Daoists always visualize the achievement of enlightenment first in terms of forming a "Spiritual Embryo" (Língtāi, 靈胎) or "Holy Embryo" (Shèngtāi, 聖胎), and then its feeding, nursing, and education until it can be independent. For many Xǐsuǐjīng lay practitioners who are looking only for longevity, this spiritual baby is considered a "baby elixir" which will lead them to longevity. It is believed that the healthy and harmonious interaction of Yīn and Yáng Qì is necessary to form this spiritual baby. Yīn is considered the mother, while Yáng is considered the father. In order to make this happen, Yīn and Yáng Qì must be abundant, and both the mother (Yīn) and father (Yáng) must be strong enough to balance each other. In order to obtain abundant Yīn Qì and Yáng Qì in your body, you must learn the methods of building up these two Qìs. In order to make Yīn and Yáng interact harmoniously, you must also learn how to adjust Kǎn (water) and Lí (fire). Therefore, in this stage, you are leading both Yáng and Yīn Qì to Huángtíng (黃庭) (i.e., Yellow Yard), and causing them to interact harmoniously. This process is called "Kǎn and Lí" (坎離) (Figure 1–22).

What, then, is the Holy Embryo or Spiritual Embryo? According to a Daoist document: "Baby Embryo means the golden elixir. To produce the golden elixir is to carry the baby embryo."[8] Elixir implies the Qì which is able to extend your life. Since elixir is precious like gold, it is commonly called "golden" elixir. Therefore, to establish a baby Embryo means to build up and store the Qì at the Huángtíng cavity. It is also stated by the Daoist Xuē, Dào-Guāng (薛道光) that: "What is the baby? It is the elixir. The elixir is unique and is the real sole Qì. It is the mother's Qì of the heaven and the earth. Mother swallows the air and belongs to the five internal (organs), thus to yield the baby's Qì. It is just like a cat keeping a mouse which cannot escape. The Qì of mother and son mutually love each other in the womb and finally combine and generate a baby. Therefore, it is said: 'The sole Grand Ultimate contains the real Qì. The way of containing the real sole Qì is just like human carries embryo, when ten months have completed, then there is a birth.'"[9]This saying implies that in order to generate life, you need the heaven Qì (Yáng Qì) and the earth Qì (Yīn Qì). When Heaven Qì and Earth Qì combine and interact, life can be produced. In the same way, a human needs the interaction of Yáng Qì and Yīn Qì

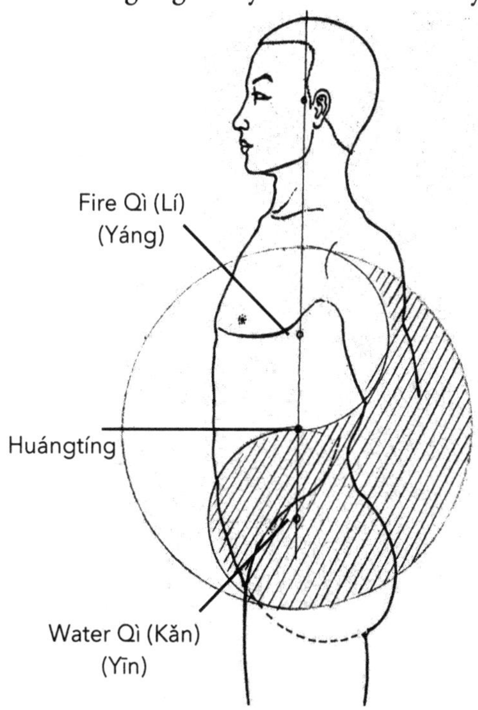

Figure 1-22. Kǎn and Lí Interaction

so the baby Embryo can be generated. This means that in order to produce the golden elixir, you must learn how to absorb the Qì from food and air (Yáng Qì or Fire Qì) and also the Qì from the Original Essence (Yuánjīng, 元精) (Yīn Qì or Water Qì). When this happens, the Qì can be stored to a high level and the foundation of longevity established.

From the scientific point of view, what you are doing is storing electric charge (i.e., Qì) in the Huángtíng, which has been recognized as the second human brain and is able to store charge.[10] This second brain is connected with the brain in our head by the spinal cord (i.e., Thrusting Vessel). The spinal cord belongs to the human central nervous system, and is composed of highly electrically conductive tissue. Because of this, the top brain and the lower brain, though appearing to be two physically, act as one in function. The top brain is able to generate thought (i.e., Electromotive Force or EMF), while the lower brain acts as a battery and supplies the charge to the entire body. Whenever EMF is generated, the charge (Qì) is led to activate the physical body, and therefore the mind and Qì are manifested into physical action.

In order to have a strong and abundant Qì circulation and supply, you must have a concentrated and powerful mind from the top brain (high EMF) and a good battery which is able to supply the Qì to an abundant level in the lower brain. When the two brains are healthy and functioning harmoniously, you may use your mind to rebuild your immune system and extend your life significantly.

In addition, once you have abundant Qì stored in Huángtíng, you can lead this Qì to the brain to nourish it and activate more brain cells, which can result in the raising of your Shén to a high level. That is what is meant by the "Holy Embryo" being formed and cultivated in the Huángtíng and then led to the brain where it matures. This is the second stage of enlightenment training, which will be discussed in the next section.

How is the Huángtíng able to store Qì and bear the Spiritual Embryo? Let us first analyze the Huángtíng. This cavity is also called "Yùhuánxué" (Jade Ring Cavity, 玉環穴). This name was first used in the book *Illustration of the Brass Man Acupuncture and Moxibustion* (*Tóngrén Yúxuè Zhēnjiǔtú*, 銅人俞穴針灸圖) by Dr. Wáng, Wéi-Yī (王唯一). The Daoist book *The Extra Comprehension of Wang Lu* (*Wánglù Shíyú*, 王錄識餘) said: "In the Illustration of the Brass Acupuncture and Moxibustion it was recorded (that) within the body's cavities of viscera and bowels, there is a Jade Ring (Yùhuán, 玉環), (but) I do not know what the Jade Ring is."[12] Later, the Daoist Zhāng, Zǐ-Yáng (張紫陽) explained the place in which the immortals form the elixir: "The heart is on the top, the kidneys are underneath, spleen is on the left, and the liver is on the right. The life door is in the front, the closed door is in the rear, they are connected like a ring, it is white like cotton with an inch diameter. It encloses the Essence and the refinement of the entire body. This is the Jade Ring."[13] Life door (Shēngmén, 生門) means "navel," which is the door connecting to the life of the fetus. The closed door (Mìhù, 密戶) implies "Mìngmén (Gv-4)" (命門), which is located between the L2 and L3 vertebrae.

From the point of view of Chinese medical science, the Huángtíng is connected with the Conception and Thrusting Vessels through Yīnjiāo (Co-7, 陰交). Through the Thrusting Vessel it is again connected with the top brain and with the Governing Vessel at the Huìyīn (Co-1, 會陰). Since the gut is considered the "second brain," similar in structure to the brain in the head, this area is able to store a great amount of charge (Qì).[11] Furthermore, the Huángtíng (黃庭) (Yellow Yard) is located between the diaphragm (Middle Dāntián), where the Yáng (Fire) Qì is stored, and the Lower Dāntián, where the Yīn (Water) Qì is stored. In addition, we know from the Yìjīnjīng training that the fasciae in the Huángtíng area are able to store an abundance of Qì. This increases the amount of Qì available to the "Holy Embryo."

The question remaining is: though the gut is considered the second brain and has a similar structure to the brain in the head, how can this lower brain create a spiritual embryo? Scientists today believe that the second brain has the capability of memory, but are not sure whether this brain is able to think. If this brain is unable to think, then no EMF can be generated. This implies that the Shén cannot be grown here and this place is only used to facilitate interaction between the Yáng and Yīn Qìs, building them to a high level. Naturally, we do not yet know whether this interaction of Yīn and Yáng can generate the seed of a "Holy Embryo."

In Yìjīnjīng training you generate Qì by converting the Original Essence in the internal Kidneys. However, this process does not provide enough Qì for the Xǐsuǐjīng training. To remedy this lack, more Essence must be drawn from the external Kidneys (testicles or ovaries) through stimulation, and converted into Qì.

From the standpoint of modern medicine, part of the health benefit of Xǐsuǐ Qìgōng comes from its use of self-stimulation to increase the production of hormones. Hormones are secretions of the endocrine glands, which include the testicles and ovaries. They are complex chemical compounds which are transported by the blood or lymph, and they have powerful and specific effects on the functions of the body.

Hormones can stimulate activity, thinking, and growth; they are directly related to the strength of your life force. They determine the length of a person's life, and whether he is healthy or sickly. They stimulate your emotions and lift your mood, or they depress you physically and emotionally. Traced back far enough, hormones are the very original source which stimulates man's thinking and ideas, and even generates the enthusiasm for energetic activity. If you know how to generate these hormones and use them properly, you can energize yourself to a degree quite impossible for the ordinary person.

Many important hormones can now be produced synthetically. However, you must understand that taking synthetic hormones is like taking vitamins: it is an unnatural and discontinuous process. However, if you generate a hormone within your own body, it is natural and continuous. In addition, when you produce the hormones yourself, your body is able to tune into and adjust to the gradual increase in production. However, if the hormones come from outside of your body, your body is subject to an abrupt change. This can produce side effects. Many hormones can be obtained from certain foods. However, these hormones will not be able to provide enough Qì to fill up the vessels. The Daoists say: "To nourish the body by using medicine is not as good as by eating food; eating food is not as good as being nourished by Qì."[14]

You can see that Xǐsuǐ Qìgōng is a way of stimulating the production of hormones in the body. These hormones are then used to increase the quantity of Qì, which in turn is used to nourish the brain and raise the Shén of Vitality.

You can only develop a healthy spiritual baby when you have sufficient Qì. To form the embryo, you will need at least one hundred days of proper diet, accurate Kǎn and Lí adjustment, correct stimulation of the sexual organ to increase the Essence (semen), and abstinence from sex in order to build up a strong Qì body combining Yīn and Yáng. In Xǐsuǐjīng Qìgōng, the process of refining Essence (semen) and converting it into Qì over the first one hundred days is considered the laying of the foundation. The process is called "hundred days to build the foundation" (Bǎirì Zhújī, 百日築基). The Spiritual Embryo will be healthy only if it has this foundation.

The testicle Essence (semen) is one of the main sources of human energy. When a person's semen is full, his vital energy is high and his lifeforce is strong. When a man loses the balance between the production and the loss of his semen, his emotions will also lose their balance. This will cause his mental body to be depressed, resulting in the speedy degeneration of his physical body. When a person has normal semen or hormone production, he will have enough Essence to stimulate his growth, thinking, and daily activities. According to the *Xǐsuǐjīng*, part of this Essence is converted into Qì and then transported to the brain. This Qì will stimulate the brain to do the thinking and energize the body for activity. When a man's semen production is insufficient, his brain will not obtain enough Qì nourishment and the Shén will be weakened in its governing of the Qì circulation in the body. This will result in sickness.

Therefore, the first step in Xǐsuǐjīng training for men is to increase the semen production and learn to convert this semen into Qì faster and more effectively than the body normally does. With the average mature man, the supply of semen will fill up naturally without any stimulation. It usually takes two to three weeks to replenish the supply of semen once it is empty. Whenever the semen and sperm are full, a hormone stimulates the brain and generates sexual desires. This hormone can sometimes energize a man, making him impatient and inclined to lose his temper, or it can make him depressed.

You should understand that the time needed for the semen to replenish itself varies from individual to individual. For example, if someone has sex frequently, his semen will be replenished faster. However, if a man refrains from sexual activity for a period of time, his testicles will start to function more slowly. If a man has sex too often, his semen level will be low most of the time, and this will affect the conversion of hormones into the

Qì which is transported to the brain. In addition to this, the four Qì vessels in the legs receive most of their Qì from the conversion of semen. If you have too much sex you will find that your legs become weak because the Qì in these vessels is deficient. It is therefore advisable to control your sexual activity.

When a boy is growing, his body produces semen during his sleep from midnight until morning. This is because Qì circulation starts in the head (Bǎihuì, Gv-20, 百會) and circulates down the front of the body, following the Conception Vessel, and reaches the Huìyīn (Co-1, 會陰) cavity in the perineum at midnight (the Huìyīn and Bǎihuì, which are connected by the Thrusting Vessel, are both major points of Qì flow at midnight). When this Qì circulation reaches the Huìyīn, it will stimulate the genitals and interact with the Original Qì from the Dāntián, generating semen Qì (Jīngqì, 精氣).

Young boys or healthy male adults usually have erections when they wake in the morning. This starts quite soon after birth. Of course, young boys cannot generate any sperm, and they do not have any sexual urge. Chinese medical society believes that once a boy is formed, his testicles continuously generate semen. This interacts with the Original Qì (Yuánqì, 元氣) which resides at the Dāntián and generates Semen Qì (Jīngqì, 精氣), which is transported to the brain (including the pituitary gland) to stimulate the boy's growth. When a boy's Yuánqì is healthy and strong, the interaction of semen and Yuánqì will also be effective and the boy will grow normally and be healthy. Once the boy reaches his teens, his testicles will also start to generate sperm. Normally, more is produced than is needed for growth, so his Qì is full and abundant, and he is therefore healthy and strong.

It is interesting to note that, starting at midnight when you are sleeping and your entire body is relaxed, the Semen Qì from the testicles (or ovaries) will naturally start to nourish the brain and rebalance its energy. It is this rebalancing which generates dreams.

In Xǐsuǐjīng training, there are two general methods for stimulating semen production. One is Wàidān, and uses physical stimulation, and the other is Nèidān, and uses mental stimulation. The more the groin is stimulated, the more semen will be produced and the longer this organ will function normally. You must also learn how to convert this semen into Qì more efficiently than is normally done automatically by your body. If you do not effectively convert the excess semen into Qì, lead it to the brain, and spread it out among the twelve channels, the abundant semen will cause your sexual desire to increase and your emotions to lose their balance.

Theoretically, the method of Essence-Qì conversion is very simple. You lead the Qì from the four vessels in the legs upward to the Huángtíng cavity, and from there to the brain. This causes the Qì in the four leg vessels to become deficient, and more Essence must be converted to replenish the supply. In this case, you are "digesting" or "consuming" the extra Essence which is generated. The process of leading the Qì upward is called "Liànqì Shēnghuá" (煉氣昇華), which means "train the Qì to sublimate." Because the

Qì is an energy form, when it is led upward, it is like the water molecules sublimated upward from ice. When the Qì is led upward and used to nourish the brain, it is called "Huánjīng Bǔnǎo" (還精補腦), which means "return the Essence to nourish the brain."

In the beginning you might not be able to convert the semen into Qì efficiently. However, the more you practice the better it will become. Generally speaking, there are two major styles of semen conversion: Buddhist and Daoist. Buddhists emphasize mainly the Nèidān conversion process, which is generally much slower than that of the Daoists, who in addition to the Nèidān also train Wàidān conversion. Buddhist priests are not allowed to get married. However, they still have sexual desires, which occur naturally because of the body's production of hormones and semen. In order to eliminate their desire, they found the way of converting the semen into Qì and using this Qì to energize the brain and reach Buddhahood. In Nèidān conversion training, the Yì and the breathing are the keys to leading the Qì upward. With the coordination of the posture and some controlling movements at the Huìyīn and anus, the Qì can be led upward to the Huángtíng and brain.

In addition to the Nèidān practice, Daoists also discovered several Wàidān conversion methods. The theory remains the same: one leads the Qì from the vessels of the legs upward to the Huángtíng and brain. Generally speaking, Wàidān methods are faster. As mentioned previously, the Daoists use primarily Wàidān methods for increasing semen production (via testicle stimulation) and for the Essence-to-Qì conversion. The exercise for stimulating semen production is called "Gāowán Yùndòng" (睪丸運動) (Testicle Exercises) or "Chílǎo Fǎnjī Yùndòng" (遲老返機運動) (Slowing the Aging and Return the Functioning Exercises). Remember, only when you have enough semen will you be able to convert it into Qì more effectively than the average person can. The more semen you have, the more Qì you can convert.

Purify Qì and Convert it into Shén (Liànqì Huàshén, 煉氣化神)—Ten Months of Pregnancy (Shíyuè Huáitāi, 十月懷胎). After a hundred days building the foundation in the first stage, the Spiritual Embryo is formed in the Huángtíng. This is the seed from which the baby grows. Now, in this second stage, you will need ten months of pregnancy (twenty-eight days for each Chinese month). During these ten months you must continue to provide purified Qì for the baby, just as a mother supplies nutrition and oxygen to the embryo. During these ten months you must train to convert the semen into Qì more efficiently while the Spiritual Embryo is growing continuously. If the conversion process is insufficient, the embryo will wither and die before its birth, or else will be born unhealthy, and may not continue to grow well. During this stage, you are growing the Embryo into a complete baby that has its own life.

In the previous stage you learned how to lead the Yīn and Yáng Qì to the Huángtíng and make them interact harmoniously. The Spiritual Embryo was formed from this interaction. In this second stage, you are continuing to build up your Qì in the

Huángtíng. Normally, it will take you ten months of Qì building to reach a high level of storage. Only then, in the third stage of the training, will you have enough Qì to activate the extra brain cells and increase the functioning of the brain. When you have done this, you can raise your Shén to a higher level.

While you are carrying the Spiritual Embryo, you must also do one important thing. As the Embryo is growing, the Shén in this Embryo is also being formed. Therefore, in this second stage of training, in addition to the Qì nourishment, you also need to lead your Shén to this Embryo. It is like a mother whose Shén and concentration must be in the Embryo while it is growing in order to obtain a spiritually healthy baby. In this stage, the mother's habits and thoughts will be passed on to the baby.

This means that, with the mother's help, the Spiritual Embryo will also grow its own Shén. That is why this stage is called "Purifying the Qì and converting it into Shén." Remember, only when the Embryo has its own Shén can it be born as a healthy, whole being. The Daoist Lǐ, Qīng-Ān (李清菴) said: "Shén and Qì combine to originate the super spiritual quality. Xīn (心) and breath are mutually dependent to generate the Holy Embryo."[15] That means that in order to grow a Holy Embryo you must first learn to combine your Shén and Qì in the Huángtíng. Only then will the Holy Embryo have a supernatural, spiritual quality. Xīn is your emotional mind, and the breathing is the strategy of the training. Only when you concentrate all of your emotion and coordinate it with your breathing in this Holy Embryo will it be able to grow and mature.

Many Qìgōng practitioners believe that once the Embryo is formed, it should be moved upward to the Upper Dāntián to grow. As a matter of fact, it does not matter where your Embryo grows. First you must have plenty of Qì, then you must learn how to use this Qì to nourish the Embryo, and finally, you must help the Embryo to build up its own Shén. As long as you are able to store an abundance of Qì to activate and energize your brain cells and raise up your Shén, where the Embryo grows is not important. It is said in a Daoist document, Real Commentaries of the Golden Elixir (Jīndān Zhēnchuán, 金丹真傳), that: "When the elixir is accomplished in ten months, the Holy Embryo is completed. (At this time,) the real person will appear."[16] After you have meditated for ten months and the Qì is abundantly stored in the Huángtíng, you then lead the Qì upward to nourish your brain. When this happens, the mask on your face drops off. You are facing your true self, the real you. This is the stage of self-recognition.

Refine Shén and Return it to Nothingness (Liànshén Fǎnxū, 煉神返虛)—Three Years of Nursing (Sānnián Bǔrǔ, 三年哺乳). After you have carried the Spiritual Embryo for ten months, it is mature enough for birth. This means that the Qì you are storing in the Huángtíng is strong enough, and your Shén has helped this Embryo to build up its own Shén. In this third stage of training you lead this Embryo upward to the Upper Dāntián to be born. According to the experience of many people, the Upper Dāntián (brain) is the place, through the Yìntáng cavity (M-HN-3, 印堂; i.e., the Third

Eye), where you can sense and communicate with natural energy and the spirit world. This place is called "Shéngǔ" (神谷) (Spiritual Valley) in Qìgōng, because the physical structure of this place looks like the entrance to a deep valley formed by the two lobes of the brain. Also, when you sense or communicate with natural energy, it seems to be happening in a deep valley which is able to reach the center of your thinking and far beyond what you can see.

Using today's science, we understand less than 12% of the functions of the brain, meaning the brain contains many mysteries which science still cannot explain. I believe that the valley formed by the two brain lobes is the key to explaining the length of brain waves. Energy resonates in this valley and is transmitted outward like waves from the antenna of a radio station. I believe that the Upper Dāntián or Third Eye is the gate which allows our thoughts to be passed to others, and allows us to communicate with nature.

If a person can activate a larger percentage of his brain cells through Qìgōng, he will probably increase the sensitivity of his brain to a wider range of wavelengths. He may be able to perceive more things more clearly, and may have a greatly heightened sensitivity to natural energy. He may even be able to sense other people's brain waves, and know what they are thinking without oral communication. At this level, when your Qì is abundant and your concentration very high, it is also possible to use your mind and Qì to cure people. This is the stage of self-awareness and awakening.

If my hypothesis is right, then the greatest obstacle to advancing your training, once you are able to lead the Qì to activate the brain cells, is learning how to open the gate of the Third Eye. Physically, beneath the skin is the skull, and underneath it is the frontal sinus. Both the skull and the skin can block much of the energy which is emitted from or received by the brain. This is why this gate is considered closed. We now know that bones are semi-conductors. This means that, through meditation (i.e., concentration), we are able to build up a significant potential difference (EMF) between the brain and outside of the head. Once this potential difference has reached the "threshold" level, the bone will become a conductor. When this happens, the energy in your brain can communicate with the outer world without blockage. In higher stages of spiritual Qìgōng this gate is called "Xuánguān" (玄關), which means "tricky gate." Through concentration, Qì can be condensed in this gate to open it, and this process is called "Kāiqiào" (開竅), or "opening the tricky gate." According to Chinese Qìgōng society, once this gate has opened, it remains open.

Another gate is located at the top of your head. It is called "Bǎihuì" (Gv-20) (百會) in acupuncture or "Níwángōng" (泥丸宮) in Qìgōng, and is also called "Gǔshén" (谷神), which means "Valley Spirit." Chinese Qìgōng does not consider it the spiritual center, but regards it as another place from which your brain can communicate with natural energy and exchange Qì with nature. This gate is commonly used to absorb heaven Qì (from the sun and stars) and earth Qì (Earth's magnetic field) to nourish the body.

If you are able to understand this discussion, then you will not be confused by the third stage of enlightenment Qìgōng training. In the third stage, you lead the abundant Qì to the brain to activate more of the unused brain cells and increase the brain's working efficiency. In addition, you are using the abundant Qì to open the gate through concentration, focus, and meditation. This means that the spiritual baby is born in the Upper Dāntián.

After you have opened this gate and have given birth to the spiritual baby, you must nurse it. Nursing means to watch, to take care of, and to nourish continuously. This process in enlightenment or brain-washing Qìgōng practice is called "Yǎngshén" (養神), or "to nurse the Shén." You can see that in this stage you are continuously nursing the baby as it grows stronger and stronger. In other words, you are increasing the Qì there so that you can sense nature more easily. When you reach this stage, since you are training your Shén to sense nature, it will gradually become accustomed to staying with the natural energy and will slowly forget the physical body. Since the natural spirit cannot be seen, it is called "nothingness." Nothingness also refers to the absence of emotional feelings and desires. This is why this stage of training is called "Refining Shén and Returning it to Nothingness." Since your spiritual body originated from physical and emotional nothingness, in this training, you are returning to nothingness. The Buddhists call this "Sìdà Jiēkōng" (四大皆空), or "Four Large are Empty." This means that the four elements (earth, fire, water, and air) are absent from the mind so that you are completely indifferent to worldly temptations.

When your spiritual baby is born, you will need to nurse it for at least three years. Just like a real baby, it needs to be protected and nurtured until it can be self-sufficient. The spiritual baby needs to stay near the mother's body to stay alive, so if it travels, it cannot go too far. It is just like a two- or three-year-old baby gradually familiarizing itself with its new environment. Normally, when you have reached this stage, you have approached the first step of enlightenment or Buddhahood.

Crushing the Nothingness (Fěnsuì Xūkōng, 粉碎虛空)—Nine Years of Facing the Wall (Jiǔnián Miànbì, 九年面壁). At this stage you begin to see the spiritual world as the more real one. Crushing nothingness means destroying the illusion which connects the physical world with the spiritual plane. According to Buddhism, your spirit cannot separate from your physical body completely, because it is still connected to the human world by emotional feelings and desires. Only if you are able to free yourself from all of these bonds of human emotions and desires will your Shén be able to separate from the physical body and be independent.

The final target of a monk is to reach enlightenment or become a Buddha. In order to become a Buddha, he must continue to develop his Shén until it can be independent and exist even after the physical body dies. When a monk has reached this level, his Qì can energize his brain so strongly that it interacts with the energy (electrical charges) in the air, generating a glow around his head. In fact, this glow or halo may even occur in earlier training stages. This glow around the head is frequently shown in pictures of the Buddha, especially when he is shown meditating in the dark. This is identical to the glow, or halo, shown in pictures of Western saints.

In order to reach this level, the spiritual baby must grow stronger and be neutral. It is called "nine years facing the wall." When you face the wall, you will overcome the temptation of external things, and you can calm down more easily. During these nine years of meditation, your spiritual baby learns how to live in the natural energy and how to continue growing even when the physical body is dead.

This stage is called "Liànshén" (煉神), or "train the Shén." At this time your Shén receives its education from the natural energy. Of course, this normally takes more than twelve years—in fact the Buddhists believe that it usually takes many lifetimes. You strengthen your Baby Shén in every lifetime, and if you continue to train, one day you can reach the level of enlightenment. However, there are also many Buddhists and Daoists who believe that the entire training depends on the individual's understanding. They believe that if a person could really understand the training process, he would be able to reach enlightenment in virtually no time at all. I am inclined to agree with these people. I have found that in virtually every area of endeavor, if a person knows the principles and studies them, he will find ways to reach the goal in a far shorter time than those who do not ponder what they are doing.

To conclude this section, I would like to point out that what this book can teach you is how to practice the first two stages of enlightenment or brain-washing Qìgōng training, which can give you a long and healthy life. There are many documents about the first two stages of training, but very little is known about the later two stages of enlightenment training. However, I believe that if your desire is sincere and you keep your mind on your goal, you will understand what you need to do in order to reach the next level. Remember: no one can understand you better than yourself.

1.6 Five Regulatings (Wǔtiáo, 五調)

No matter what kind of Qìgōng you practice, either Internal Elixir (Nèidān, 內丹) or External Elixir (Wàidān, 外丹), there are normally five regulating processes involved in reaching the final goal of practice. These are: regulating the body (Tiáoshēn, 調身), regulating the breathing (Tiáoxí, 調息), regulating the emotional mind (Tiáoxīn, 調心), regulating the Qì (Tiáoqì, 調氣), and regulating the spirit (Tiáoshén, 調神). These Five Regulatings are commonly called "Wǔtiáo" (五調).

Before we discuss them you should first understand the word Tiáo (調) which I translate as "regulating." Tiáo (調) is constructed of two words, Yán (言) which means "speaking" or "negotiating" and Zhōu (周) which means "to be complete," "to be perfect," or "to be round." Therefore, the meaning of Tiáo is to adjust or tune a thing until it is complete and each part is harmonious with the others. It is just like tuning a piano string-by-string until every note is in mutual harmony. Tiáo means to coordinate, to cooperate, and to harmonize with others by continual adjustment. That means all of the five items—body, breathing, mind, Qì, and Shén—need to be regulated with each other until the final harmonious stage is reached.

The key to regulating is through self-feeling. You should know that feeling is the language of the mind and body. Without feeling, we will not know if there is anything wrong with the body. The deeper and the more sensitively you are able to feel, the more profoundly you are able to regulate. Conversely, the deeper you are able to regulate, the more profoundly you can feel. Naturally, it will take a lot of time and effort to practice until your feeling is profound and your regulating can reach the finest stage. This kind of inner-feeling training is called Gōngfū of Self-Internal-Observation (Nèishì Gōngfū, 內視功夫) (i.e., internal feeling or awareness). The higher your Gōngfū is, the deeper and more finely you can harmonize with others.

At the beginning of regulating, your mind is absorbed in regulating to make the regulating happen. Therefore, it is not natural and smooth. The final stage of regulating is "regulating without regulating." In Chinese Qìgōng society, it is said: "The real regulating is without regulating."[17]It is just like when you are learning how to drive a car: at first your mind is on the road, the steering wheel, the accelerator, the clutch, etc. This is the stage of regulating. However, after you have driven for a long time, your mind does not have to be regulating. In this stage, you are driving without "driving." Everything will happen naturally and smoothly. It is the same for all Five Regulatings in Qìgōng. You must keep practicing until regulating is unnecessary. When this happens, your feeling can be profound.

Next, we will review these Five Regulatings briefly. We will also point out the importance of mutual coordination and harmonization. For more detail about these five regulatings, you may refer to the book: *The Root of Chinese Qìgōng*, published by YMAA Publication Center.

1.6.1 Regulating the Body (Tiáoshēn, 調身)

If the posture in meditation practice is incorrect, the body will be tense. This will affect the smooth circulation of Qì and also disturb the mind. "(When) shape (i.e., body posture) is not correct, then the Qì will not be smooth. (In turn, when) the Qì is not smooth, the Yì (i.e., Wisdom Mind) will not be at peace. (When) the Yì is not at peace, then the Qì is disordered."[18]

From this, you can see that the purposes of regulating the body are:

1. **To find the most natural, relaxed, and comfortable posture or position for meditation.** This will allow the Qì to flow freely, with the breathing natural and smooth, and with the mind relaxed and focused, so the Shén can be raised to a higher level.
2. **To provide the best conditions for self-internal-feeling.** When your physical body is regulated correctly, your feeling can reach to a deep and profound level. Your judgment will be more accurate. The efficiency of your mind-body communication will increase to a high level. It is through this profound feeling that your mind is able to lead the Qì to circulate effectively in the body.
3. **To coordinate and harmonize the physical center and mental center.** By using the Yì (意) (Wisdom Mind) and correct feeling, you can bring your physical center and mental center to a high degree of coordination and harmony.

1.6.2 Regulating the Breathing (Tiáoxí, 調息)

When you have relaxed your body to the stage of "regulating without regulating," then you should pay attention to the breathing. Breathing is considered the strategy in Qìgōng practice. When the breathing methods are correct, the mind can lead the Qì efficiently and effectively. Therefore, Qìgōng breathing methods have been studied and practiced since ancient times. In many cases, the methods were kept top-secret in each style. For example, "Embryonic Breathing" (Tāixí, 胎息) is the crucial key to storing Qì at the Real Lower Dāntián (Zhēn Xiàdāntián, 真下丹田). However, the actual training techniques have only been passed down orally. Since breathing is the main subject of this book, I will explain in more detail the general concepts of regulating the breathing, including its purpose, theory, and some techniques in this section.

Purposes of Regulating the Breathing:

1. **To take in oxygen sufficiently and smoothly, and to expel carbon dioxide efficiently.** Approximately one trillion cells die every day in a healthy person.[19] In order to slow down the aging process, the same number of healthy new cells must be produced each day. We also know that oxygen is one of the necessary elements in the production of the new cells. Without an ample supply of oxygen, the new cells constructed will be deformed or unhealthy. In addition, dead cells in the body must be excreted to prevent problems in the body. The task of supplying sufficient oxygen and expelling the dead cells (i.e., carbon) falls to our respiratory system. Therefore, if you are able to inhale and exhale deeply, you will have reached this goal, which allows the smooth replacement of cells.
2. **To serve the strategic purpose in Qìgōng practice of regulating the body's Yīn and Yáng.** As mentioned earlier, breathing has Kǎn (water, 坎) and Lí (fire, 離), and so is able to adjust the body's Yīn and Yáng. Inhalation can make the body more Yīn, while exhalation can make the body more Yáng. Therefore, the methods of breathing correctly have become one of the major subjects of study in Chinese Qìgōng society.
3. **To coordinate and harmonize with the body, mind, Qì, and Shén.** Since breathing is one of the five important regulatings in which a Qìgōng practitioner must reach a profound level of practice, it plays an important role in coordination and harmonization. For example, concentrating during a deep and profound inhalation can make you more calm, and the Shén can be more condensed. If you focus during exhalation, the body's energy can be increased, the mind will be aroused, and the Shén can be raised. In addition, with correct breathing, the Qì can be led by the mind to the desired place more efficiently.

Breathing and Qìgōng

First, let us analyze how Qì circulation relates to your breathing. As mentioned earlier, there are eight Qì vessels (Mài, 脈) which function like reservoirs in your body, and twelve primary Qì channels (Jīng, 經) which function like rivers. In addition, there are millions of tiny secondary channels called "Luò" (絡), which branch out from the twelve channels to the surface of the skin to generate a shield of Guardian Qì (Wèiqì, 衛氣). This Qì is responsible for hair growth and for defending against negative outside influences. These tiny channels also deliver Qì into the bone marrow (Suǐqì, 髓氣) (i.e., Marrow Qì) to keep it healthy so blood cells can be produced properly.

Generally speaking, Qì circulation happens naturally and automatically in people who do not have Qìgōng training. However, an experienced Qìgōng practitioner can use his mind, coordinated with the breath, to generate an EMF (Electromotive Force) and control the Qì circulation more efficiently. Normally, when the average person exhales, he expands the Qì and leads it from the primary channels to the skin, and the body becomes more Yáng (Lí). When he inhales, he draws in the Qì, leading it from the primary channels to the bone marrow, and the body becomes more Yīn (Kǎn) (Figure 1–23). When inhalation and exhalation are balanced, Yīn and Yáng will be balanced.

As you get older, the length of your breath becomes shorter and shorter, causing less Qì to be led to the skin and the bone marrow. As Qì stagnates in the skin and marrow, the skin starts to wrinkle and the hair turns gray or falls out. In addition, fewer blood cells are produced, and these are not as healthy as those produced when you were young. Since blood cells carry nutrition and oxygen to the entire body, problems start to occur. In other words, you get sick more often and age faster.

You can see that the first key to maintaining your youth is learning to regulate your breathing. This enables you to control Kǎn and Lí, and consequently the Yīn and Yáng of your body. Next I would like to summarize how these Kǎn and Lí affect the body's Yīn and Yáng.

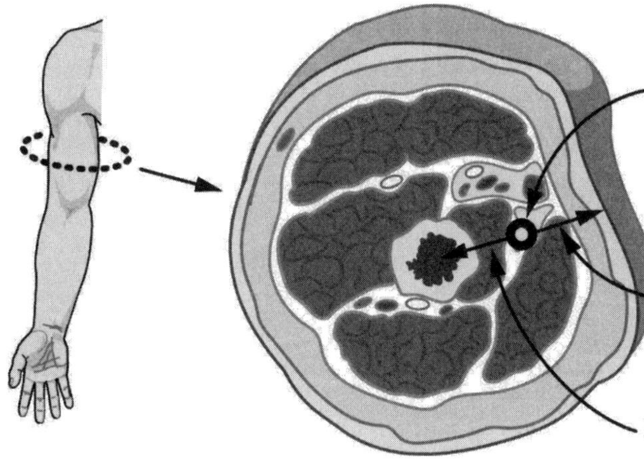

Figure 1-23. The Expansion and Condensing of Qì during Breathing

General Rules of Breathing's Kǎn-Lí and Yīn-Yáng

Kǎn-Lí	Method	Consequence
Kǎn	Inhalation	Yīn
Lí	Exhalation	Yáng
Kǎn	Inhale, then Hold the Breath	Yīn
Lí	Exhale, then Hold the Breath	Yáng
Kǎn	Soft, Slow, Calm, and Long Breathing	Yīn
Lí	Heavy, Fast, and Short Breathing	Yáng
Kǎn	Normal Abdominal Breathing (Buddhist Breathing)	Yīn
Lí	Reverse Abdominal Breathing (Daoist Breathing)	Yáng

Yīn and Yáng are relative, not absolute. After defining a reference standard, we can then compare them to each other. Yīn: Cold, Calm, Physical Body Relaxed and Qì Body Energized. Yáng: Hot, Excited, Physical Body Tensed and Energized.

Breathing Methods

1. **Normal Breathing** (Píngcháng Hūxī, 平常呼吸)

"Normal Breathing" is also called "Chest Breathing" (Xiōngbù Hūxī, 胸部呼吸), in which the breathing behavior is normally controlled by emotion. First you should learn how to regulate your normal chest breathing, inhaling and exhaling smoothly with the lungs relaxed. The mind must concentrate on the practice until it is neutral, calm, and peaceful. Then you will find that the breathing can be long and deep and the body can remain relaxed. When you have done this, the heart beat will slow down. You may practice in any comfortable position.

You should practice until the "real regulating" has been reached, meaning "regulating without regulating" (Wútiáo Értiáo, 無調而調). When this happens you will be practicing your breathing all the time, since you have built a natural habit. You should understand that the best and most powerful result of Qìgōng practice is to bring it into your lifestyle as a habit.

2. **Normal Abdominal Breathing** (Zhèng Fùhūxī, 正腹呼吸)

"Normal Abdominal Breathing" is also commonly known as "Buddhist Breathing" (Fójiā Hūxī, 佛家呼吸). After you have completed the above training, you then learn how to control your abdominal muscles and coordinate them with the breathing. When you inhale, your abdomen expands, and when you exhale it withdraws. You should practice until the process becomes smooth and the entire body remains relaxed. Naturally, at first your mind must concentrate on your abdomen in order to control the abdominal muscles. After practicing for some time, you will find the entire breathing process becoming natural and smooth. This will mean that you are ready to build up Qì at the Lower Dāntián (Xiàdāntián, 下丹田) (i.e., Qìhǎi, Co-6, 氣海).

Once you have reached this level, you should then coordinate your breathing with the movements of your Huìyīn (Co-1, 會陰) (Perineum) and anus. When you inhale, relax the Huìyīn and anus, and when you exhale hold them up (Figure 1–24). Remember, you are gently holding up the Huìyīn and anus, not tightening them. When you hold them up, they can still remain relaxed. If you tighten them, you will impede the Qì circulation. Tensing them also causes tension in the abdomen and stomach, which can generate other problems. At the beginning, naturally you will need to use your mind to control the muscles of the abdomen. However, with practice, you will realize that your mind does not have to be there to make it happen. That means you are regulating it without regulating. When you have reached this stage, you will feel a wonderful, comfortable feeling in the area of the Huìyīn and anus. You will also feel that the Qì is led more strongly to the skin than when you practiced Chest Breathing. It will feel as though your entire body is breathing with you.

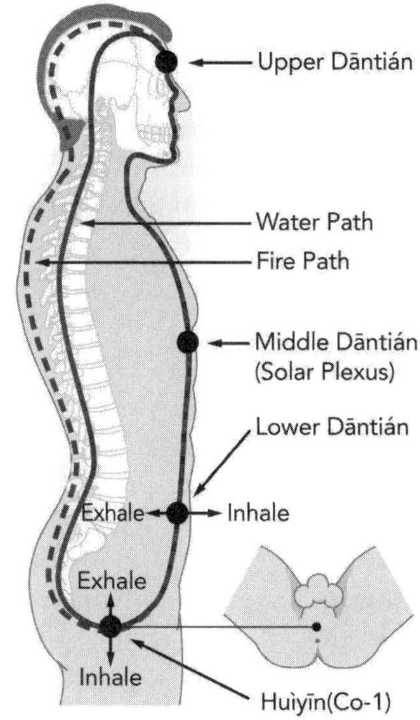

Figure 1-24. Normal Abdominal Breathing

Normal Abdominal Breathing

Neutral (inhalation and exhalation equal length)

Yīn –Inhalation (Abdomen Expands, Huìyīn Pushed Out Gently)

Yáng –Exhalation (Abdomen Withdraws, Huìyīn Held Up Gently)

Body Yīn (inhalation longer than exhalation)

–Inhalation (Abdomen Expands, Huìyīn Pushed Out Gently)

–Exhalation (Abdomen Withdraws, Huìyīn Relaxed)

Body Yáng (exhalation longer than inhalation)

–Inhalation (Abdomen Expands, Huìyīn Pushed Out Gently)

–Exhalation (Abdomen Withdraws, Huìyīn Held Up Strongly)

3. Reverse Abdominal Breathing (Fǎn Fùhūxī. Nì Fùhūxī, 反腹呼吸・逆腹呼吸)

"Reverse Abdominal Breathing" is also commonly called "Daoist Breathing" (Dàojiā Hūxī, 道家呼吸). After you have mastered Buddhist Breathing, you should then start this breathing. It is called Reverse Abdominal Breathing because the movement of the abdomen is the reverse of Buddhist Breathing. In other words, the abdomen withdraws when you inhale and expands when you exhale (Figure 1–25). Relatively speaking, Buddhist breathing is more relaxed compared with Daoist breathing, which is more aggressive. As a result, Daoist breathing can make the body more Yáng (tense and excited), while Buddhist breathing makes the body more Yīn (calm and relaxed).

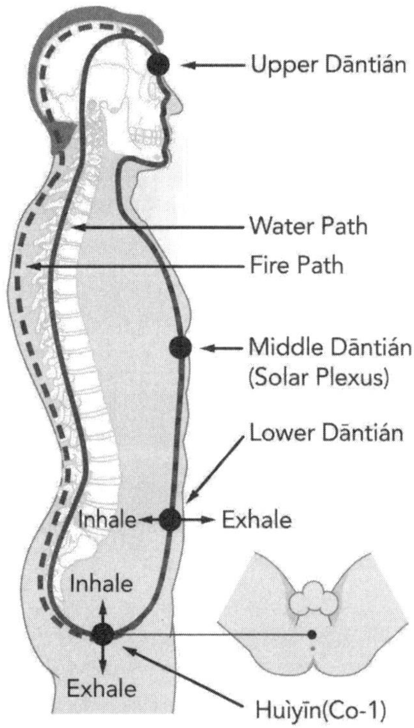

Figure 1-25. Reverse Abdominal Breathing

Many people today falsely believe that the reverse breathing technique is against the Dào, or nature's path. This is not true. If you observe your breathing carefully, you will realize that we use reverse breathing in two types of situations.

First, when we have an emotional disturbance, we often use reverse breathing. For example, when you are happy and laugh with the sound "Hā, Hā, Hā..." (哈) you are using reverse breathing. While you are making this sound, your stomach or abdominal area is expanding. When this happens, your exhalation is longer than your inhalation, your Guardian Qì expands, and you become hot and sweaty. This is the natural way of releasing the excess energy in your body caused from excitement or happiness.

Also, when you are sad and you cry, making a sound of "Hēng" (哼) while inhaling, your abdominal area is withdrawn. When this happens, your inhalation is longer than your exhalation, your Guardian Qì shrinks, and you feel cold and chilly. This is the natural way of preventing energy loss from inside your body. When you are sad, your Shén and your body's energy are low.

The second occasion in which we use reverse breathing is when we intend to energize our

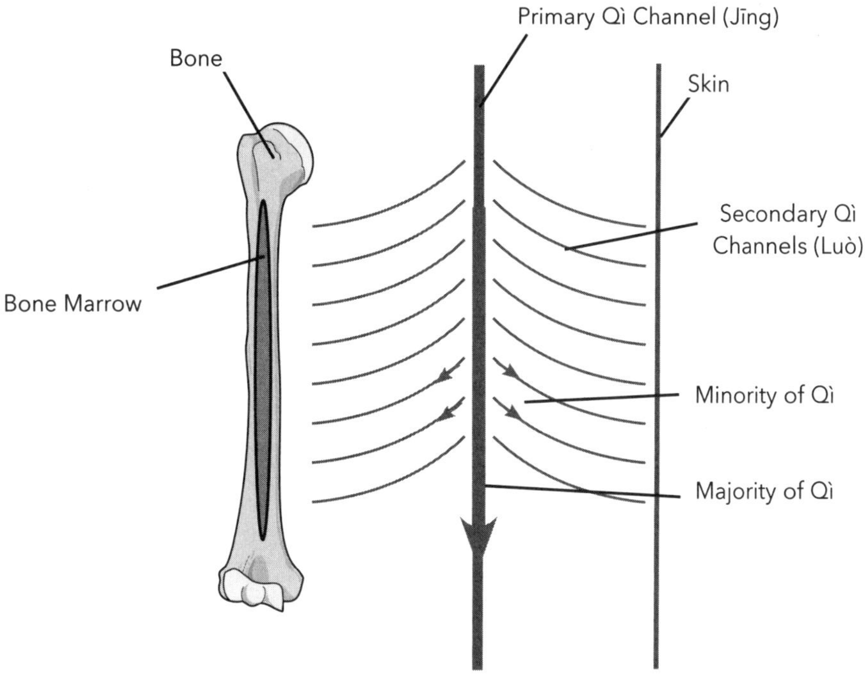

Figure 1-26. In Normal Abdominal Breathing, a Majority of the Qì Circulates in the Primary Qì Channels

physical body, for example when pushing a car or lifting some heavy weight. In order to exert strenuous effort, you first must inhale deeply, and then exhale while pushing the object. If you pay attention, you will again see that you are using reverse breathing.

From the above discussion, we can generally conclude that when we are disturbed emotionally, or when we have a focused intention in our mind, for example to energize our physical body, we use reverse breathing naturally.

After you have practiced for a while, you may discover that you can now lead the Qì to the skin more efficiently when you exhale than with the Buddhist method. Not only that, you may also discover that you are able to lead the Qì to the bone marrow. To help you understand this more clearly, let us take a comparison of the Normal Abdominal Breathing with the Reverse Abdominal Breathing and see how the Qì can be led in these two different breathing strategies.

In Normal Abdominal Breathing, the majority of Qì circulates in the primary Qì channels (Jīng, 經) which connect the internal organs to the extremities. Some Qì also spreads out through the secondary Qì channels (Luò, 絡) and reaches the skin and bone marrow (Figure 1–26). Since the majority of Qì is not led away from the primary Qì channels, the physical body is not energized and therefore the body remains relaxed. Therefore, Normal Abdominal Breathing is able to bring a beginning practitioner to a

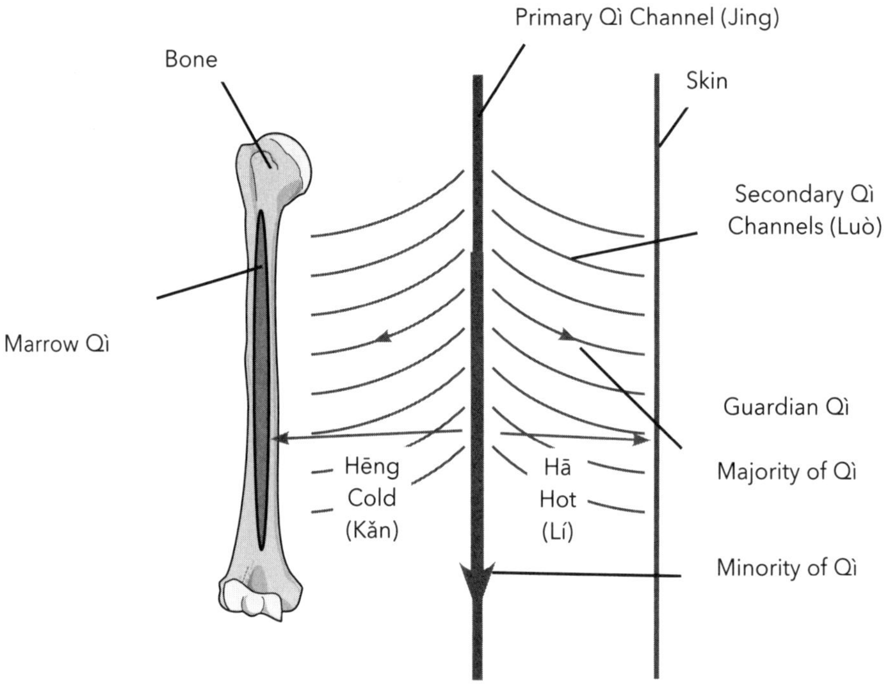

Figure 1-27. In Reverse Abdominal Breathing, a Majority of the Qì is Led to the Skin Surface and Bone Marrow

state of deep relaxation. Normal Abdominal Breathing (Kǎn) is able to make the body Yīn, while Reverse Abdominal Breathing (Lí) will cause the body to be Yáng.

However, in Reverse Abdominal Breathing, the majority of Qì has been led sideways through the secondary Qì channels to the skin and also to the bone marrow, with the minority of Qì circulating in the primary Qì channels (Figure 1–27). As mentioned earlier, normally these Qì-circulating behaviors are influenced by the emotional mind or Intentional Mind. Generally, patterns of Qì circulation related to the mind can be distinguished according to the breathing and emotional behavior. When you are excited and generate a sound of "Hā," exhalation is longer than inhalation. The Qì is led strongly outward to the skin surface from the primary Qì channels, the muscles are energized, and you sweat. The Guardian Qì (Wèiqì, 衛氣) is strengthened and this will result in your body's becoming more Yáng. However, if you are scared or sad while making the Hēng sound, your inhalation will be longer than your exhalation. The Qì is led inward to the marrow from the primary Qì channels and the Guardian Qì is weakened. You will feel cold. Naturally, this will result in the body's being more Yīn.

From this brief discussion, you can see that Skin Breathing (or Body Breathing) (Tǐxí, Fūxí, 體息・膚息) can be done much more effectively and efficiently through Reverse Abdominal Breathing. Naturally, the Marrow Breathing (Suǐxí, 髓息) can be reached more aggressively through Reverse Abdominal Breathing as well. Next, let us summarize some important concepts of Reverse Abdominal Breathing.

Reverse Abdominal Breathing

(Emotionally Disturbed, or the Mind has Intention of Yīn or Yáng)

Neutral (inhalation and exhalation equal length)
Yīn –Inhalation (Abdomen Withdraws, Huìyīn Held Up Gently)
Yáng –Exhalation (Abdomen Expands, Huìyīn Pushed Out Gently)

Body Yīn (inhalation longer than exhalation)
–Inhalation Longer (Abdomen Withdraws, Huìyīn Held Up Firmly)
–Exhalation (Abdomen Expands, Huìyīn Relaxed)

Body Yáng (exhalation longer than inhalation)
–Inhalation (Abdomen Withdraws, Huìyīn Held Up Gently)
–Exhalation (Abdomen Expands, Huìyīn Pushed Out Firmly)

4. **Embryonic Breathing** (Tāixí, 胎息)

Embryonic Breathing has always been a huge subject in Qìgōng practice. This is because it is the breathing method that allows you to store the Qì in the Real Lower Dāntián (Zhēn Xiàdāntián, 真下丹田). In other words, through Embryonic Breathing, you are able to charge your bio-battery to a high level. Then your vital energy will be raised, the immune system will be strengthened, and the physical body can be re-conditioned. However, the most important aspect of Embryonic Breathing is that once your Qì storage is built up to a high level, you are able to raise the Qì up through the spinal cord (Chōngmài, 衝脈) to nourish the brain and raise the Shén. This is the crucial key to spiritual enlightenment. Not only that, Embryonic Breathing is also a crucial key to Skin Breathing and Marrow Breathing that is closely related to our immune system and longevity. We will discuss this topic in detail in Chapter 5.

5. **Skin-Marrow Breathing** (Fū-Suǐxí, 膚髓息)

"Skin Breathing" (Fūxí, 膚息) is sometimes called "Body Breathing" (Tǐxí, 體息) Actually, Body Breathing involves breathing with the entire body, not just the skin. That means when you exhale you lead the Qì to the muscles and the skin, and when you inhale you lead the Qì to the marrow and the internal organs. Once you have reached a profound level, you should feel that your entire body is transparent to Qì. That means you feel your physical body disappear.

In fact, Skin-Marrow Breathing is closely related to Embryonic Breathing. When the Qì is led to the Real Lower Dāntián, you are also leading Qì to the bone marrow. When the Qì is led to enhance and expand the Qì in the Girdle Vessel, you are also leading Qì to the skin. Since Skin-Marrow Breathing is related to Embryonic Breathing, we will discuss it together with Embryonic Breathing in Chapter 5.

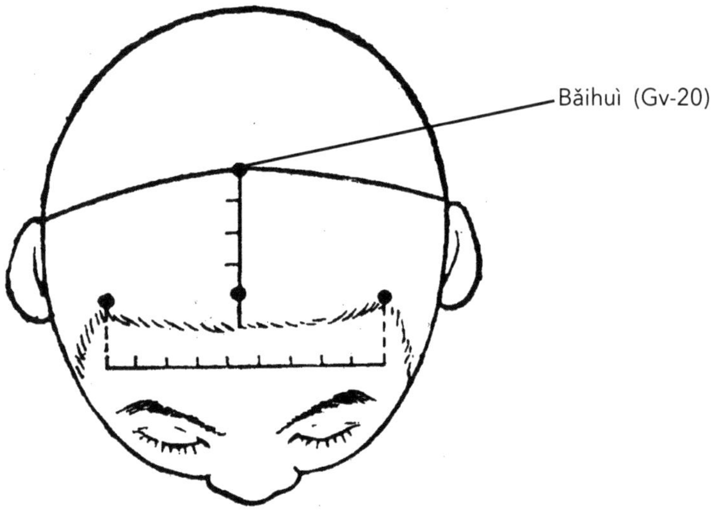

Figure 1-28. The Băihuì (Gv-20) Cavity

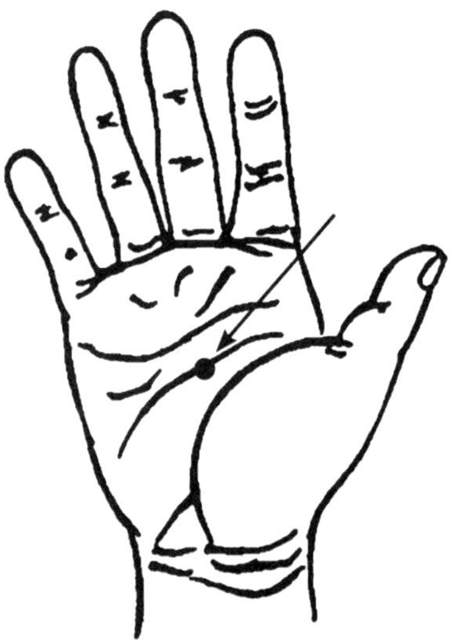

Figure 1-29. The Láogōng (P-8) Cavity

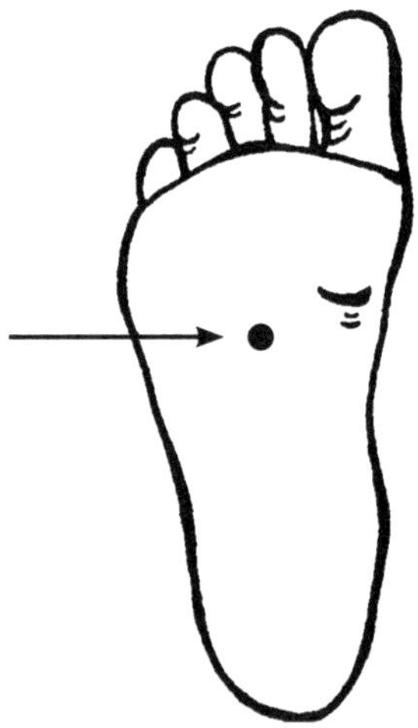

Figure 1-30. The Yǒngquán (K-1) Cavity

6. **Five Gates Breathing** (Wǔxīn Hūxī, 五心呼吸) (Wǔxīnxí, 五心息)

The Five Gates or Five Centers are the head (including the Upper Dāntián or The Third Eye and Băihuì, Gv-20, 百會) (Figure 1–28), the two Láogōng (P-8, 勞宮) cavities on the palms (Figure 1–29), and the two Yǒngquán (K-1, 湧泉) cavities on the soles of the feet (Figure 1–30). Beginners use the Băihuì gate on the crown, from where it is easier

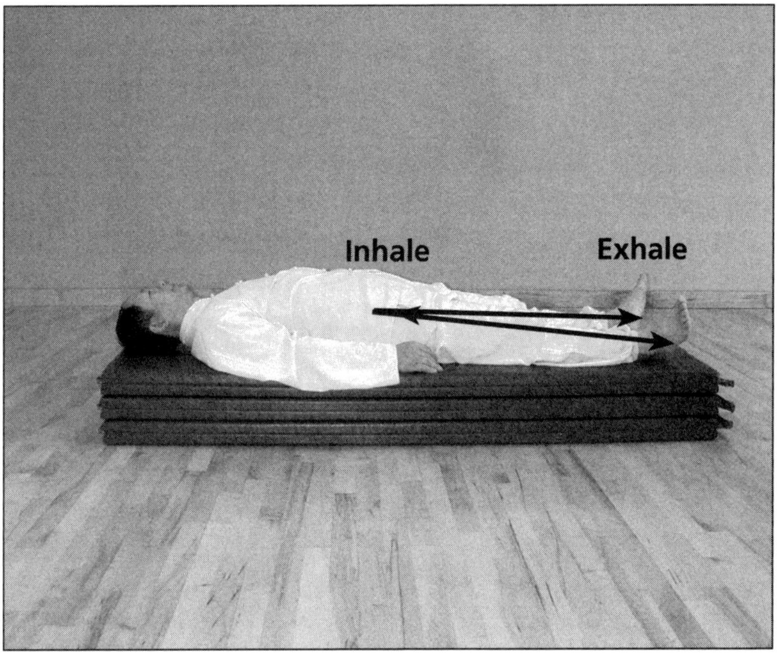

Figure 1-31. Yǒngquán Breathing with Normal Abdominal Breathing

for them to communicate with the natural Qì. Later, the Upper Dāntián (Third Eye) will be used instead. When you practice, you first learn Yǒngquán Breathing, and then add two Láogōng to make it Four Gates Breathing. Once you have included the Bǎihuì in your breathing, it is classified as one type of Spiritual Breathing.

Therefore, after you have learned how to build up the Qì at the Lower Dāntián, you will learn how to coordinate your breathing with the mind to lead the Qì to the Yǒngquán cavities on the bottom of the feet. In this practice, you may choose any desired position. If you wish to practice Yǒngquán breathing (Yǒngquánxí, 湧泉息) in a more relaxed way, you may simply lie down and use Normal Abdominal Breathing. When you inhale, use your mind to lead the Qì from the Yǒngquán to the Lower Dāntián, and when you exhale, lead the Qì from the Lower Dāntián to the Yǒngquán cavities (Figure 1–31). Naturally, when you inhale, the abdomen is expanded while the Huìyīn (Co-1, 會陰) cavity is gently pushing out and when you exhale, the abdomen is withdrawn while the Huìyīn cavity is gently held up. Even though the mind is involved in this practice, relaxation remains the major concern. The mind is not aggressively involved in leading the Qì.

However, if you wish to lead the Qì to the the Yǒngquán strongly, then the intention is strong, and naturally Reverse Abdominal Breathing is more effective. Daoist Qìgōng practitioners and Chinese martial artists favor this practice. The best posture for this is standing. First, inhale and use your mind to lead the Qì from the Yǒngquán cavities to

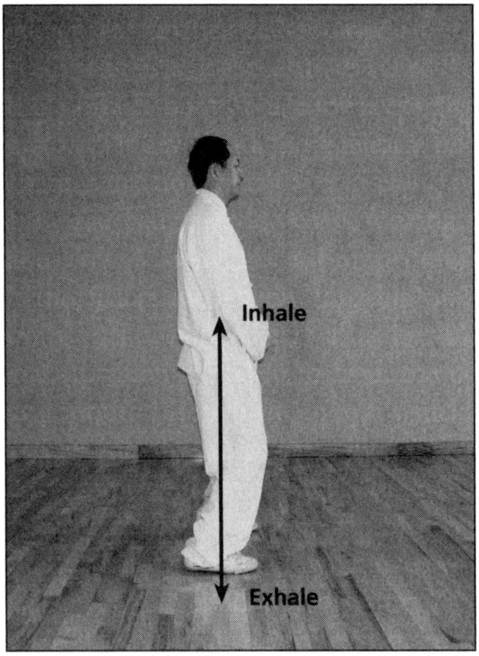

Figure 1-32. Yǒngquán Breathing with Reverse Abdominal Breathing

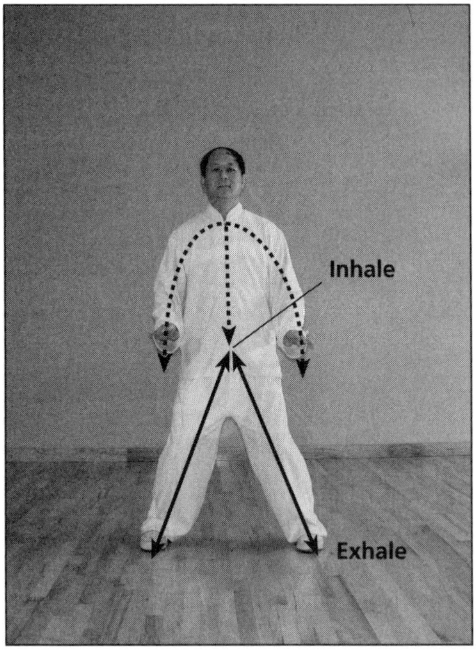

Figure 1-33. Four Gates Qì Breathing

the Lower Dāntián, and when you exhale, lead the Qì to the Yǒngquán cavities while slightly squatting down, imagining you are pushing your feet down into the ground (Figure 1–32). Naturally, in this practice, when you inhale the abdomen is drawn inward while the Huìyīn cavity is held up, and when you exhale, the abdomen expands while the Huìyīn cavity is pushed out.

Yǒngquán cavity breathing is also called "Sole Breathing" (Zhǒngxí, 踵息) as described by the well-known Daoist scholar Zhuāngzi (莊子) during the Warring States Period (戰國, 403–222 BCE). He said: "The ancient truthful persons (i.e., persons who have attained the Dào), ... their breathing was deep and profound. The real persons use the soles to breathe while the laymen use the throat to breathe."[20] From this, you can see that Yǒngquán breathing has been practiced for more than two thousand years. From medical Qìgōng, it is well-known that Yǒngquán breathing is one of the most effective breathing methods to regulate abnormal Qì levels in the three Yīn organs: Liver, Kidneys, and Spleen.

After you have practiced Yǒngquán Breathing for a long time and have reached the real regulating, you should then add the Láogōng cavities at the centers of your palms. These two gates are used to regulate the heart and lungs. Again, you can use either Normal Abdominal Breathing or Reverse Abdominal Breathing. When you inhale, you lead Qì from the Four Gates to the Lower Dāntián, and when you exhale, you lead the Qì from the Lower Dāntián back to the Four Gates (Figure 1–33).

By now, you may have realized that Four Gates Breathing is actually a common breathing method for Grand Qì Circulation (Dàzhōutiān, 大周天). Once you are able to reach a profound level of four gates breathing, then you learn the fifth gate. This is also commonly known as "Spiritual Breathing" (Shénxí, 神息) and will be discussed next.

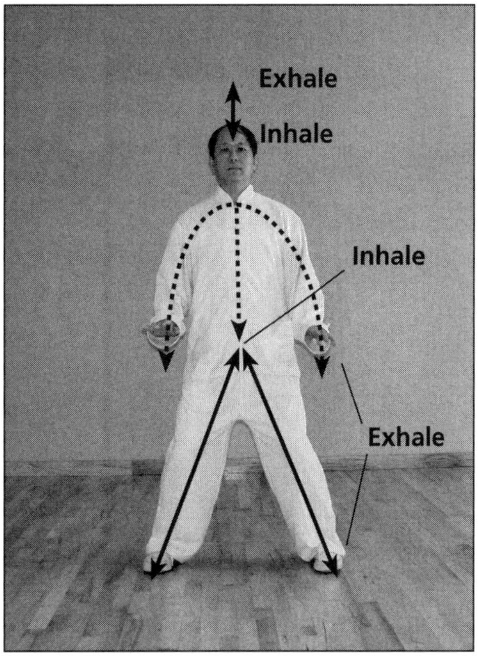

Figure 1-34. Five Gates Qì Breathing

7. **Spiritual Breathing** (Shénxí, 神息)

There are two definitions of Spiritual Breathing. One is the harmonization and unification of the Shén and the Breathing in Embryonic Breathing so the Spiritual Embryo can be conceived. This kind is commonly used for Marrow/Brain Washing, which aims for spiritual enlightenment. The other definition is the so-called "Fifth Gate Breathing," which is used to raise the Spirit of Vitality so that Four Gates Breathing can reach its maximum efficiency. This is generally used to increase the manifestation of the physical body for Muscle/Tendon Changing practice, and is commonly used in martial arts society. Since we are going to discuss Spiritual Breathing in Parts II and III of this book, we will not explain too much here. Instead, we will briefly discuss the "Fifth Gate Breathing" in this sub-section.

"Fifth Gate Breathing" (Dìwǔxīn Hūxī, 第五心呼吸) is also called "Bǎihuì Breathing" (百會呼吸), or "Upper Dāntián Breathing" (Shàngdāntián Hūxī, 上丹田呼吸), which means breathing through the Third Eye. This is the crucial key to raising the Spirit of Vitality.

Once you have reached a profound level of Four Gates Breathing, you will learn how to lead the Qì upward through the spinal cord (Thrusting Vessel, Chōngmài, 衝脈) to nourish the brain and energize it. This allows the Shén to be raised and the energy potential to reach a high level (Figure 1–34). When this happens, physical power can be manifested to its maximum efficiency. If you are interested in this ancient practice, you should refer to the book, *Qìgōng—The Secret of Youth*, published by YMAA Publication Center.

When you have reached the level of Spiritual Breathing, it implies that you have already regulated your body, breathing, mind, and Qì, and are now in the process of regulating the Shén. This means your Qìgōng practice and the search for spiritual enlightenment has reached the final stage in approaching maturity. It is said in *The Complete Book of Principal Contents of Human Life and Temperament* (*Xìngmìng Guīzhǐ Quánshū*, 性命圭旨全書): "What is spiritual breathing? It means the maturity of cultivation."[21] That means the cultivation of the interaction of Kǎn (water) and Lí (fire) has reached the stage of "regulating without regulating." In this case, all the cultivations have become natural.

There are some other breathing methods trained in Daoist Qìgōng such as Turtle Breathing (Guīxí, 龜息) and Hibernation Breathing (Dōngmiánxí, 冬眠息), but we will not discuss them here.

1.6.3 Regulating the Mind (Tiáoxīn, 調心)

Regulating the Mind means to regulate and control the emotional mind (Xīn, 心). This practice has always been the most difficult subject to understand and train in Nèidān Qìgōng (內丹氣功) practice. Here you are dealing with your own mind. Each person has his own unique thinking and emotional disturbance, thus, it is also the most difficult subject to explain.

The methods of regulating the mind have been widely studied, discussed, and practiced in all Chinese Qìgōng societies, which include scholar, medical, religious, and martial arts groups. In this section, we will study the conclusions of these four schools. We will define the mind, and the purposes of regulating the mind. Then, we will discuss the thinking process from the Buddhist point of view. Finally, we will analyze the methods of regulating the mind.

Two Minds—Xīn and Yì 心・意. To regulate the mind is actually to regulate the "heart" (Tiáoxīn, 調心). The Chinese believe that the "heart" is closely related to our emotional thinking and reaction.

As explained before, in Chinese society, it is commonly recognized that we have two minds. The mind that is related to our emotional feeling is called "Xīn" (心) (heart). This mind is Yáng and makes you confused, scattered, depressed, and excited. The other mind, related to our rational and logical thinking, is called "Yì" (意) (intention). This mind is Yīn and makes you calm, concentrated, and able to feel and ponder deeply. The Chinese word "Yì" (意) is constructed of three words: "立" on the top means "to establish," "曰" in the middle means "to speak," and "心" at the bottom means the "heart." From this you can see that the meaning of Yì is "to establish communication (an opinion) with the heart (emotional mind) under control." This means logical thinking and judgment.

Purposes of Regulating the Mind (Diàoxīn Zhī Mùdì, 調心之目的). There are many different purposes or goals for regulating the mind. These purposes can be varied from one school to another. For example, practitioners in scholar and medical Qìgōng societies are aiming for a calm, peaceful, and harmonious mind so the emotional mind will not disturb the body's Qì circulation. As discussed earlier, it is believed that our thinking can seriously influence the normal, healthy Qì circulation of the body. For instance, if you are happy and excited, the Qì status in your heart will be too Yáng and can trigger a heart attack. If you are angry, the Qì level in your liver will be abnormal and affect the liver's healthy functioning. In the same way the Qì circulation in kidneys is related to fear, while that of the lungs is related to sadness. Therefore, if you are able to regulate your emotional mind to a harmonious and peaceful state, you will be healthy.

However, for Daoist and Buddhist religious groups, in addition to regulating the emotional mind to a calm and peaceful state, they are also aiming for Buddhahood and enlightenment. Therefore, once they have controlled the emotional mind and developed their Wisdom Mind to a profound stage, they will ponder and search for the meaning of life and of nature.

Finally, the martial Qìgōng practitioners aim to raise their Spirit of Vitality and build up a highly concentrated mind to develop a sense of enemy. This is critical in battle. While your mind is calm and clear, your Shén must be raised to a state of high alertness.

However, it does not matter what goals each school is aiming at, the basic training rules and principles remain the same. In order to reach their goals, they must follow the same training path. To conclude, the purposes of regulating the mind are:

1. **To harmonize the body and the mind** (Shēnxīn Pínghéng, 身心平衡).

In order to have a calm meditative mind, you must first regulate the condition of your physical body. When your body is tense and energized, your mind will be excited and the breath will be faster. Therefore, the body and the mind must coordinate and harmonize with each other. This is called "The balance of the body and the Xīn" (Shēnxīn Pínghéng, 身心平衡). *The Complete Book of Principal Contents of Human Life and Temperament* (*Xìngmìng Guīzhǐ Quánshū*, 性命圭旨全書) said: "(When) the body is not moving, then the Xīn will be peaceful. (When) the Xīn is not moving (disturbing), then the Shén can abide by itself."[22] Therefore, the first step in regulating the mind is to calm the body. Once the body is calm, the mind can then be calm. When the emotional mind is calm, then the Wisdom Mind can function efficiently. Only once the mind is calm and peaceful, can the Spirit of Vitality be raised.

2. **To harmonize the breathing and the mind** (Xīnxí Xiāngyī, 心息相依).

As mentioned earlier, to regulate the emotional mind is to learn how to use the Wisdom Mind to control the function of the emotional mind. In Chinese Qìgōng society, the emotional mind (Xīn) is compared to an ape, while the Wisdom Mind (Yì) is compared to a horse. It is commonly said "Xīn (is) an ape, Yì (is) a horse" (Xīnyuán Yìmǎ, 心猿意馬). An ape is not powerful but, by being unsteady and disturbing, generates confusion and excitement. Yet a horse, though powerful, can be calm, steady, and controllable.

In Qìgōng society, through thousands of years of studying the method of regulating the mind, it is understood that in order to lead an ape into a cage and restrain it, you need a banana. Our "banana" is Regulating the Breathing. As long as you are able to concentrate on your breathing, sooner or later your emotional mind will be restrained and calm down. That means when your breathing is long, slender, soft, and calm, your mind will be calm. Naturally, in order to make your breathing long, slender, soft, and calm, you must also keep your mind calm. Both the mind and breathing mutually affect each other. They must work together harmoniously in order to reach a high mental state of meditation. Therefore, it is said that "The Xīn and the breathing mutually rely on each other" (Xīnxí Xiāngyī, 心息相依).

The *Complete Book of Principal Contents of Human Life and Temperament* (*Xìngmìng Guīzhǐ Quánshū*, 性命圭旨全書) said: "To conform with the real person's (i.e., person who has reached the real truth or Dào) deep profound breathing, then the Xīn and the breathing can be relying on each other mutually. (When) the breathing is regulated, the Xīn can then be calm."[23] This short paragraph clearly states that in order to have a calm emotional mind, you must first regulate your breathing. The way of regulating the breathing is to conform with the real person's breathing methods. The real people (i.e., Zhēnrén, 真人) are those who have already reached the real truth of the Dào.

It was also explained in the book *Questions From A Buddhist Guest About Listening to the Heart* (*Tīngxīn Zhāikè Wèn*, 聽心齋客問), "The Xīn has been relying on the affairs and objects for a long time; once separated from its residence, it cannot be independent. Therefore, (we must) use the Gōngfū of regulating the breathing to restrain this Xīn. The Xīn and the breathing can then mutually rely on each other. The word of regulating is also not to use the Yì. It is only a thought of one inhalation and one exhalation. Once the Xīn has separated from its residence, then it is (free) without others and without self. In this case, there is no breathing which can be regulated. Only (keep the breathing) soft and continuous as if it is existing and not existing (i.e., regulating without regulating). After a long time, it will be become proficient naturally."[24] This paragraph explains that our emotional mind is attracted to human affairs and the objects around us, and is influenced by them. When this happens, the emotional mind will be confused and unsteady, and consequently cannot be independent. The way to restrain this emotional mind is to regulate the breathing until the emotional mind and the breathing are mutually dependent on each other. When you regulate the breathing, you should not have an intention (Yì). Should you have this intention, your mind would cause tension in the breathing. Simply pay attention to the breathing. After you have practiced for a period of time, you can breathe softly, naturally, smoothly, and continuously. When you have reached this stage, the Xīn will be staying at its residence without disturbance.

3. Use the mind to build up, store, and lead the Qì.

In religious and martial arts Qìgōng groups, one of the main goals of practicing Qìgōng is using the mind to build up the Qì, to store it, and also to lead its circulation. In order to build up and store Qì in the Real Lower Dāntián (Zhēn Xiàdāntián, 真下丹田), you must practice Embryonic Breathing (Tāixí, 胎息). The crucial key to this practice is keeping your mind in this Qì residence and center. Once your mind is away from this center, your Qì will be led away from it and consumed. Therefore, the Qì will never build up and store in the body to a higher level. That is why it is said: "Keep the Yì at the Dāntián" (Yìshǒu Dāntián, 意守丹田). This is the practice of storing the Qì. Once you have stored Qì to an abundant level, you learn how to use your mind to lead the Qì. It is said: "Use the Yì to lead the Qì" (Yǐyì Yǐnqì, 以意引氣). Normally, in Nèidān practice, first you learn to lead the Qì to circulate in the Conception (Rènmài, 任脈) and Governing Vessels (Dūmài, 督脈) to complete Small Circulation (Xiǎozhōutiān, 小周天). After this, you learn to lead the Qì to the extremities, skin, bone marrow, and brain for Grand Circulation (Dàzhōutiān, 大周天). Since these are the main subjects of this book and the next, we will not discuss them further here.

4. **To raise up the Spirit of Vitality for enlightenment.**

To Buddhists and Daoists, the final goal of Qìgōng practice is to reach enlightenment or Buddhahood. Once you have learned how to store the Qì at the Real Lower Dāntián, you then lead it upward, following the Thrusting Vessel (Chōngmài, 衝脈) (spinal cord) to the brain to nourish the Shén. The goal is to reopen the Third Eye. It is believed that through thousands of years, since we learned to lie and cheat to protect our secrets, we closed our Third Eye so that other people would be unable to see the truth behind our mask. In so doing, we lost the power of telepathy and communication with natural Qì and Shén. In order to reopen this Third Eye, we must first be truthful to the point where there is nothing to hide. Then, we learn how to accumulate Qì in the front of the brain. Accounts of past experience tell us that the Third Eye can be reopened.

In practice, in order to raise the Shén to an enlightened level, you must first regulate your Xīn until it has reached an extremely calm state. When you are in this state, your mind is clear and not wandering. It is said in the Dào Scriptures (Dàozàng, 道藏) that: "The Xīn is the master of the entire body, the commander of a hundred spirits. (When it is) calm, then the wisdom is generated, (when it is) acting, then confusion is originated. Its complacency (goal of steadiness) and confusion are within the movement and the calmness."[25]

1.6.4 Regulating the Qì (Tiáoqì, 調氣)

Different Qìgōng schools have different purposes for regulating the Qì. To the medical Qìgōng group, regulating the Qì means: 1. Improving the Qì circulation, thereby maintaining health; 2. Removing existing Qì stagnation in the body (healing); 3. Bringing the Qì circulation in the internal organs to a harmonious and balanced state.

To the scholar Qìgōng group, regulating Qì means: 1. Calming down excitement due to the manifestation of Qì; and 2. Bringing the Qì in the internal organs to a harmonious and balanced state.

To the martial Qìgōng group, regulating the Qì means: 1. Improving the flow of Qì to a desired area for higher efficiency and stronger physical manifestation; 2. Enhancing the level of Qì circulation so the manifestation of Qì can reach a higher level (i.e., power); and 3. Increasing Qì storage in the Lower Dāntián and the Qì vessels.

However, to the religious Qìgōng group, regulating the Qì includes many goals: 1. Producing extra Qì at the False Lower Dāntián (Jiǎ Xiàdāntián, 假下丹田); 2. Storing Qì at the Real Lower Dāntián (Zhēn Xiàdāntián, 真下丹田); 3. Leading the Qì to circulate in the Conception and Governing Vessels (i.e., Small Circulation); 4. Increasing the Qì level in the Qì vessels; 5. Enhancing the strength of Guardian Qì (Wèiqì, 衛氣) and expanding it (i.e., strengthen the immune system); 6. Washing the bone marrow and maintaining its healthy functioning (i.e., longevity); 7. Achieving Grand Circulation (Dàzhōutiān, 大周天) of the Twelve Primary Qì Channels (Jīng, 經) to condition the sensitivity of the entire body; 8. Exchanging Qì with partners and the natural environment (i.e., Grand Circulation with nature); 9. Leading the Qì upward through the Thrusting Vessel (Chōngmài, 衝脈) to nourish the brain for spiritual enlightenment; and finally, 10. Reunifying the human spirit and Qì with the natural spirit and Qì (i.e., Unification of Heaven and Human).

You can see that regulating the Qì in religious society (espcially in Daoist society) covers a much wider variety of practice, depending on the level of cultivation. This is also the main reason that religious Qìgōng has been recognized as the highest level in Qìgōng society. Embryonic Breathing is one of the practices in this society that teaches you how to produce Qì at the False Lower Dāntián and how to store it at the Real Lower Dāntián. Only if a practitioner is able to comprehend the profound theory and grasp the keys of practice can he then proceed to other Qì-regulating practices. That is the reason Embryonic Breathing is considered the root or essence of Internal Elixir (Nèidān, 內丹) practice.

Both in theory and practice, in order to reach a highly efficient level of Qì regulation, you naturally must already have regulated the body, breathing, and mind to a profound level. As mentioned earlier, regulating the body, regulating the breathing, and regulating the mind cannot be separated. They are mutually related and interact with each other. Only when these three are harmoniously coordinated can the Qì be led by the clear and calm mind.

Since regulating the Qì is the main goal of Qìgōng practice, each purpose mentioned above is a huge subject for discussion. It would take a few books just to cover Qì regulation in any one of the medical, scholar, or martial schools, but the coverage of Qì regulation in the religious group is even larger and much deeper. Therefore, you should keep your mind open and continue to search for the training theory and methods. This is the way of searching for the Dào. Those who follow this way, the Chinese call "Xúndàozhě" (尋道者), meaning "Dào Seeker."

In this book, we will cover only those practices related to Embryonic Breathing. Through these practices, you will have built a firm foundation for all the other practices.

1.6.5 Regulating the Spirit (Tiáoshén, 調神)

In general, there are four major tasks to learn in regulating your spirit (Shén, 神): 1. How to raise your Shén; 2. How to keep it at its residence and strengthen it; 3. How to coordinate it with your breathing; and finally, 4. How to use your Shén to direct and manifest your Qì effectively. All of these are called "Liànshén" (煉神) by Daoist Qìgōng practitioners. Liàn (煉) means to refine, to train, or to discipline. In religious Qìgōng, there is another ultimate goal in regulating the Shén, and that is to train it to be independent enough to leave the physical body (i.e., spiritual immortality).

1. **Raising up the Shén** (Yǎngshén, 養神)

Yǎng (養) means to nourish, to raise, or to nurse. Yǎngshén has been the main task for scholars and Buddhists in their training to regulate the Shén. Shén needs to be nourished by Qì. Normally, the Fire Qì from food and air is able to raise up the Shén easily. However, this Fire Qì also increases emotional disturbance and therefore leads the Shén away from its residence. Raising your Shén using your Yì, which is nourished by Water Qì, is more difficult. However, if you are able to do it, this Shén can be stronger and more concentrated than when you use Fire Qì. In Qìgōng practice, you are learning to adjust your Xīn and Yì to raise your Shén. If you are able to use your Xīn and Yì properly, your Shén will be raised but not excited, and can remain at its residence.

Raising the Shén the right way is almost like raising a child: you need a great amount of patience and perseverance. One way to raise a child is to help him resist his attraction to the seven emotions and six desires; another way is to let him maintain contact with his human nature, educating him and helping him develop the wisdom to make clear judgments. It is a long process, and demands a lot of understanding and patience. In Qìgōng, raising the Shén is not a question of increasing your emotional excitement. This would scatter the Yì, and your Shén would become confused and lose its center. Yángshén training builds a strong center for your Shén, and helps the Shén take control over a larger part of your life.

2. **Keeping Shén in Its Residence and Training it** (Shǒushén Yǔ Liànshén, 守神與煉神)

After raising your Shén, you must learn how to keep it at its residence and train it. As with a child of a certain age, you must be able to keep his attention within the home, where you can educate him, instead of letting him stray outside and run wild. In Qìgōng training, to keep and train the Shén includes four major steps:

A. **To Protect the Shén** (Shǒushén, 守神)

"Shǒu" (守) means "to keep and to protect." The very beginning of the training involves learning how to keep your Shén at its residence. While it is relatively easy to raise your Shén, it is much harder to keep it in its residence. In Shǒushén training, in order to keep the Shén in its residence you must use your regulated mind to direct, nurse, watch, and keep the Shén there. You must be patient and control your temper (regulate your mind). You can see, therefore, that the first step in regulating your Shén is to regulate your Xīn (emotional mind) and Yì (Wisdom Mind). If you lose your patience and temper, you will only make the child want to leave home again. Only when you have regulated your Xīn and Yì will you be able to guard and keep your Shén effectively.

B. **To Firm the Shén** (Gùshén, 固神)

"Gù" (固) means "to solidify and to firm." After you can keep your Shén in its residence, you then learn how to firm and solidify it. Gùshén means to train your Shén to stay at its residence willingly. After you are able to control your child in the house, you must make him sincerely want to stay. Only then will his mind be steady and calm. Naturally, in order to reach this stage, you will need a lot of love and patience to educate him until he understands how important it is for him to stay home and grow up normally and healthily. Qìgōng training operates on the same principle. In order to do this, your mind must be able to regulate all emotional thoughts. Only then will your Shén be able to stay in its residence in peace.

C. **To Stabilize the Shén** (Dìngshén, 定神)

"Dìng" (定) means "to stabilize and to calm." When you have brought your child into the stage of peace, he will not be as excited and attracted to outside emotional distractions. In regulating your Shén, you must learn to calm the Shén so that it is energized but not excited. Then the mind will be peaceful and steady.

D. **To Focus the Shén** (Níngshén, 凝神)

"Níng" (凝) means "to concentrate, to condense, to refine, to focus, and to strengthen." You can see from the above three processes that keeping, firming, and stabilizing are the foundations of the cultivation of your Shén. It is like a child who is able to stay at home willingly with a calm and steady mind. Only then will you be able to teach and train him. In Qìgōng, once you have passed these three initial steps, you will learn to focus and condense your Shén into a tiny spot. The "condensing the Shén" stage is where you can train the Shén to a higher spiritual state. When the Shén is focused into a tiny point, it is like a sunbeam focused through a lens: the smaller the point, the stronger its beam.

3. **Combining Shén with Breathing** (Shénxì Xiāngyī, 神息相依)

After the Shén has been trained to a high degree, you can put it to work. The first assignment for your Shén is coordination with your breathing. Remember, in Qìgōng training your breathing carries out your strategy. When this strategy is directed by your Shén, it can obtain maximum results. This is called "Shénxí Xiāngyī" (神息相依), which means "the Shén and the breathing are mutually dependent." In Qìgōng training, this is called "Shénxí" (神息) which means "Shén breathing." At this stage, your Shén and breathing have united into one. When you have accomplished this, your Qì will be led most efficiently. Naturally, this is not an easy task. In order to reach this stage, you must have regulated your body, breathing, and mind.

4. **Combining Shén with Qì** (Shénqì Xiànghé, 神氣相合)

The last stage of regulating Shén involves learning to use the Shén to direct the circulation and distribution of Qì in the most efficient way. In Qìgōng society, this stage is called "Shénqì Xiànghé" (神氣相合), which means "the Shén and Qì combine together." In a battle, if the Shén of the soldiers is kept high, their fighting ability and efficiency will be increased, and the strategy will be carried out more thoroughly.

In Chapter 3, you will see that there are many ancient documents discussing the "regulation of the Shén." The reason for this is that in order to reach the final goal of Embryonic Breathing, other than "regulating the breathing" and "regulating the mind," it is "regulation of the Shén" which plays the important role in reaching a successful Embryonic Breathing practice.

1.7 Muscle/Tendon Changing and Marrow/Brain Washing Qìgōng (Yìjīnjīng Yǔ Xǐsuǐjīng qìgōng, 易筋經與洗髓經氣功)

Embryonic Breathing is the root and essence of the Internal Elixir Qìgōng (Nèidān Qìgōng, 內丹氣功) practice. From this root, the physical body (Yáng) and the energy body (Yīn) can be cultivated and developed. The physical body includes tissue such as skin, muscle, tendon, ligament, bone, marrow, etc. The Qì body supplies energy to the physical body to maintain life. This includes nourishing the brain to generate thought (mental action).

However, Chinese people often view the Yīn body as the mental body instead of as the energy body. In this case, Qì is considered to be neutral, supplying energy to the physical body and also to the brain for mental activity. Since Thought is connected to and associated with spiritual cultivation, the spiritual body is commonly considered the Yīn body in Chinese religious societies. The physical body is called "Mìng" (命), which means "life," while the spiritual body is called "Xìng" (性), meaning "human temperament," i.e., the natural spirit we were born with.

Muscle/Tendon Changing Qìgōng and Marrow/Brain Washing Qìgōng are the two halves of a religious Qìgōng training passed down by an Indian monk, Dámó, in a Chinese Buddhist monastery, the Shàolín Temple (少林寺). Dámó's classic emphasizes that in order to achieve spiritual enlightenment, we must have a strong and long physical life, which allows us more time for spiritual cultivation. Therefore, Muscle/Tendon Changing Qìgōng teaches a practitioner how to condition his physical body. In addition, in order to reach the final goal of spiritual enlightenment, you must also have abundant Qì to nourish the brain and promote the brain's functioning to a higher level. When this happens, then spiritual enlightenment can be reached. In one of the prefaces to Dámó's classic, there is a section about this:

> *The* Xǐsuǐjīng *says a man's body (is) touched by love and desire, and formed with shape, contaminated by sediment and dirtiness. If you wish to cultivate the real meaning of Buddhism, (Shén) moving and stopping at will, (then) the five viscera and six bowels, four limbs and hundreds of bones must be completely washed clean individually. (When they are) pure and (you) are able to see the calmness and peace, then (you) can be cultivated and enter the domain of Buddhahood. (If you) do not cultivate this (way), (obtaining the Dào) will not have foundation and origin. Read till here, then know that the believers thought that "acquiring the marrow" was not a comparison.*
>
> 洗髓經者，謂人之生，感於愛慾，一落有形，悉皆滓穢；欲修佛諦，動障真如，五臟六腑，四肢百骸，必先一一洗滌淨盡，純見清虛，方可進修，入佛智地，不由此經進修，無基無有是處；讀至此，然後知向者所謂得髓者，非譬喻也。

> *The* Yìjīnjīng *says that outside of the bone and marrow, under the skin and meat (i.e., muscles), (there is) nothing but the tendons and vessels which connect the entire body and transport the blood and Qì. All of these are post-birth body, (and) must be promoted (i.e., trained); borrow them to cultivate the real (Dào). If you do not assist and promote them, (you will) see weakening and withering immediately. (If you) see (this training) as ordinary (training), how could you reach the final goal? (If you) give up and do not train them, then there is no strength for cultivation, and nothing can be achieved.*

易筋者，謂髓骨之外，皮肉之內，莫非筋聯絡周身，通行血氣，凡屬後天，皆其提挈，借假修真，非所贊勷，立見頹靡，視作泛常，曷臻極至？舍是不為，進修不力，無有是處；讀至此，然後知所謂皮肉骨者，非譬喻，亦非漫語也。

From these two paragraphs, you can see that Muscle/Tendon Changing is for physical life, while Marrow/Brain Washing is for spiritual life. This concept was very important to religious Qìgōng meditators. The ultimate goal of both Buddhist and Daoist study is to reach Buddhahood or enlightenment. According to their theory, it would normally take hundreds of lifetimes to cultivate your Shén and gradually reach the final destination. Therefore, if you have a long life in each life time, then you will have a longer period for cultivation. This is most critical, especially as the best period for spiritual cultivation is after the age of forty. This is because, normally, before you are thirty you are still looking for the meaning of your life and your mind is still learning how to fit in and survive in the new environment. During this period, the Shén of your new life is not yet mature enough to establish contact with the Pre-Birth Shén. If you die before you are thirty, you will only have a short period of time to cultivate your Shén to a higher level. However, if you are able to live long, then you will have a long time to promote your Shén. Essentially, the longer life you have, the better your Shén is able to develop. Naturally, you have also become wiser.

From the section quoted, it seems the concept of longevity has been well understood by the Daoists but not by many of the Buddhists. Daoists believed that the physical body and spiritual body are equally important, and should be cultivated together. This is called "dual cultivation of spiritual virtue (human temperament) and physical life" (Xìngmìng Shuāngxiū, 性命雙修) in Daoist society. This is not the case in Buddhist society. In fact, many Buddhists believed that our physical body is only used temporarily for the Shén to reside there. For them, spiritual cultivation is more important than physical cultivation, and spending time building physical strength is a waste of time.

Kǎn and Lí in Yìjīnjīng and Xǐsuǐjīng (Yìjīnjīng Yǔ Xǐsuǐjīng Zhī Kǎn-Lí, 易筋經與洗髓經之坎離). When you try any style of Qìgōng, you must balance Yīn and Yáng by controlling Kǎn (坎) (water) and Lí (離) (fire). For example, when you practice Tàijíquán, you learn the slow, meditative physical movements that are Lí, which may cause your body to become too Yáng. You must also learn still meditation, which is Kǎn and neutralizes the excessive Yáng. Again, within the moving Tàijíquán form itself there is also Kǎn and Lí adjustment. While the physical movement is Lí (which causes Yáng), the calm mind is Kǎn (and may neutralize the Yáng). In still meditation, while the stillness of the physical body is Kǎn and causes Yīn, the Qì must be actively led by the mind to circulate in the body. This is Lí and results in Yáng, which balances the Yīn. This means that in all Qìgōng practices, if there is Yīn, there must be Yáng to balance it, and vice versa.

It is the same with the Yìjīnjīng and Xǐsuǐjīng training. They are based on this Yīn and Yáng concept. The Yìjīnjīng is Lí because it generates Qì and manifests it as physical strength, thus generating Yáng. The Xǐsuǐjīng is Kǎn, because it utilizes and stores the Qì in the marrow/brain and generates Yīn. The Yìjīnjīng deals with the muscles/tendons and skin, which are visible externally, while the Xǐsuǐjīng deals with the marrow and brain, which must be felt internally. While the Yìjīnjīng training emphasizes the physical body, the Xǐsuǐjīng training focuses on the spiritual body. Therefore, Yīn and Yáng are balanced and coexist harmoniously.

In the *Yìjīnjīng*, the physical stimulation and exercises are considered Lí and cause the body to become Yáng, while the still meditation of the Small Circulation is Kǎn, which counterbalances the Lí and makes the body more Yīn. Again, in the physical stimulation Lí training, external strength is Lí while internal mental strength is Kǎn. In still meditation, the physical body is still and is Kǎn, while the Qì moving inside and led by the mind is Lí.

The same theory prevails in Xǐsuǐjīng training. The physical stimulation to increase the Original Essence production is Lí, while the techniques of internal cultivation (which are used to lead the Qì to the marrow and brain) are Kǎn.

You can see from this discussion that the basic key to successful Qìgōng training is Yīn and Yáng balance, and the trick to reaching this goal is Kǎn and Lí adjustment. Once you understand this fundamental theory, you will not have too much difficulty understanding the foundation of Qìgōng practice.

If you are interested in knowing more about Muscle/Tendon Changing and Marrow/Brain Washing Qìgōng, please refer to the book: *Qìgōng—The Secret of Youth*, published by YMAA Publication Center.

1.8 Small Circulation, Grand Circulation, and Enlightenment Meditation (Xiǎozhōutiān, Dàzhōutiān, Yǔ Xiāndào Wùzhēn Jìngzuò, 小周天、大周天、與仙道悟真靜坐)

In order to understand the relationship between Embryonic Breathing and various spiritual meditations in the next section, I would like to review three of the most important Daoist meditation practices: Small Cyclic Heaven Meditation (Xiǎozhōutiān, 小周天) (Small Circulation or Microcosmic Meditation), Grand Cyclic Heaven Meditation (Dàzhōutiān, 大周天) (Grand Circulation or Macrocosmic Meditation), and Divine Enlightenment Meditation (Xiāndào Wùzhēn Jìngzuò, 仙道悟真靜坐).

Let us first discuss the three common Qì paths in spiritual Qìgōng meditation practice (Figure 1–35). From this discussion, it will be easier for you to grasp the definitions of Small Circulation, Grand Circulation, and Enlightenment Meditation. Naturally, each of these three paths has its own training theory, purposes, and methods.

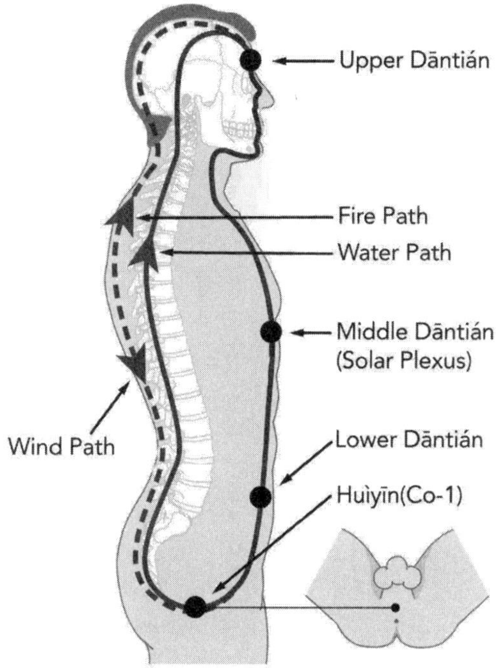

Figure 1-35. The Fire, Water and Wind Paths of Qì Circulation

1.8.1 Three Meditation Paths (Jìngzuò Sānlùjìng, 靜坐三路徑)

FIRE PATH (SMALL CIRCULATION MEDITATION) (XIǍOZHŌUTIĀN, 小周天)

This Fire Path is also commonly known as Small Cyclic Heaven or Small Circulation Meditation. In Fire Path circulation, you first build up an abundance of Qì in your Real Lower Dāntián (Zhēn Xiàdāntián, 真下丹田) through Abdominal Breathing. Then you use your mind to lead the Qì down to the Huìyīn (Co-1) (會陰) following the natural Qì circulation of the Conception Vessel (Rènmài, 任脈) and then upward along your back by following the natural Qì circulation of the Governing Vessel (Dūmài, 督脈). Finally, lead the Qì down the Conception Vessel to complete the cycle.

The purposes of this meditation are to bring the Qì in these two reservoirs up to a higher level, and to improve the flow of the Qì circulation. When the Qì is able to circulate in these two vessels smoothly and strongly, then the Twelve Primary Qì Channels (Jīng, 經) can be regulated efficiently. This can therefore strengthen your physical body and enhance your Guardian Qì (Wèiqì, 衛氣). However, it also energizes your physical body and makes it more Yáng. This is because the Fire Path is the natural Qì circulation path. When you use your mind to lead the Qì to circulate in this natural path, you are enhancing the Qì circulation. From this, you can see that the Fire Path meditation is Lí (離) (fire), which generates the vital force and fire in the body. We will discuss this subject in the next book: Qigong *Meditation Small Circulation*.

WATER PATH (ENLIGHTENMENT MEDITATION) (XIĀNDÀO WÙZHĒN JÌNGZUÒ, 仙道悟真靜坐)

To those meditatiors whose goal is enlightenment or Buddhahood, this Water Path is recognized as a core of the practice. Though this path is also considered one of the Grand Circulation practices, it is far deeper than many other Grand Circulation practices. To help you grasp it better, I will summarize those common Grand Circulation practices later in this section.

The Water Path is the hardest but most effective method of Kǎn (坎) (water) to neutralize the body's Yáng. This is the method of Marrow/Brain Washing Qìgōng (Xǐsuǐjīng, 洗髓經), and focuses the training on the "Central Energy Line." This line is known as the Thrusting Vessel (Chōngmài, 衝脈) (i.e., the spinal cord). In Water Path training, Qì is led by the mind from the Real Lower Dāntián directly upward through the Thrusting Vessel to nourish the brain. When the brain is nourished to a higher level, the Shén can also be raised to a higher level for enlightenment. From this, you can see that the Water Path makes you calm physically and mentally, and leads the Qì inward to the center of the body (marrow), as well as to the brain for nourishment. Since the bone marrow is the factory of white and red blood cells, when the Qì is abundant in the marrow, the production of blood cells is normal and healthy. Red blood cells are the carriers of the oxygen and nutrients required for cellular metabolism. When cellular replacement is smoothly carried out, the degeneration process of your physical body will slow down. Therefore, Marrow Washing Qìgōng is the key to longevity. In addition, when the white blood cells are abundant and healthy, the immune system is strong. Water Path Qìgōng meditation is for enlightenment or Buddhahood. We will discuss this subject in the book *Qigōng—Grand Circulation for Spiritual Enlightenment*.

WIND PATH (KǍN-LÍ MEDITATION) (KǍN-LÍ JÌNGZUÒ, 坎離靜坐)

This Wind Path is considered a reversed Small Circulation. In the Wind path, the Water Qì accumulated in the Real Lower Dāntián is led by the mind to circulate in the path which exactly reverses the Fire Path Qì circulation. There are many reasons for this Wind Path Qì circulation. First, by reversing direction you are moving against the natural Qì circulation, slowing it down. This can cool down your over-excited mental and physical body. Second, through the Wind Path you can lead the Water Qì from the Real Lower Dāntián upward to cool down the Fire Qì accumulated in the Middle Dāntián (Zhōngdāntián, 中丹田) (diaphragm). In this way, the mental and physical body can also be cooled down. This process is commonly called "Kǎn-Lí" (坎離). However, to Enlightenment Meditation practitioners, there is another meaning. The Wind Path is crucial for them to conceive a Spiritual Embryo (Língtāi, 靈胎) at the Huángtíng (黃庭) cavity (located between the Middle Dāntián and Real Lower Dāntián). As mentioned earlier, in this practice the Water Qì is led up the Wind Path from the Real Lower Dāntián, the Fire Qì is led downward from the Middle Dāntián, and the two meet at the Huángtíng. This process is also called "Kǎn-Lí" which causes the interaction of the Yīn and Yáng. From this Yīn-Yáng interaction, with the focused attention of the Shén, a new Spiritual Embryo can be produced.

1.8.2 What is Grand Circulation? (Héwèi Dàzhōutiān?, 何謂大周天？)

The original meaning of "Grand Circulation" implies the natural Qì circulation between the heavens and the earth. Later, this concept was adapted for meditation and became Grand Circulation meditation. This is because the head is considered "heaven" while the abdominal area is considered "earth." Huìyīn (Co-1) (會陰) (Perineum) is considered as "sea bottom" (Hǎidǐ, 海底). Like Small Circulation, as long as you are alive, Grand Qì Circulation always exists. The purpose of Grand Circulation meditation is to enhance the Qì circulation for different reasons. Next, we will discuss the different general concepts of Grand Circulation. A detailed theory and methods of practice will be discussed in the book *Qigōng—Grand Circulation for Spiritual Enlightenment*.

Self Grand Circulation Meditation (Zìwǒ Dàzhōutiān Jìngzuò, 自我大周天靜坐)

The main purpose of Self Grand Circulation meditation is learning how to use the mind to transport the Qì to any place of the body. Naturally, first you must build up a sensitive feeling for the entire body, from the surface to deep inside. If you are not able to feel the body, how would you able to lead Qì there? Therefore, the deeper the state your meditative mind is able to reach, the more profound the achievements you can aspire to.

Once you are able to feel the body precisely and clearly, you can lead the Qì to the tiniest place in the body for self-healing. If your Qì is strong, you may also use your Qì to heal or nourish other people. This kind of healing is commonly called "Qì Massage" (Qìànmó, 氣按摩) or "External Qì Healing" (Wàiqì Liáofǎ, 外氣療法). To Chinese martial artists, the purpose of Grand Circulation meditation is learning how to lead the Qì to energize the body to a stage of high efficiency. Consequently, the Shén can be raised to a higher state of alertness and the power manifested can reach its maximum.

Next, we will briefly explain some of the common Self Grand Circulation meditation practices.

A. **Self Primary Qì Channel Circulation Meditation** (Zìwǒ Shíèrjīng Dàzhōutiān Jìngzuò, 自我十二經大周天靜坐)
The main purpose of this Grand Circulation is to enhance the Qì circulation in the twelve primary Qì channels. When this happens, the twelve internal organs become stronger and healthier. Not only that, the Qì distribution to the arms and legs is increased, making the physical body stronger as well.

B. **Joint Grand Circulation Meditation** (Guānjié Dàzhōutiān Jìngzuò, 關節大周天靜坐)
The purpose of the Joint Grand Circulation Meditation is learning how to use the mind, coordinated with the breathing, to lead the Qì to circulate between the joints. This includes the circulation in the primary channels and in the bone marrow. If you are able to do so, you can transport the Qì from one section of your body to another as you wish. Naturally, you will also be able to lead the Qì to the bone marrow for nourishment (marrow washing).

C. **Four Gates Breathing Circulation** (Sìxīn Hūxī Dàzhōutiān Jìngzuò, 四心呼吸大周天靜坐)
As explained earlier, Four Gates Breathing is one of the Grand Circulations in Qìgōng practice. The purpose of Four Gates Breathing Circulation is learning how to use the mind, coordinated with the breathing, to lead the Qì from the Real Lower Dāntián to the Four Gates: two "Láogōng" (P-8) (勞宮) (Labor Palace) and two "Yǒngquán" (K-1) (湧泉) (Bubbling Well). This breathing technique can be effectively practiced through still meditation.
From Chinese medicine, it is understood that these four cavities are the main gates which regulate the Qì level of the heart and the kidneys. When Qì can be led to these four gates strongly and smoothly, not only will the body be healthy, but the power generated from the limbs will also be stronger. For this reason, Four Gates Meditation has become one of the crucial practices in Chinese martial arts, especially the internal arts. Four Gates Breathing practices have been discussed in the books: *The Essence of Tàijí Qìgōng*, *Qìgōng—The Secret of Youth*, and The Essence of Shàolín White Crane, published by YMAA Publication Center.

D. **Skin/Marrow Breathing Circulation** (Fū/Suǐxí Dàzhōutiān Jìngzuò, 膚髓息大周天靜坐)
The purpose of Skin/Marrow Breathing Circulation is to expand the abundant Qì to the surface of the skin, to enhance and expand your "Guardian Qì" (Wèiqì, 衛氣), and to strengthen the storage of "Marrow Qì" (Suǐqì, 髓氣) by condensing your extra Qì into the bone marrow. When the Guardian Qì

is strong, your immune system will function efficiently, and you will not get sick easily. When the Marrow Qì is strong, the function of the bone marrow in blood cell production will be normal and healthy, slowing the aging process. If you are interested in this subject, please refer to the book: *Qìgōng—The Secret of Youth*, published by YMAA Publication Center.

Grand Circulation Meditation with a Partner (Shuāngxiū Dàzhōutiān Jìngzuò, 雙修大周天靜坐)

If you are able to store the Qì abundantly in your Real Lower Dāntián, and are also capable of using your mind to lead the Qì circulation strongly in your body, then you may use your Qì to nourish or heal other people. In addition this practice allows two healthy persons to nourish each other and raise the Shén of training significantly. In Daoist Qìgōng practice, this Qì-exchange practice is called "Dual Cultivation" (Shuāngxiū, 雙修). To many Daoists, Dual Cultivation practice is one of the most effective ways to speed up the process of spiritual enlightenment. To Qìgōng healers, Dual Cultivation is the best way of cultivating the Qì mutually, and the most efficient way of training Qì exchange with another person. In fact, Dual Cultivation is the foundation of Qì healing.

There are many methods of Dual Cultivation Qì exchange practice, ranging from basic Palm Qì exchange to a deep and profound Central Qì exchange. We will discuss this subject in more detail in the book: *Qigōng—Grand Circulation for Spiritual Enlightenment*.

Grand Circulation Meditation with Great Nature (Tiānrén Héyī Dàzhōutiān Jìngzuò, 天人合一大周天靜坐)

A. **Grand Circulation Meditation with the Earth** (Dìrén Dàzhōutiān Jìngzuò, 地人大周天靜坐)

The main purpose of this practice is to extend your Qì beyond your body and exchange Qì with the surrounding natural objects such as the earth, trees, animals, or even the air. It is believed that all natural objects, and especially living things, also have Qì. If you know how, you can use them to regulate and harmonize the Qì circulation in your body. It is also possible to absorb Qì from your surroundings and increase your Qì level. In China, trees are the most common objects used for regulating Qì.

The difference between this Qì exchange and Qì exchange with a human partner is that these objects do not have mind, or the mind is weak, and therefore they are not able to use their mind to lead their Qì to handle the exchange with you.

B. **Grand Circulation Meditation with the Heavens** (Tiānrén Dàzhōutiān Jìngzuò, 天人大周天靜坐)

Grand Circulation Meditation with the Heavens is also called the "Fifth Gate" meditation. The purpose of Grand Circulation with Heaven is to try to reach the final spiritual unification between the human and the universe. This is called "Tiānrén Héyī" (天人合一) (unification of heaven and human). In order to reach this stage, you must first learn how to lead the Qì upward along the Thrusting Vessel (Chōngmài, 衝脈) to the brain to nourish and energize it to a higher state. In order to do so, you must learn the Water Path mentioned earlier. When this happens, the Shén will grow and The Third Eye can be reopened. This stage is called "enlightenment" (Wùzhēn, 悟真). Once you have opened The Third Eye, there is no obstacle to communication between your brain and the surrounding energy. Suddenly, you are able to comprehend many things which cannot be understood by others. You are able to communicate with other humans or animals without speaking. Your telepathic capability will return. Through this meditation, you will comprehend the meaning of life and of nature.

1.9 Definition of Embryonic Breathing (Tāixí Zhī Dìngyì, 胎息之定義)

Before you study and practice Embryonic Breathing, you must first know what it is. How is it defined, and how is it related to spiritual cultivation in Qìgōng society? Only then can you have a better understanding of what goal you are aiming for. Without knowing this, the entire practice will be in vain.

According to the available ancient documents, there are two Embryonic Breathings defined. One is to search for the spiritual center and the Qì center, then unite Shén and Qì together at the Lower Dāntián. These two centers are the two poles of a human energy body. After you have located them, then you will bring the Shén (神) (Spirit) down to meet and unite with the Qì at the Qì center (Real Lower Dāntián) (Figure 1–36). Thus you have returned to the Wújí state of life (the origin of life). Since this place (Real Lower Dāntián or Center of Gravity) is the place where the fetus is conceived, you are searching for the beginning formation of your fetus life. Once you have returned to this Wújí state, you have returned your being to nature.

The earliest document in which the concept of this Embryonic Breathing was propounded is Lǎozi's *Dào Dé Jīng* (*Classic on the Virtue of the Dào*) (老子・道德經). In Chapter 16 of the *Dào Dé Jīng*, it says: "Approaching the nihility (nothingness or emptiness) to its extremity and maintaining the calmness with sincerity. Millions of objects (lives) are in actions which allow me to observe their cyclic repetitions. Though there are so many objects, each individual must repeatedly return to its root (origin). When it returns to the root, it means 'calmness.' When it is calmed, then it means 'repetition of a life.' When the life repeats, it means 'constant natural routine.'"[26] From this document, we can see that the purpose of this kind of Embryonic Breathing is to trace back the root of our lives and to observe and understand the cyclic repetition of nature. That means to return our spiritual being to the Wújí state (無極) (No Extremity or neutral state) of human life, and thus be able to reach the origin of our human spiritual nature.

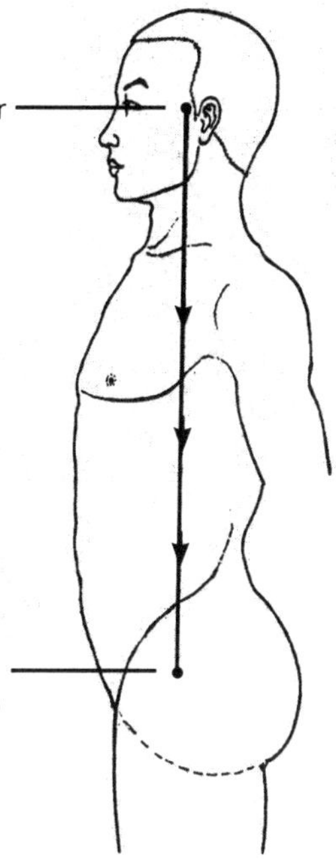

Figure 1-36. Unification of Shén and Qì at the Wújí Center

Therefore, the first step in reaching this Embryonic Breathing is to regulate the Shén, through the cultivation of the mind, to its empty (neutral) state. When this happens, the Shén will be able to find its center and stay at its residence. Without reaching this neutral spiritual state, we will remain locked in the human emotional matrix. Consequently, our mind will not be clear and calm enough to see through to the root of our spiritual nature. In addition, without this calm and peaceful mind, we will not be able to lead the Qì to its residence (Real Lower Dāntián) and preserve it there. From this, you can see that the very beginning of Embryonic Breathing is the search for the spiritual origin in the center of the brain (Upper Dāntián), as well as the Qì origin located at the center of physical gravity (Real Lower Dāntián).

In reference to regulating the Shén, it is said in Chapter 6 of Dào Dé Jīng: "The Valley Spirit (Gǔshén, 谷神) does not die, then it is called 'Xuánpìn' (玄牝). The door (key) of reaching this 'Xuánpìn' is the root of heaven and earth (nature). It is very soft and continuous as if it exists. When it is used, it will not be exhausted."[27] Shén is called "Valley Spirit" (Gǔshén, 谷神) because it resides in the "Spiritual Valley" (Shéngǔ, 神谷) (The space between the two hemispheres of the brain). "Xuánpìn" (玄牝) means "the marvellous and mysterious Dào, the mother of creation of millions of objects." That means the goal of regulating the Shén is to keep it at the Spiritual Valley, the Shén residence.

Once you have firmed and condensed your Shén to a high level, you lead this Shén down to meet and unite with the Qì at the Real Lower Dāntián, the very origin of your life, so you can return your being to its origin. In order to reach this final goal, besides firming the Shén at the "Spiritual Valley," you must also know how to find the root of the Qì (bio-battery) so you can conserve it. In addition, in order to attain longevity and reach the goal of spiritual enlightenment, you must also learn to increase the quantity of Qì stored at the Qì residence (Real Lower Dāntián or Second Brain).

This means breathing softly, slenderly, and deeply like a newborn baby. That is why it is said in Chapter 10 of Dào Dé Jīng that: "When bearing and managing the Pò (魄) (Vital Spirit) and embracing (maintaining) it to a state of singularity (singleness) (Bàoyī, 抱一), can it be not separated (from its residence)? When concentrating the Qì to reach its softness, can it be as (soft as) a baby? When cleansing thought to reach its purity, can it be flawless?"[28] The Daoist document Língjiànzi's Dàoyīn Zǐ-Wǔ Recording (Língjiànzi Dǎoyǐn Zǐwǔ Jìzhù, 靈劍子導引子午記注) said: "What is Embryonic Breathing? It is a method of Embracing Singularity (Bàoyī, 抱一) (Wújí center) and keeping it in the neutral state."[29]

We can summarize that Embryonic Breathing means to regulate the mind and Shén to their calm and concentrated state, to preserve and regulate the Qì at the Lower Dāntián to an abundant level, and then to unite the Shén and Qì so as to return the being to its origin. Embryonic Breathing has always been a huge subject in Chinese Qìgōng practice, because it is the breathing method which allows you to store Qì in the Real Lower Dāntián. In other words, through Embryonic Breathing, you are able to charge your bio-battery to a high level. Then your vital energy will be raised, the immune system will be strengthened, and the physical body can be reconditioned. However, to Buddhists and Daoists, the final goal and most important part of Embryonic Breathing is the achievement of enlightenment or Buddhahood.

According to Buddhist and Daoist documents, the definition of Embryonic Breathing is to conceive a Spiritual Embryo (Shéntāi, 神胎) at the Huángtíng (黃庭) cavity. Once this Spiritual Embryo has matured, it is led up to the Upper Dāntián for its birth (i.e., the reopening of the Third Eye). In order to reach this goal, you must first build up an abundance of Water Qì (Shuǐqì, 水氣) (Original Qì) at the Real Lower Dāntián. You will then lead this Qì upward, also leading the Fire Qì (Huǒqì, 火氣) (Post-Heaven Qì) downward from the Middle Dāntián, and the two meet at the Huángtíng (黃庭) cavity. This process is called "intercourse of dragon and tiger" (Lónghǔ Jiāogòu, 龍虎交媾) which means "the interaction of Yīn and Yáng," commonly called "Kǎn-Lí" (坎離). This will result in the conception of life. Then, you will lead the Shén downward to meet this life (Qì). This process is called "Mutual Dependence of Mother and Son" (Mǔzǐ Xiāngyī, 母子相依) ("Mother" refers to the Qì, and "Son" to the Shén). Once this happens, a new Shén can develop on this conceived embryo (Figure 1–37).

When this Spiritual Embryo has matured, it will be led upward through Chōngmài (衝脈) (spinal cord) to nourish the brain. When the energy has reached a high level, the "Heaven Eye" (Tiānyǎn, 天眼) (Third Eye) can be reopened.

1.10 Embryonic Breathing and Cultivation of Dào (Tāixí Yǔ Xiūdào, 胎息與修道)

In this section, I would like to put into two charts what I have come to understand about the relationship between Embryonic Breathing and spiritual cultivation. Almost all of the concepts are compiled and concluded from the ancient documents translated and commented upon in Chapter 3. Therefore, if you do not understand these two charts after you have read and pondered them, do not be disappointed. They are placed here to summarize the entire concept of spiritual cultivation relations and procedures. After you have read through the entire book, I highly recommend you refer back to these charts. When the time is right, you will see that everything has come to make logical sense.

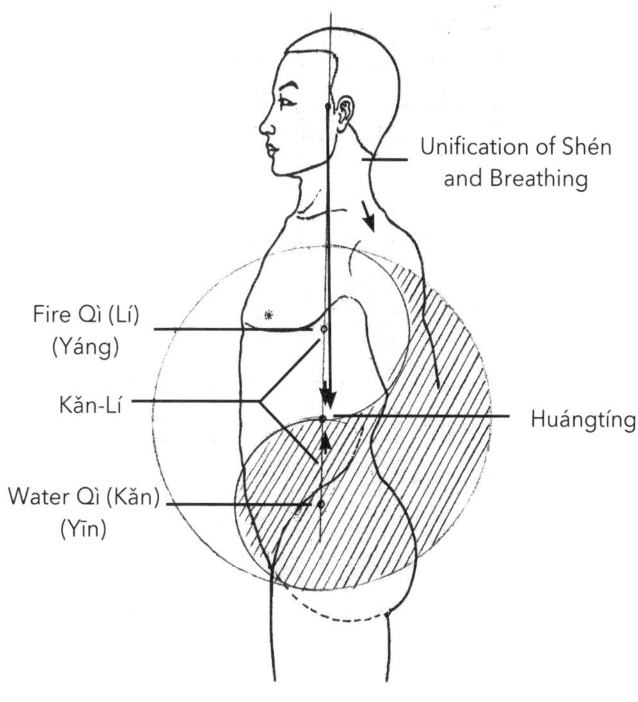

Figure 1-37. Conceiving the Spiritual Embryo

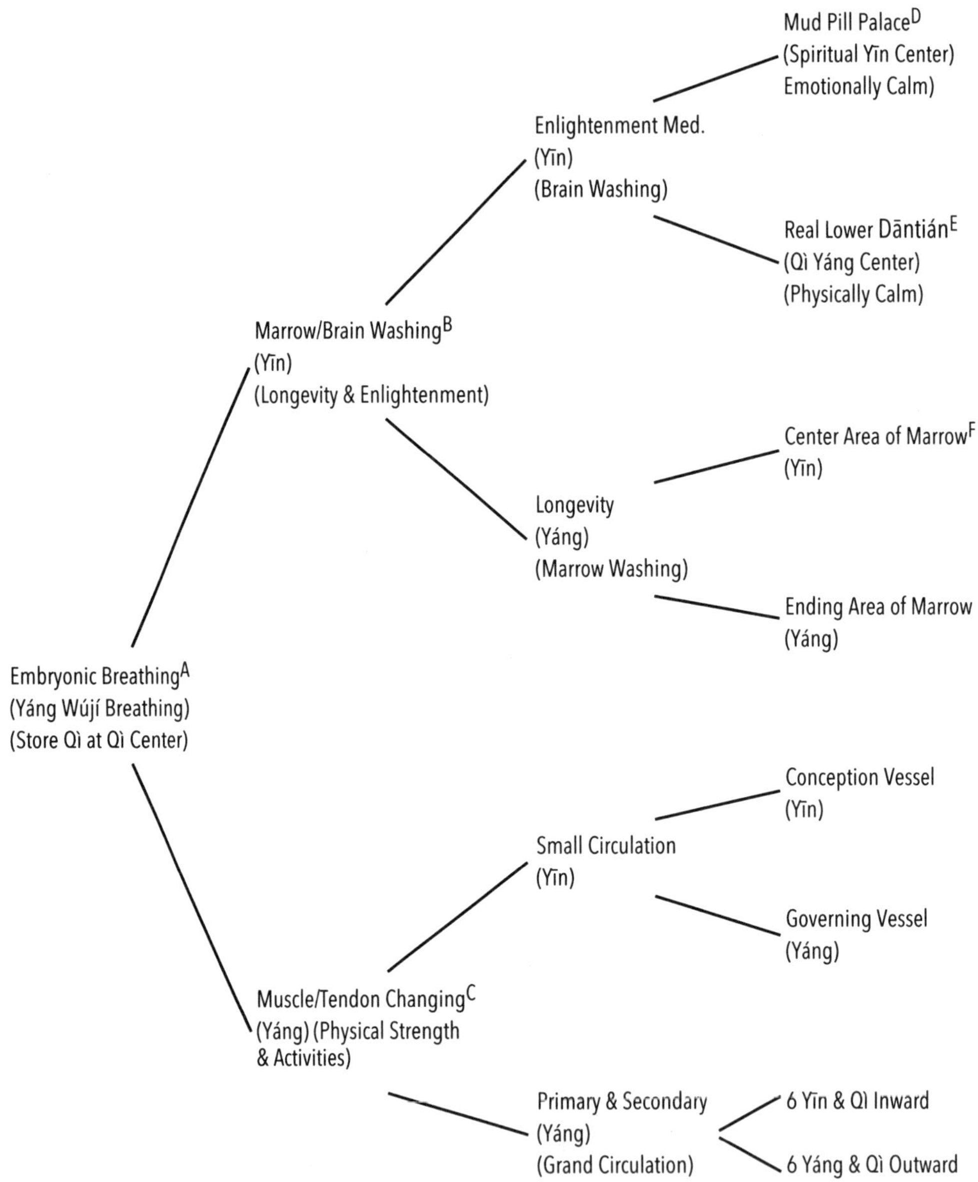
Embryonic Breathing[A]
(Yáng Wújí Breathing)
(Store Qì at Qì Center)
Marrow/Brain Washing[B]
(Yīn)
(Longevity & Enlightenment)
Enlightenment Med.
(Yīn)
(Brain Washing)
Mud Pill Palace[D]
(Spiritual Yīn Center)
Emotionally Calm)
Real Lower Dāntián[E]
(Qì Yáng Center)
(Physically Calm)
Longevity
(Yáng)
(Marrow Washing)
Center Area of Marrow[F]
(Yīn)
Ending Area of Marrow
(Yáng)
Muscle/Tendon Changing[C]
(Yáng) (Physical Strength
& Activities)
Small Circulation
(Yīn)
Conception Vessel
(Yīn)
Governing Vessel
(Yáng)
Primary & Secondary
(Yáng)
(Grand Circulation)
6 Yīn & Qì Inward
6 Yáng & Qì Outward

Table 1-2. Yáng Physical Cultivation Chart

A. Through Embryonic Breathing, the Qì is stored at the Real Lower Dāntián to an abundant level. Since this Qì storage is used to manifest physical life and Shén, it is considered Yáng. That is why it is called "Yáng Wújí Center." The way to reach this goal is to bring the concentrated Shén downward to the Real Lower Dāntián so the mind can stay there. This is called the "harmonization of the Shén and the Qì" (Shénqì Xiànghé, 神氣相合). When this happens, the mind is calm, the Shén is condensed, and the Qì is stored. When the Qì is stored to an abundant level, it can be used to wash the marrow/brain (Yīn) and also to condition the physical body (Yáng).

B. Through Marrow/Brain Washing, spiritual enlightenment can be achieved (Yīn), as well as longevity (Yáng). When the Qì is led upward through the spinal cord (Chōngmài, 衝脈) to the brain, the brain Qì status can reach a higher level. Consequently, the sensitivity to spiritual vibration (i.e., spiritual resonant energy) will be enhanced. In addition, when the Qì is led inward to the bone marrow (i.e., blood cell factory), longevity can be attained.

C. Through Muscle/Tendon Changing, physical health and strength can be improved. This includes the practice of Small Circulation (Xiǎozhōutiān, 小周天) through circulation of Conception and Governing Vessels (Renmài, Dūmài; 任脈・督脈) (Yīn). The Qì can be led to the Twelve Primary Qì Channels (Shíèrjīng, 十二經) to nourish the internal organs, and also to countless Secondary Qì Channels (Luò, 絡) (Yáng) (Grand Circulation) for nourishing skin (Yáng) (Qì outward) and marrow (Yīn) (Qì inward). Remember, when the Qì is led outward from the primary Qì channels to the skin, the Guardian Qì (Wèiqì, 衛氣) (immune system) will be enhanced. When the Qì is led inward from the primary Qì channels to the bone marrow (Suǐqì, 髓氣), production of blood cells is enhanced.

D. The Mud Pill Palace (Níwángōng, 泥丸宮) located at the center of the Spiritual Valley (Shéngǔ, 神谷) (i.e., site of pineal and pituitary glands) is the spiritual Yīn center and the residence of the Shén. When the Shén is kept here, it can be focused and the mind can be calm and concentrated. When the Shén is led away from this center, then Qì will be manifested and Shén turns into Yáng. Please refer to Chapter 2 for more discussion.

E. The Real Lower Dāntián is the Qì Yáng center where the Qì is produced and stored. It is understood that through the absorption of food essence and exercises of the abdominal area, Qì can be produced in the body. When the Qì is kept at this center, it is not led out and manifested. Therefore, the physical body can be relaxed.

F. In a piece of long bone, the center of the bone marrow area is considered Yīn while the ending of the bone marrow area is considered Yáng. Normally, due to the manifestation of Qì at the ends of the bone (joint areas), the Qì is depleted faster and marrow degenerates here first. However, from the point of view of physical manifestation, the centers of bones and muscles are Yáng, while the ligaments and tendons at the joints are considered Yīn. The electric conductivities of tendons and ligaments are higher than that of the midsection of muscles. In addition, the central area of bone (Yáng) is stronger than that of the ends (Yīn) (Figure 1-38). This can be seen in that the structure of the central area of a long bone is stronger and more compact than that of the ends.

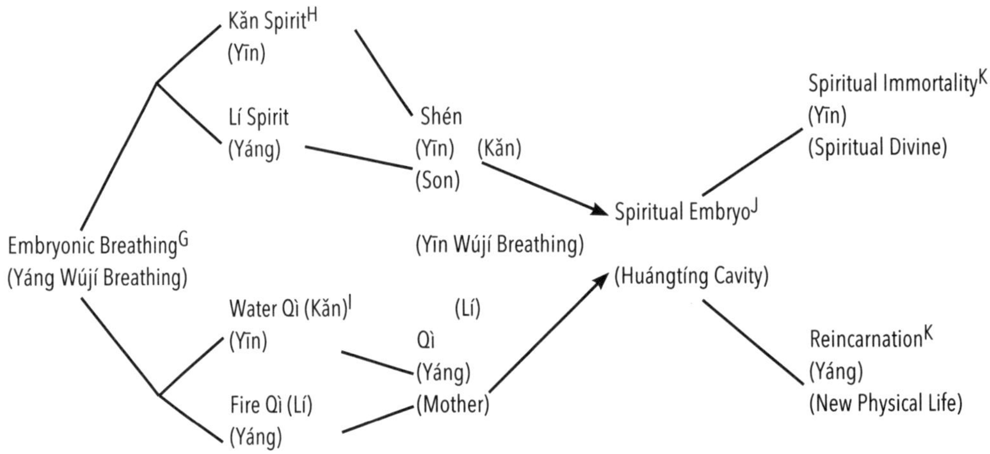

Table 1–3. Yīn Spiritual Cultivation Chart

G. When you have achieved Embryonic Breathing (Yáng Wújí Breathing), your mind is calm, Shén focused, physical body relaxed, and the Qì stays at its residence (Real Lower Dāntián). From this, you have returned to the beginning of life.

H. In order to conceive your Spiritual Embryo, you must first cultivate and harmonize your Yángshén and Yīnshén. If you have too much Yīnshén (Kǎn, 坎), though your Shén is condensed, your physical manifestation of life will be weak, and mentally you will be depressed. However, with too much Yángshén (Lí, 離), though your physical life will be strong due to strong Qì manifestation, your mind will be scattered, excited, and emotionally disturbed. The key to raising the Shén while maintaining control is to keep the Shén strong, yet focused. That means both Yīnshén and Yángshén must harmonize with and balance each other.

I. In addition, in order to conceive a Spiritual Embryo, you must also have an abundant Qì storage. To conceive a new spiritual life, you need to let the Water Qì (Shuǐqì, 水氣) from the Real Lower Dāntián interact with the Fire Qì (Huǒqì, 火氣) from the Middle Dāntián. Water Qì is also called "Original Qì" (Yuánqì, 元氣), or "Pre-Heaven Qì" (Xiāntiānqì, 先天氣). Fire Qì is also called "Post-Heaven Qì" (Hòutiānqì, 後天氣). When you move the Fire Qì downward and Water Qì upward, uniting them at the Huángtíng cavity (黃庭) (inner area behind navel), it is called "Kǎn and Lí" (坎離) or "Small Tripod and Furnace" (Xiǎodǐnglú, 小鼎爐). Huángtíng is a tripod while the Real Lower Dāntián is a furnace (Figure 1–39).

J. The final stage of conceiving a Spiritual Embryo at the Huángtíng cavity is to unite the Shén in the head with the Qì at the Huángtíng. In order to do so, you must move your Shén downward from your Upper Dāntián. This process is again called Kǎn (坎) (water) and Lí (離) (fire). Kǎn means the Shén (son) at your Upper Dāntián while the Lí is the Qì (mother) at the Huángtíng. This process is also called "Large Tripod and Furnace" (Dàdǐnglú, 大鼎爐) (Figure 1–40).

K. Once the Spiritual Embryo is conceived, you will need nine months of pregnancy. This Spiritual Embryo is then led upward to be born through the Heaven Eye (Tiānyǎn, 天眼) (the Third Eye). Once the spiritual baby is born, you will then need three years of nursing, followed by nine years of facing the wall (spiritual independence training). Once the Shén has gained its independence, you will have an eternal spiritual life. This spiritual life can either remain in a spiritual form or re-enter into a physical life through reincarnation.

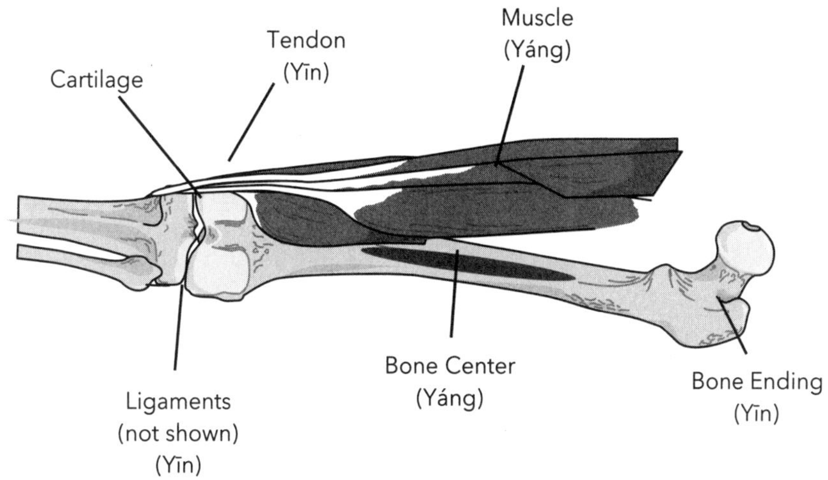

Figure 1-38. The Yin and Yang Status of a Section of Limb

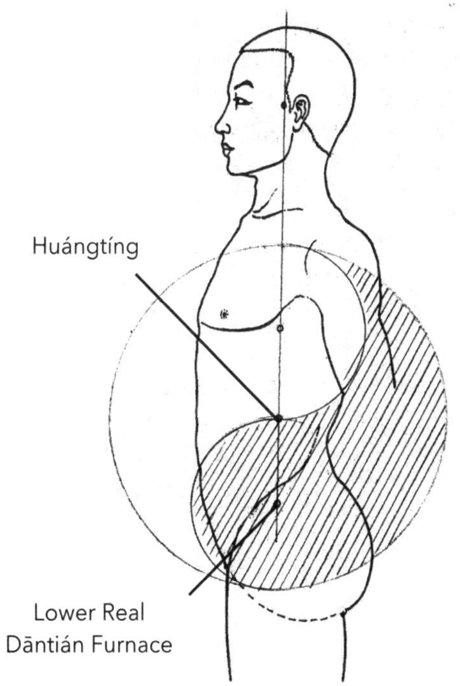

Figure 1-39. Small Tripod and Furnace

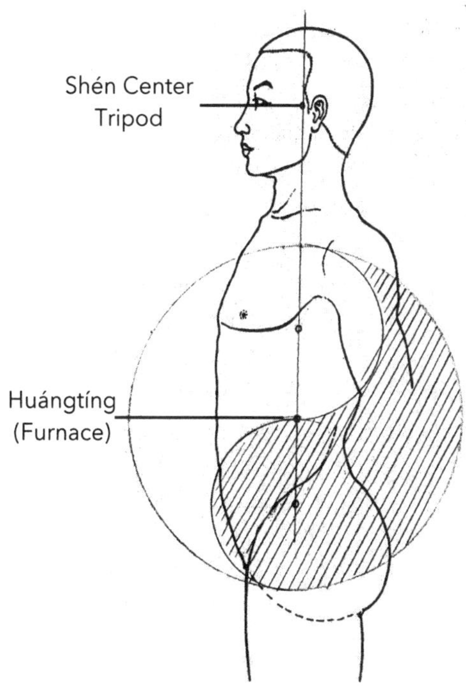

Figure 1-40. Large Tripod and Furnace

1.11 About This Book (Guānyú Zhèběnshū, 關於這本書)

Qìgōng science and knowledge is like exploring a huge garden which contains everything in Nature, on both the material and spiritual planes. Since we have never had a detailed map of this garden, we have been left to wonder about ourselves and about Nature. In the past, each Qìgōng master, through a lifetime of pondering and experience, has discovered some of the passages which could lead us to a new understanding of this spiritual garden. Gradually, many mysterious and hidden places were discovered which manifest the truth and the beauty of Nature. These masters passed down their understanding and experience, either through teaching students or through writing. Though each one of these writings may provide only a little clue about reaching a tiny area of the garden, it took a Qìgōng master's lifetime to obtain this information. Each piece of passed-down information is a road sign, marking a way which could possibly lead to our goal—the true face of this garden. When much of this knowledge is combined, we can obtain a map of this Qìgōng garden. By studying the map and pondering the structure of nature, we can arrive at a theory which might take us to parts of the Qìgōng garden where nobody has gone before. It will probably take humans many thousands of years of effort to obtain a detailed map of this garden.

However, what we have accomplished so far is only limited information about the material side of nature, while very little is known about the spiritual aspect. For this reason we are still confused about the meaning of our life and of Nature. Naturally, we are still very far away from a full understanding of Nature.

In order to improve ourselves both materially and spiritually, we need an open mind which can allow us to set ourselves free from the traditional brainwashing and bondage (matrix). Therefore, we should be unafraid to face the challenge, and willing to accept the truth and the mistakes we have already made. Only then, will we be able to create our dream of the future correctly.

Once we have created this correct attitude, then we can think with an open mind. Even though nobody is able to prove it, we should dare to make an assumption and formalize a possible theory and explanation (i.e., hypothesis). Naturally, most of this is generated from the imaginary mind. From this assumed theory, we will then try to prove it. If the result has been proven wrong, then we go back to modify the theory and try again. This is no different from Einstein or any other great physicists who assume their theory first and later their followers try to prove it. The attitude of study and research is to dare to dream, dare to accept the challenge, and dare to accept the facts.

When you read this book, if you have a different cultural and intellectual background, you must keep reminding yourself to keep your mind open. If you are interested in cultivating your mind and Shén, this book is a necessary book that can provide you with a solid foundation for the ultimate goal of spiritual enlightenment cultivation.

When you read this book, you will see that many explanations originate from my personal understanding and are based on my scientific background. I cannot guarantee what I have assumed about the theory in the explanation is completely correct. However, through these theories and assumptions, I am able to offer you a possible logical and scientific explanation for the experience of the past. It is quite possible that, once humans have understood this subject better, someone may step in to modify or even completely change my theory. That is the natural course and attitude of scientific study. After the assumed theory has been tested repeatedly, we can confirm what is correct and what is wrong. When the theory is proven correct, the map will become clear. From the correct guidance of the map, we can create and advance further.

Next, you should understand that all of the theory and methods of practice introduced in this book originated only from the study of Chinese sources. If you are wise, you should also keep your mind open and study the same subject from other different cultures. Only then will you have a different angle of viewing the same topic which could lead you to a clear and wise judgment. This is especially true for spiritual cultivation. We are still at the beginning stage of understanding this subject. Any source or past experience could offer you a piece of more information and direct you to a better path of reaching the goal. Therefore, this book is not an authority on this subject. This book can only offer you one angle of viewing this subject.

You should always remember that even though we cannot prove the existence of the spirit in this universe with today's infant science, it does not mean it does not exist. We should keep our minds open and continue our pondering and research. Only then will we be able to untie the knot and open the gate of spiritual science which has been experienced by humans in all different cultures in the past.

Once you have understood the theory and the practice of this book, you should then learn how to adopt it into your thinking and living. Only then will you be able to reunite the feeling originated from both material and spirit.

In the second chapter of Part I, I will offer you a possible scientific theoretical foundation of Embryonic Breathing. When you read this chapter, you should always remember that the theoretical foundation in this practice is just like a map which could lead you to the final goal. Therefore, you should study this map and understand it clearly. If you rush into the practice without first comprehending the theory, you may enter the wrong path and become confused. Next, in Part II, precious related ancient documents will be translated and commented upon. Since Part II is the core of this book, you should always return to it to read and ponder every sentence. Remember that these road signs are the keys to lead you to the correct path of pondering and practice. Finally, the actual training method of Embryonic Breathing will be introduced in Part III.

References

1. "Life's Invisible Current," by Albert L. Huebner, East West Journal, June 1986.
2. 《莊子刻意》：〝吹呴呼吸，吐故納新，熊經鳥伸，為壽而已矣。此導引之士，養形之人，彭祖壽考者之所好也。〞
3. 李時珍《奇經八脈考》：〝蓋正經猶夫溝渠，奇經猶夫湖澤，正經之脈隆盛，則溢于奇經。〞
4. 人生七十古來稀。
5. 一百二十謂之夭。
6. 《達摩大師住世留形內真妙用訣》：〝若不知子母相守，氣雖呼吸於于內，神常勞役于外，遂使神常穢濁而神不清，神既不清，即元和之氣漸散，而不能相守也。〞
7. 《性天風月通玄記．師徒傳道》：〝論性命，要雙修，將鉛汞，兩下投，這消息，難參透，修性即煉己，修命即還丹。心是神之舍，身是氣之宅。命即氣也，修性之人，把身心混作一家，精氣神打成一片。修命之能事備矣。〞
8. 胎指金丹，產金丹喻為懷胎。
9. 薛道光《悟真篇》註：〝嬰兒者，即丹也。丹是一，一是真一之氣，天地之母氣也。以母咽氣歸五內，以伏子氣，猶貓伏鼠而不走也。子母之氣相戀于胞胎之中，結成嬰兒之一。故曰：太一含真氣。言含真一之氣。如人懷胎，十月滿足，然後降生。〞
10. "Complex and Hidden Brain in the Gut Makes Stomachaches and Butterflies," by Sandra Blakeslee, *The New York Times*, Science, January 23, 1996.
11. *The Second Brain: The Scientific Basis of Gut Instinct and a Groundbreaking New Understanding of Nervous Disorders of the Stomach and Intestine*, Michael D. Gershon, New York: Harper Collins Publications, 1998.
12. 王錄識餘云：〝銅人針灸圖，載臟腑一身俞穴有玉環，余不知玉環是何物。〞
13. 張紫陽玉清金華祕文，論神仙結丹處曰：〝心上腎下，脾左肝右，生門在前，密戶居後，其連如環，其白如綿，方圓徑寸，密裹一身之精粹，此即玉環。〞
14. 藥補不如食補，食補不如氣補。
15. 李清菴詩云：〝神氣和合生靈質，心息相依結聖胎。〞
16. 《金丹真傳．溫養》：〝丹成十月聖胎完，自有真人出現。〞
17. 真調為無調而自調。
18. 形不正，則氣不順。氣不順，則意不寧。意不寧，則氣散亂。
19. *A Study of Anatomic Physiology Physiology* (解剖生理學)，李文森編著。華杏出版股份有限公司。Táipěi, 1986.
20. 《莊子．大宗師》：〝古之真人，．．．其息深深。真人之息以踵，眾人之息以喉。〞
21. 《性命圭旨全書．火候》：〝神息者，火候也。〞指文火安神定息，任其自如，謂之神息。即〝不得勤，不得怠者，是皆神息之自然火候之微旨也。〞
22. 《性命圭旨全書．亨集》：〝身不動而心自安，心不動而神自守。〞

23. 《性命圭旨全書・蟄藏氣穴，眾妙歸根》：〝合真人深深之息，則心息相依，息調心靜。〞

24. 《聽心齋客問》：〝心依著事物已久，一旦離境，不能自立。所以用調息功夫，拴系此心，便心息相依。調字亦不是用意，只是一呼一吸系念耳。至心離境，則無人無我，更無息可調，只綿綿若存，久之，自然純熟。〞

25. 《道藏・坐忘論》：〝夫心者一身之主，百神之帥，靜則生慧，動則生昏，欣迷動靜之中。〞

26. 《道德經・十六章》：〝致虛極，守靜篤；萬物并作，吾以觀其復。夫物芸芸，各復歸其根。歸根曰靜，靜曰復命。復命曰常。〞

27. 《道德經・六章》：〝谷神不死，是謂玄牝。玄牝之門，是謂天地根，綿綿若存，用之不勤。〞

28. 《道德經・十章》：〝載營魄抱一，能無離乎？專氣致柔，能如嬰兒乎？滌除玄鑒，能無疵乎？〞

29. 胎息者，抱一守中之法也。

CHAPTER 2

Theoretical Foundations of Embryonic Breathing

2.1 INTRODUCTION (JIÈSHÀO, 介紹)

Before discussing the theory of Qìgōng, let us first analyze the Chinese concept of the Dào (道). Dào has been commonly translated as the "Natural Way." How then do we define the "Natural Way?"

First, it is stated in *Yìjīng* (易經) (*Book of Changes*) (1122–1115 BCE) that: "One Yīn and one Yáng is called Dào."[1] From this statement, we can see that the fundamental concept of Dào is the coexistence of Yīn and Yáng aspects of nature. Later, this concept was re-defined by Lǎozi (老子) (604–531 BCE). In his book *Dào Dé Jīng* (*Classic on the Virtue of the Dào*) (道德經), Chapter 42, he stated: "Dào begets one, one produces two, two generates three, and from three derive millions of objects."[2] From this, you can see that Dào is the natural cause which creates the first single object from emptiness, and later this object (i.e., Wújí State of No Discrimination) divides into two aspects, and continues to derive into millions of objects and lives.

In addition, in Chapter 25 of *Dào Dé Jīng* (道德經), Lǎozi states: "There is an undiscriminating thing formalized (in the space), (born) before the heaven and the earth (Yáng and Yīn). Extremely quiet and extremely few, existing alone and without change, repeat with cycle without end, it is able to be the mother of heaven and earth. I do not know its name and forceful wording as Dào."[3] This explains that Dào existed even before the heavens and the earth were discriminated. The Dào exists quietly and alone, and does not change its original virtue. When the Dào caused the Wújí (無極) (No Extremity or No Discrimination) to derive into Yīn and Yáng, the pattern of opposing forces or aspects (polarities) came into existence and the natural cycles formalized. This derivation from Wújí into Yīn and Yáng is the origin of millions of things and therefore, is the mother of lives.

Lǎozi held the Dào responsible for the creation of all life. Therefore, he said Dào is: "the most mysterious of the mysterious, and is the door (origin) of all marvelousness" (Chapter 1).[4] Also: "When the Dào is born, natural virtues are raised, objects are formalized, and the natural state will be completed" (Chapter 51).[5] This implies that millions of variations of nature are derived from the Dào. Once this natural pattern is completed, then the natural cycles are established and repeated. Therefore, in order for humans to fit into this nature, Lǎozi believes: "Human copies the earth, the earth patterns the heaven, the heaven models after the Dào, the Dào follows the natural" (Chapter 25)[6] This passage explains that it does not matter how big (such as heaven) or how small (such as an insect), all follow the same energy pattern and the same Dào. Dào follows nature.

From these statements, we can conclude that Dào is the major force in nature, which creates from nothing a single object, and from this single object, divides into Yīn and Yáng. When Yīn and Yáng interact with each other harmoniously, millions of lives are created and derived. It is said in Huáinánzi (淮南子): "Dào begins from one, one does not beget, therefore dividing into Yīn and Yáng. When Yīn and Yáng harmonize with each other, the millions of objects are born."[7]

In addition, Lǎozi points out that the variation from Wújí to Yīn and Yáng can also be reversed. That means Wújí can derive into Yīn and Yáng Two Poles, and the Yīn and Yáng Two Poles can be united and become Wújí. This implies that the influence of the Dào is not one way only. Lǎozi said in Chapter 1 of *Dào Dé Jīng* (道德經): "Nothing, is the beginning of the Pre-Heaven (Wújí state); having, is the mother of millions of objects (Yīn and Yáng). Always keep nothingness, so to observe the marvelousness (of nature). Always having, so observe the returning (recycling or ending) of millions of objects." [8] This means the Dào goes from nothing to something, and also from something to nothing, always changing from one to the other. Dào is the natural force which makes all of these occurrences. That is why the Dào was later re-defined as: "the oppositional consistent rules which divide the object of matter from one into two and re-unify the objects from two to one."[9] If we trace back the oldest Chinese philosophy related to the development of nature, especially human nature, *Yìjīng* (易經) (*Book of Changes*; 1122–1115 BCE) can be said to be the first book that offers a detailed and clear discussion. It was from this book that the Dào of nature (natural way) was followed by Chinese people.

From *Yìjīng*, it is said:

> *Yì Great Biography said: "Ancient person, Bāoxī, was a king of the heaven and the earth. Look up to observe (different) phases (variations) of heaven, and look down to inspect the rules (patterns) of the earth. Behold the behavior of birds and animals (living styles) and its relationship with the earth. Close, use own body (to experiment) and far, adopt the phenomenon of the object's (variations). Then, begin to create Bāguà (trigram) which is used to transport (understand) the virtue of the (natural) spirit and the divine, and also to classify the behaviors of the millions of objects."*

易大傳曰："古者包義氏之王天下也。仰則觀象於天，俯則觀法於地。觀鳥獸之文，與地之宜。近取諸身，遠取諸物。於是始作八卦，以通神明之德，以類萬物之情。"

Bāoxī (包義) (2852–2737 BCE) was the ruler of China. The heaven and the earth means the kingdom. According to *Yìjīng*, after Bāoxī carefully observed the natural cyclic patterns and the behaviors of natural lives (both plants and animals), he created the Eight Trigrams (Bāguà, 八卦) which can be used to interpret and to trace the patterns of nature. Since then, the theory of trigrams has significantly influenced Chinese culture.

From these statements, we can see that *Yìjīng* was written based on the understanding of nature by observing its routine cycles. From this, the Yīn and Yáng theory was developed.

Therefore, it is also said in *Yìjīng*:

> *Therefore, Yì (Change) has Tàijí (Grand Ultimate), and thus begets Two Poles (Yīn and Yáng). Two Poles produce Four Phases. Four Phases give rise to Bāguà (Eight Trigrams). Bāguà is able to define good or bad luck (fortune), (from) good or bad luck, the great career (creations of variation of nature) is created.*
>
> 是故易有太極，是生兩儀，兩儀生四象，四象生八卦，八卦定吉凶，吉凶生大業。

From this statement, you can understand that it is because there is a Tàijí (太極) (Grand Ultimate), that there is change. Without Tàijí, there is no change. Through Tàijí, the Two Poles are created from Wújí (無極) (No Extremity) and with the influence of Tàijí, the Two Poles again derive into Four Phases (Sìxiàng, 四象). Again, Four Phases produce the Eight Trigrams (Bāguà, 八卦). From Eight Trigrams, the natural cyclical patterns can be calculated. From this, good or bad fortune can be calculated (predicted). Therefore, in order to be prosperous in your business, you must follow the natural patterns of good luck and avoid those of bad luck. From here, you can see that all of the derivations originate from Tàijí. Therefore, Tàijí is the Dào or the natural force which makes division and unification happen.

In a Daoist classic, *Records of Recent Pondering* (*Jìnsīlù*, 近思錄), it is said:

> *Wújí begets Tàijí, (when) Tàijí moves (initiates an action), the Yáng is born; (when) movement reaches its extremity, again calm; (when) calm, generates the Yīn. (When) calmness reaches its extremity, again moving. One moves and one calm, mutually as the root (origin of generation). Yīn and Yáng are discriminated and the Two Poles are completed.*

無極生太極，太極動而生陽，動極復靜；靜而生陰，靜極復動。一動一靜，互為其根，分陰分陽，兩儀至焉。

It is through the action of this repeated Yīn and Yáng cycle that the millions of lives are begotten. The originating force of this Yīn and Yáng division is called Tàijí. An ancient Daoist classic, *Glossary Talking of Zhūzi* (*Zhūzi Yǔlèi*, 朱子語類), said: "What is called Tàijí, is what is the root of the millions of things in heaven and earth."[10]

Later, Tàijí was again interpreted and clarified by Wáng, Zōng-Yuè (王宗岳) (c. 1750 CE). In *Tàijíquán Classic*, he said:

> *What is Tàijí? It is generated from Wújí and is a pivotal function of movement and stillness. It is the mother of Yīn and Yáng. When it moves (in action), it divides. At rest it reunites.*
>
> 太極者，無極而生，動靜之機，陰陽之母也。動之則分，靜之則合。

From this statement, you can see that Tàijí is neither Wújí nor Yīn and Yáng, but the natural force or Dào which makes the divisions and unifications happen (Figure 2–1). It is the cause and origin of all life's creation and death. It is the way of the natural cycle.

From the above, we can see that the origin of Chinese culture was based on the philosophy of Tàijí and Yīn-Yáng theory. This has therefore become the traditional empirical foundation for the development of Chinese culture. Naturally, this also includes Qìgōng.

When the Yīn and Yáng theory is applied to Qìgōng, the first important goal of Qìgōng practice is the harmony and balance of Yīn and Yáng (Yīnyáng Xiétiáo, 陰陽諧

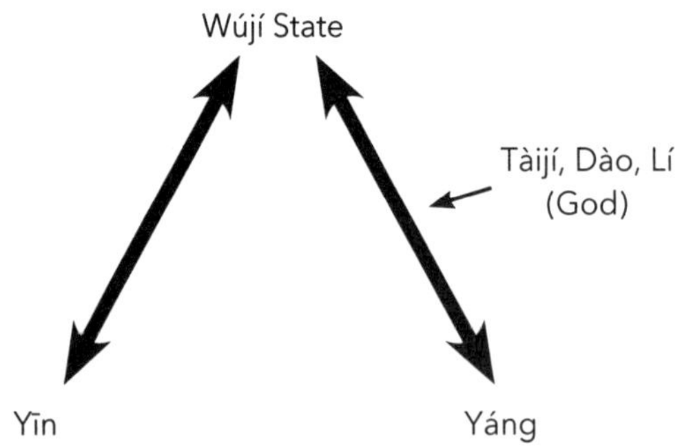

Figure 2-1. The Meaning of Tàijí

調). In order to reach this harmonious stage of balance, you must know the method of adjusting Yīn and Yáng, namely the methods and theory of Kǎn (坎) (Water) and Lí (離) (Fire). Therefore, you should thoroughly comprehend the meaning of Yīn and Yáng, and Kǎn and Lí, which has been discussed in Chapter 1.

When these Yīn-Yáng and Kǎn-Lí theories are applied to human health, the physical body is considered Yáng while the mental and spiritual bodies are considered Yīn. In order to have a healthy and long life, you must not only be concerned with your physical health but also with your spiritual condition. Mental and spiritual condition are the foundation of life. Though they cannot be seen, they are the origins and the causes of the physical manifestation. When this foundation is firm and strong, the manifestation of life can be strong. Therefore, the method of reaching health and longevity is the cultivation of both mental body and physical body. It is called "dual cultivation of the human nature and life" (Xìngmìng Shuāngxiū, 性命雙修). Here, human nature (temperament) means the internal nature, or the original human sense and spirit (mental mind) which has been carried with us since we were born. Life here means the physical life, which is limited.

When you know how to adjust yourself into a harmonious state of both internal and external, it is called "balance of the body and mind" (Shēnxīn Pínghéng, 身心平衡). Once you have gained this balance, you will be able to live long, which allows you to have a longer time for your spiritual cultivation. Spiritual cultivation is considered the way of reaching enlightenment or Buddhahood, the final goal or meaning of human life.

We are very fortunate that we have developed our material science over the last few centuries to a level which today allows us to verify and explain many phenomena that were previously inexplicable. Nevertheless, many mysteries and unknowns remain, and we are still waiting for further understanding from the scientific point of view. We are in the most exciting and challenging era, in which ancient mysterious experience can finally be resolved by today's science.

The theory is like a map of a city: it can direct you to the correct path to reach your goal, and practice is the act of transportation which takes you there. From this, you can see that a correct theory is crucial to reaching the goal. If the theory is wrong, all action will be in vain.

Fortunately, the documents passed down by thousands of Qìgōng experts, written from lifetimes of experience, have provided us with many road signs. Each of these signs offers a tiny piece of information about the whole map. When all of these pieces of information are gathered and compiled, many useless ones will be put aside while others become crucial keys to drawing the map.

I am just someone putting together a puzzle. In front of me are thousands of puzzle pieces that have been revealed to us regarding Qìgōng practice. Some of them are useful and very valuable, while many others may mislead us. From my collections, I try to make judgments and choose those which are useful and relevant. From many years of compiling, studying, and understanding, I will finally be able to make the hidden map of Qìgōng appear. Though it is not as detailed as I would like it to be, I have nevertheless obtained a clear direction for reaching my goal, without being afraid of confusion or of getting lost.

After so many years of study and research, I deeply realize that a clear and detailed map is necessary for those people who are interested in the study of the Dào of Qìgōng. However, it is not easy to accomplish this great task by myself in a single lifetime. There are a few reasons:

1. Since there are thousands of ancient documents which need to be translated, interpreted, and explained, we will first need a group of qualified Chinese scholars who are not only familiar with the Qìgōng practice, but are also masters of ancient Chinese writing. If a person does not have these two requirements, he or she will not be able to understand some special terminology used in ancient Qìgōng society.
2. We will also need a group of experienced Qìgōng practitioners who are able to translate these ancient documents into other languages with the correct meaning. Naturally, this is not an easy task since a Chinese word can convey many different meanings depending on where, how, and when it is used.
3. We will need a group of open-minded modern scientists and medical experts to offer their opinions of these ancient practices. This group will not only challenge and try to verify the ancient experience, but also offer possible scientific explanations of the remaining mysteries.

In order to reach this goal, we will need a foundation with strong financial support. In this foundation, all the experts—both on the past and on the present—should sit together and discuss every subject of Qìgōng practice. The information from these conferences will be compiled, researched, and experimented on, and the results presented to the public. Naturally, it is not an easy task — nearly impossible for any one person to accomplish without government support or the interest of academic society.

In this chapter, I will try to explain many mysteries in Qìgōng practice based on my limited personal scientific background. Naturally, all of these possible explanations still need to be scientifically verified. However, until then, these remain the most probable explanations.

In the second section of this chapter, possible scientific explanations and definitions of Qì and Qìgōng will be given. In addition, the relationship between respiration, Qìgōng, and health will be discussed. To help a beginner understand the documents of

Embryonic Breathing, the definition of the three Dāntiáns will be offered. Then, I will offer a theoretical and scientific understanding of Embryonic Breathing in Section 2–3. Finally, I will summarize the meaning and purposes of meditation in Section 2–4.

2.2 Human Qìgōng Science (Rénlèi Qìgōng Kēxué, 人類氣功科學)

In this section, I would like to interpret Chinese Qìgōng from a scientific point of view. However, since the West has just begun to accept Eastern Qìgōng concepts, there is still a long way to go before modern science reaches a profound understanding of this subject. All of the explanations in this section are based on the available published information and my personal understanding of science. In order to have a reasonable and satisfactory explanation, many theoretical assumptions are given. Naturally, when you read this section, you should keep a neutral mind to understand the subject, and use your logical and scientific mind to make a wise judgment. You should always place a doubt in your mind about all of these assumptions and explanations. Only in the future, when we have verified the theories discussed in this section, can we then trust them fully.

In this section, first I would like to explain the concepts of Qì and Qìgōng from the modern scientific point of view. After this, a hypothetical human electric network will be presented to compare with the ancient Chinese medical concept. Then we will define the human bio-battery, both from the traditional Chinese concept and also in view of Western scientific discoveries.

A Modern Definition of Qì (Qì Zhī Xiàndài Dìngyì, 氣之現代定義). It is important that you know about the progress made by modern science in the study of Qì. This will keep you from getting stuck in the ancient concepts and level of understanding.

In ancient China, people had very little knowledge of electricity. They only knew from acupuncture that when a needle was inserted into acupuncture cavities, some kind of energy other than heat was produced that often caused a shock or a tingling sensation. It was not until the last several decades, when the Chinese people became more acquainted with electromagnetic science, that they began to recognize that this energy circulating in the body, which they called Qì, might be the same thing as what today's science calls "bioelectricity."

It is understood now that the human body is constructed of many different electrically conductive materials, and that it forms a living electromagnetic field and circuit. Electromagnetic energy is continuously being generated in the human body through the biochemical reaction in food and air assimilation, and circulated by the electromotive forces (EMF) generated within the body.

In addition, you are constantly being affected by external electromagnetic fields such as that of the earth, or the electrical fields generated by clouds. When you practice Chinese medicine or Qìgōng, you need to be aware of these outside factors and take them into account.

Countless experiments have been conducted in China, Japan, and other countries to study how external magnetic or electrical fields can affect and adjust the body's Qì field. Many acupuncturists use magnets and electricity in their treatments. They attach a magnet to the skin over a cavity and leave it there for a period of time. The magnetic field gradually affects the Qì circulation in that channel. Alternatively, they insert needles into cavities and then run an electric current through the needle to reach the Qì channels directly. Although many researchers have claimed a degree of success in their experiments, none has been able to publish any detailed and convincing proof of the results, or give a good explanation of the theory behind the experiment. As with many other attempts to explain the How and Why of acupuncture, conclusive proof is elusive, and many unanswered questions remain. Of course, this theory is quite new, and it will probably take a lot more study and research before it is verified and completely understood. At present, there are many conservative acupuncturists who are skeptical.

To untie this knot, we must look at what modern Western science has discovered about bioelectromagnetic energy. Many reports on bioelectricity have been published, and frequently the results are closely related to what is experienced in Chinese Qìgōng training and medical science. For example, during the electrophysiological research of the 1960s, several investigators discovered that bones are piezoelectric; that is, when they are stressed, mechanical energy is converted to electrical energy in the form of electric current.[11] This might explain one of the practices of Marrow Washing Qìgōng in which the stress on the bones and muscles is increased in certain ways to increase the Qì circulation.

Dr. Robert O. Becker has done important work in this field. His book *The Body Electric*[12] reports on much of the research concerning the body's electric field. It is presently believed that food and air are the fuels which generate the electricity in the body through biochemical reaction. This electricity, which is circulated throughout the entire body by means of electrically conductive tissue, is one of the main energy sources which keep the cells of the physical body alive.

Whenever you are sick or have an injury, your body's electrical circulation is affected. If this circulation of electricity stops, you die. But bioelectric energy not only maintains life, it is also responsible for repairing physical damage. Many researchers have sought ways of using external electrical or magnetic fields to speed up the body's recovery from physical injury. Richard Leviton reports: "Researchers at Loma Linda University's School of Medicine in California have found, following studies in sixteen countries with over 1,000 patients, that low-frequency, low-intensity magnetic energy has been successful in treating chronic pain related to tissue ischemia, and has also worked in clearing up slow-healing ulcers, and in 90 percent of patients tested, raised blood flow significantly."[13]

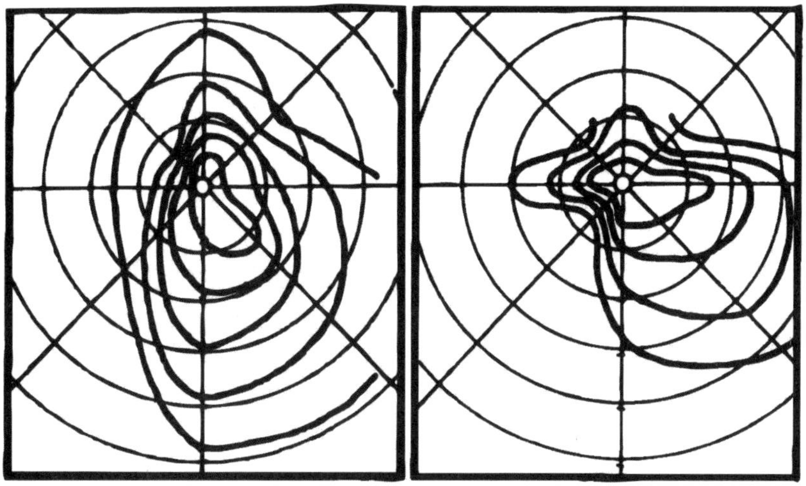

Figure 2-2. Electric Conductivity Maps of the Skin Surface over Acupuncture Points

Mr. Leviton also reports that every cell of the body functions like an electric battery and is able to store electric charge. He reports that: "Other biomagnetic investigators take an even closer look to find out what is happening, right down to the level of the blood, the organs, and the individual cell, which they regard as 'a small electric battery'."[13] This has convinced me that our entire body is essentially a big battery which is assembled from millions of small batteries. All of these batteries together form the human electromagnetic field.

Furthermore, much of the research on the body's electrical field relates to acupuncture. For example, Dr. Becker reports that the conductivity of the skin is much higher at acupuncture cavities, and that it is now possible to locate them precisely by measuring the skin's conductivity (Figure 2–2).[12] Many of these reports prove that the acupuncture practiced in China for thousands of years is reasonable and scientific.

Some researchers use the theory of the body's electricity to explain many of the ancient "miracles" attributed to the practice of Qìgōng. A report by Albert L. Huebner states: "These demonstrations of body electricity in human beings may also offer a new explanation of an ancient healing practice. If weak external fields can produce powerful physiological effects, it may be that fields from human tissues in one person are capable of producing clinical improvements in another. In short, the method of healing known as the laying on of hands could be an especially subtle form of electrical stimulation."[11]

Another frequently reported phenomenon is that when a Qìgōng practitioner has reached a high level of development, a halo would appear behind and/or around his head during meditation. Halos are commonly seen in paintings of Jesus Christ, the Buddha, and various Oriental immortals. Frequently the light is pictured as surrounding the whole body. This phenomenon may again be explained by the body electric theory. When a person has cultivated their Qì (electricity) to a high level, the Qì may be led to accumulate in the head. This Qì may then interact with the oxygen molecules in the air and ionize them, causing them to glow.

Although the link between the theory of *The Body Electric* and the Chinese theory of Qì is becoming better-proven and more accepted, there are still many questions to be answered. For example, how actually does the mind generate an EMF (electromotive force) to circulate the electricity in the body? Is bioelectricity circulating in the animal body a direct current or an alternating current? How is the human electromagnetic field affected by the multitude of other electric fields that surround us, such as radio wiring or electrical appliances? How can we readjust our electromagnetic fields and survive in outer space or on other planets, where the magnetic field is completely different from Earth's? You can see that the future of Qìgōng and bioelectric science is a challenging and exciting one. It is about time that we start using modern technology to understand the inner energy world which has, for the most part, been ignored by Western society.

A Modern Definition of Qìgōng (Qìgōng Zhī Xiàndài Dìngyì, 氣功之現代定義). If you accept that the inner energy (Qì) circulating in our bodies is bioelectricity, we can now formulate a definition of Qìgōng based on electrical principles.

Let us assume that the circuit shown in Figure 2–3 is similar to the circuit in our bodies. Unfortunately, although we now have a certain degree of understanding of this circuit from acupuncture, we still do not know, in detail, exactly what the body's circuit looks like. We know that there are Twelve Primary Qì Channels (Qì rivers) (Shíèrjīng, 十二經) and eight vessels (Qì reservoirs) (Bāmài, 八脈) in our body. There are also thousands of small Qì channels (Luò, 絡) which allow the Qì to reach the skin and the bone marrow. In this circuit, the twelve internal organs are connected and mutually related through these channels. Finally, there is a Dāntián (丹田) (Elixir Field) (bio-battery) which produces and stores the Qì.

If you look at the electrical circuit in the illustration, you will see that:

1. The Qì channels are like the wires, which carry electric current.
2. The internal organs are like the electrical components, such as resistors and solenoids.
3. The Qì vessels are like capacitors, which regulate the current in the circuit.
4. The Dāntián is like a battery, which stores the charge and provides the EMF in the circuit.

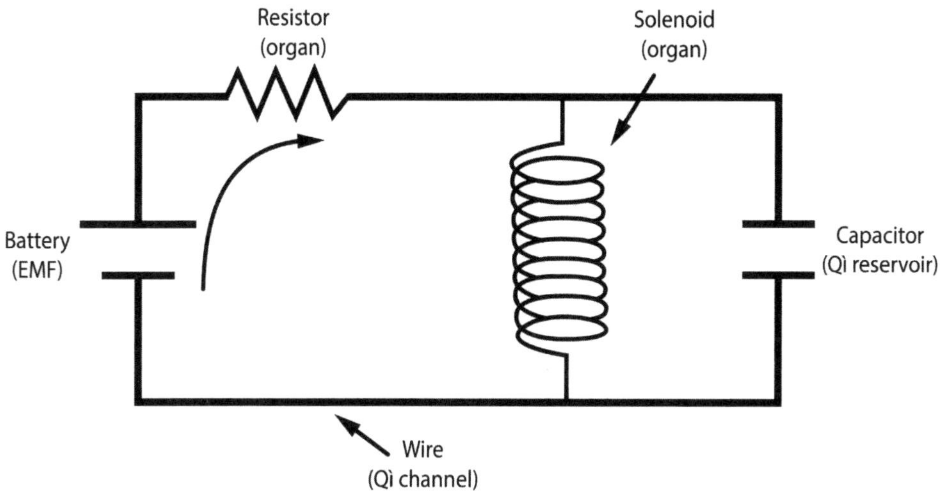

Figure 2-3. The Human Bioelectric Circuit is Similar to an Electric Circuit

How do you keep this electrical circuit functioning most efficiently? Your first concern is the resistance of the wire which carries the current. In a machine, you want to use a wire which has a high level of conductivity and low resistance; otherwise heat may be generated and the wire may melt. Therefore, the wire should be of a material like copper or perhaps even gold. In your body, you want to keep the current flowing smoothly. This means that your first task is to remove anything which interferes with the flow and causes stagnation. Fat has low conductivity, so you should use diet and exercise to remove excess fat from your body. You should also learn how to relax your physical body, because this opens all the Qì channels. This is why relaxation is the first goal in Tàijíquán and many Qìgōng exercises.

Your next concern in maintaining a healthy electrical circuit is the components—your internal organs. If you do not have the correct level of current in your organs, they will either burn out from too much current (Yáng), or malfunction because of a deficient level of current (Yīn). In order to avoid these problems in a machine, you use a capacitor to regulate the current. Whenever there is too much current, the capacitor absorbs and stores the excess, and whenever the current is weak, the capacitor supplies current to raise the level. The eight Qì vessels are your body's capacitors. Qìgōng is concerned with learning how to increase the level of Qì in these vessels so that they will be able to supply current when needed, and keep the internal organs functioning smoothly. This is especially important as you get older when your Qì level is generally lower.

In addition, in order to have a healthy circuit, you must be concerned with the components themselves. If any of them are not strong and of good quality, the entire circuit may malfunction. This means that the final concern in Qìgōng practice is how to maintain or even rebuild the health of your internal organs. Before we go any further, we should point out that there is an important difference between the circuit shown in the diagram and the Qì circuit in our bodies. This difference is that the human body is alive, and, with proper Qì nourishment, all of the cells can be regrown and the state of health improved. For example, if you are able to jog three miles today, and you keep jogging regularly and gradually increase the distance, eventually you will easily be able to jog five miles. This is because your body rebuilds and readjusts itself to fit the circumstances.

This means that, if we are able to increase the Qì flow through our internal organs, they can become stronger and healthier. Naturally, the increase in Qì must be slow and gradual so that the organs can adjust to it. In order to increase the Qì flow in your body, you need to work with the EMF (electromotive force) in your body. If you do not know what EMF is, imagine two containers filled with water and connected by a tube. If both containers have the same water level, then the water will not flow. However, if one side is higher, the water will flow from that container to the other. In electricity, this potential difference is called electric potential difference or electromotive force. Naturally, the higher the EMF is, the stronger the current will flow.

You can see from this discussion that the key to effective Qìgōng practice is, in addition to removing resistance from the Qì channels, learning how to increase the EMF in your body. Now let us see what the sources of EMF in the body are, so that we may use them to increase the flow of bioelectricity. Generally speaking, there are six major sources:

1. **Natural Energy.** Since your body is constructed of electrically conductive material, its electromagnetic field is always affected by the sun, the moon, clouds, the earth's magnetic field, and by the other energies around you. The major influences are the radiation of the sun and moon, the moon's gravity, and the earth's magnetic field. These affect your Qì circulation significantly, and are responsible for the pattern of your Qì circulation since you were formed. We are now also being greatly affected by the energy pollution generated by modern technology, such as electromagnetic waves generated by radio, television, microwave ovens, computers, and many other devices.

2. **Food and Air.** In order to maintain life, we take in food and air essence through our mouths and noses. These essences are then converted into Qì through biochemical reaction in the chest and digestive system (called the Triple Burner in Chinese medicine). When Qì is converted from the essence, an EMF is generated that circulates the Qì throughout the body. Consequently, a major part of Qìgōng is devoted to getting the proper kinds of food and fresh air.

3. **Thinking.** The human mind is the most important and efficient source of bioelectric EMF. Any time you move, you must first generate an idea (Yì, 意). This idea generates the EMF and leads the Qì through the nervous system to energize the appropriate muscles to carry out the desired motion. The more you can concentrate, the stronger the EMF you can generate, and the stronger the flow of Qì you can lead. Naturally, the stronger the flow of Qì you lead to the muscles, the more they will be energized. Because of this, the mind is considered the most important factor in Qìgōng training.
4. **Exercise.** Exercise converts the food essence (fat) stored in your body into Qì, and therefore builds up the EMF. Many Qìgōng styles have been created which utilize movement for this purpose.
5. **Converting Pre-Birth Essence into Qì.** The hormones produced by our endocrine glands are referred to as "Pre-Birth Essence" or "Original Essence" (Yuánjīng, 元精) in Chinese medicine. They can be used to regulate the biochemical reaction which converts the food or fat into Qì. Hormones act as catalysts in our body's biochemical reaction process (metabolism). Thus, hormones are able to stimulate the functioning of our physical body, thereby increasing our vitality. Balancing hormone production when you are young and increasing its production when you are old are important subjects in Chinese Qìgōng.
6. **Artificial Stimulation.** The enhancement or the adjustment of Qì circulation can also be done artificially. In fact, this is the basic theory of Chinese medicine such as acupuncture and Qìgōng massage. From external artificial Qì stimulation, the Qì can be brought to a state of balance, thus preventing or curing sickness.

From the foregoing, you can see that within the human body, there is a network of electrical circuitry. In order to maintain the circulation of bioelectricity, there must be a battery (or power supply) to store and supply charge. Where then, is the battery in our body?

Chinese Qìgōng practitioners believe that there is a place that is able to store Qì (bioelectricity). This place is called the Dāntián (丹田) (Elixir Field). According to such practitioners, there are three Dāntiáns in the human body. One is located at the abdominal area, one or two inches below the navel, called the "Lower Dāntián" (Xiàdāntián, 下丹田). The second is in the area of the lower sternum which is connected to the diaphragm, and is called the "Middle Dāntián" (Zhōngdāntián, 中丹田). The third is the center of the brain, which connects to the lower center of the forehead (or the Third Eye), and

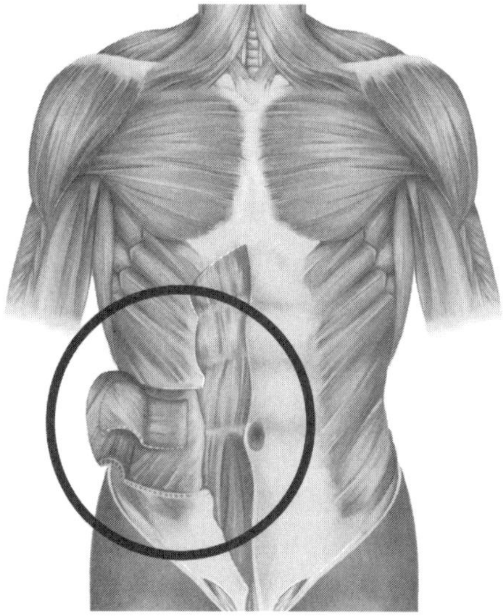

Figure 2-4. Anatomic Structure of the Abdominal Area
(Illustration by Shutterstock)

is called the "Upper Dāntián" (Shàngdāntián, 上丹田). In fact, often the entire brain is considered to be the Upper Dāntián.

The Lower Dāntián is considered to be the residence of the Water Qì, or the Qì which is generated from the "Original Essence" (Yuánjīng, 元精). Therefore, Qì stored here is called "Original Qì" (Yuánqì, 元氣). According to Chinese medicine, in this same area there is a cavity called "Qìhǎi" (Co-6) (氣海), which means "Qì ocean." This is consistent with the conclusions drawn by Qìgōng practitioners, who also call this area the "Lower Dāntián" (Lower Elixir Field). Both groups agree that this area is able to produce Qì or elixir like a field, and that here the Qì is abundant like an ocean.

In Qìgōng practice, it is commonly known that in order to build up the Qì to a higher level in the Lower Dāntián, you must move your abdominal area (Lower Dāntián) up and down through abdominal breathing. This kind of up-and-down abdominal breathing exercise is called "Qǐhuǒ" (起火) and means "start the fire." It is also called "back to childhood breathing" (Fǎntóng Hūxī, 返童呼吸). Normally, after you have exercised the Lower Dāntián for about ten minutes, you will have a feeling of warmth in the lower abdomen, which verifies the accumulation of Qì or energy. Therefore, Daoists called the abdominal area the "Dānlú" (丹爐) which means the "elixir furnace."

Theoretically and scientifically, what is happening when the abdominal area is moved up and down? If you look at the structure of the abdominal area, you will see that there are about six layers of muscle and fasciae sandwiching each other in this area (Figure 2–4). In fact, what you actually see is the sandwich of muscles and fat accumulated in the fasciae layers. When you move your abdomen up and down, you are actually using your

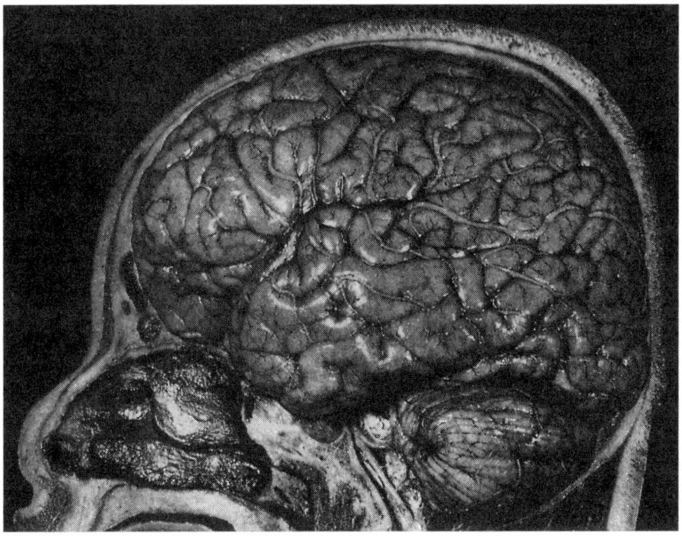

Figure 2-5. The Upper Dāntián–The Human Brain

mind to move the muscles, not the fat. Whenever there is a muscular contraction and relaxation, the fat slowly turns into bioelectricity. When this bioelectricity encounters resistance from the fasciae layers, it turns into heat. From this, you can see how simple the theory might be for the generation of Qì. Another thing you should know is that, according to our understanding today, fat and fasciae are poor electrical conductors, while the muscles are relatively good electrical conductors.[11,12,13] When these good and poor electrical materials are sandwiched together, they act like a battery. This is why, through up and down abdominal movements, the energy can be stored temporarily and warmth generated.

However, understanding the Dāntiáns is not a simple task. In fact, they are more complicated than most people thought. Next, we will discuss the "Three Dāntiáns" (Sāntián, 三田) more clearly.

Upper Dāntián (Shàngdāntián, 上丹田). Generally, the entire brain is considered to be the Upper Dāntián. We already know that the brain and the spinal cord are considered the central nervous system, in which the electrical conductivity is highest in our body. If we examine the brain's structure, we can see that it is segregated by the arachnoid mater (mater is a kind of membrane in the body; "arachnoid mater" is a delicate membrane of the spinal cord and brain, lying between the "pia mater" and "dura mater") into separate portions (Figure 2–5). It is reasonable to assume that these materials are tissue of low electrical conductivity. If the good conductors have been sandwiched by poor conductive material, then this system is able to store some electricity. However, we should also know that the brain does not produce Qì, but consumes a great amount of it. From Western science, we already know that each brain cell consumes at least twelve times more oxygen than other cells. Since, in the biochemical reaction, oxygen is proportional to the production of energy (Qì) in the body, it is reasonable to assume that each brain cell also consumes at least twelve times more Qì than regular cells.

Middle Dāntián (Zhōngdāntián, 中丹田). Next, let us examine the structure of the Middle Dāntián area. This is located at the lower section of the sternum, which is connected to the diaphragm (Figure 2–6). We know that the diaphragm is a membranous muscular partition separating the abdominal and the thoracic cavities. It functions in respiration and is a good electrically conductive material. On the top and the bottom of the diaphragm are the fasciae, which isolate the internal organs from the diaphragm. We see, once again, a good electrical conductor isolated by a poor electrical conductor. This means that it is capable of storing electricity or Qì. Since this place is between the lungs and the stomach, and they absorb the Post-Birth Essence (air and food) and convert it into energy, the Qì accumulated in the Middle Dāntián is classified as Fire Qì (Huǒqì, 火氣). In other words, Qì converted from the contaminated air and food can affect Qì status and make it Yáng. Naturally, this Fire Qì can also agitate your emotional mind. Some documents believe that the heart is the Middle Dāntián. However, it makes more sense that the diaphragm is the Middle Dāntián, since it is able to store Qì. I personally believe that the "heart" is related to our emotion. Our emotion is associated with the air and food we absorb. Thus, the heart is related to the Qì status in the Middle Dāntián, but not to the Middle Dāntián itself.

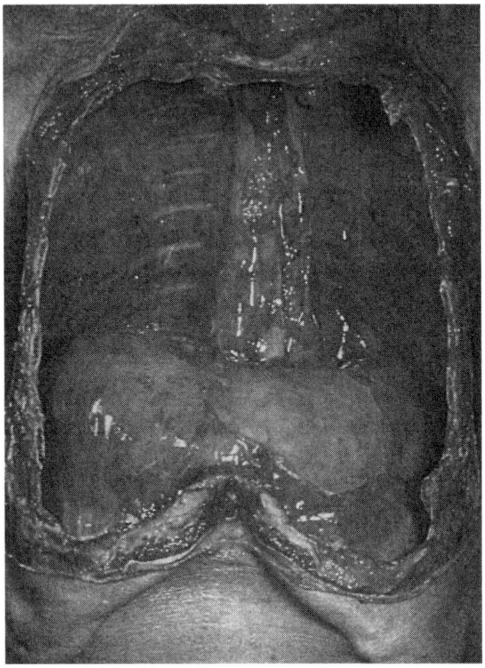

Figure 2-6. The Middle Dāntián is Connected to the Diaphragm

Lower False Dāntián and Real Dāntián (Xià Jiǎ Dāntián, Zhēn Dāntián; 下假丹田・真丹田). Through nearly two thousand years of experience, Daoists have said that the front abdominal area is not the Real Dāntián, but is in fact a "False Dāntián" (Jiǎ Dāntián, 假丹田). Their argument is that, although this Lower Dāntián is able to generate Qì and build it up to a higher level, it does not store it for a long time. This is because it is located on the path of the Conception Vessel (Rènmài, 任脈), so that whenever Qì is built up, it will circulate in the Conception and Governing Vessels (Rènmài, Dūmài; 任脈・督脈). This Lower Dāntián therefore cannot be a battery as we understand the term. A real battery should be able to store the Qì to an abundant level. Where then, is the "Real Lower Dāntián" (Zhēn Xiàdāntián, 真下丹田)? We will discuss this later. First, let us clarify the function of the False Lower Dāntián.

False Lower Dāntián (Jiǎ Xiàdāntián, 假下丹田). As mentioned earlier, through abdominal movement coordinated with breathing, the fat accumulated at the abdominal area can be converted into Qì. This kind of abdominal exercise is called "back to childhood breathing" (Fǎntóng Hūxī, 返童呼吸). Consequently, the amount of Qì can be increased in the body. From this, we see something at variance with the ancient teachings. It is said that through abdominal breathing, the Original Essence (Yuánjīng, 元精) can be converted into Original Qì (Yuánqì, 元氣). Today, we know that Original Essence is hormones. If we look closely, we can see that the Qì is actually converted from the fat stored in the abdominal area. Fat is the extra food essence stored in our bodies for an emergency. Fat is a material which has been filtered by the liver and has a very high content of calories. Therefore, it can be converted into Qì efficiently.

We can trace this back to a very long time ago, before humans knew how to grow food and raise cattle. At that time, we were no different from other animals. When we had food we ate a lot, and when we did not have food, we starved. However, like animals, we did not die in a short time from starvation. This is because the body has different places to store the extra food essence—fat—in the body. When we lack food, this extra food essence will be converted naturally into energy to supply our needs. The abdominal area is the main area for the storage of fat. There are six layers of muscle and six layers of fasciae sandwiched between each other. Wherever there are fasciae, there is a stagnation of Qì and blood circulation, and consequently fat can be deposited. Through abdominal exercises, this fat can be converted into Qì efficiently.

From this we can see that it is not Original Essence (hormones) which is converted into Qì. However, due to the hormones' function, the Qì can be converted more efficiently, whether from food essence or fat stored in the body. This is simply because the hormones act as catalysts in the body's biochemical reaction. One of the possible causes of increased hormone production via the abdominal up-and-down exercises is the stimulation of islets of Longerhans in the pancreas.

Real Lower Dāntián (Zhēn Xiàdāntián, 真下丹田). Daoists teach that the Real Lower Dāntián is at the center of the abdominal area, at the physical center of gravity located in the large and small intestines (Figure 2–7). Now, let us analyze this from two different points of view.

First, let us take a look at how life begins. It starts with a sperm from the father entering an egg from the mother, thus forming the original human cell (Figure 2–8).[14] This cell next divides into two cells, then four cells, etc. When this group of cells adheres to the internal wall of the uterus, the umbilical cord starts to develop. Nutrition and energy for further cell multiplication is absorbed through the umbilical cord from the mother's body. The baby keeps growing until it develops a more mature body. During this nourishing and growing process, the baby's abdomen is moving up and down, acting like a pump drawing in nutrition and energy into his or her body. Later, immediately after birth, air and nutrition are taken in from the nose and mouth through the mouth's sucking action and the lungs' breathing. As the child grows, it slowly forgets the natural movements of the abdomen. This is why the abdomen's up and down movement is called "back to childhood breathing."

Think carefully: if your first human cell were still alive, where would it be? Naturally, this cell has already died a long time ago. It is understood that approximately one trillion cells die in a human body each day.[15] However, if we assume that this first cell is still alive, then it should be located at our physical center, that is, our center of gravity. If we think carefully, we can see that it is from this center that the cells could multiply evenly outward until the body was fully constructed. In order to maintain this even multiplication physically, the energy or Qì must be centered at this point and radiate outward. When we are in an embryonic state, this is the center of gravity and also the Qì center. As we grow after birth, this center remains.

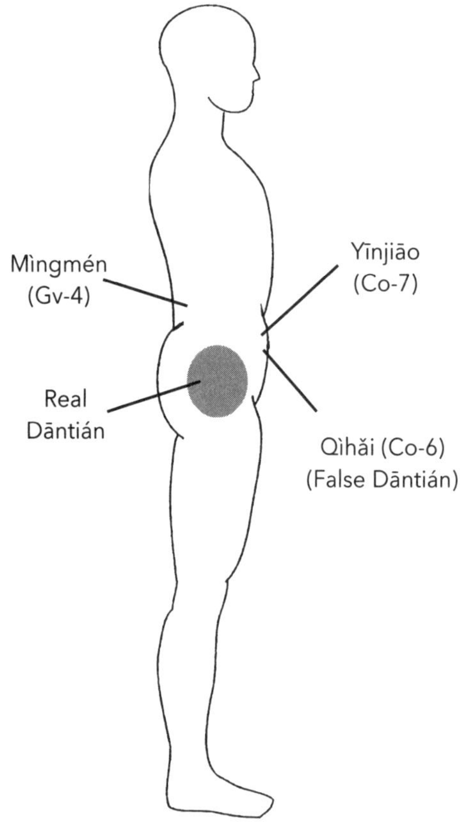

Figure 2-7. The Real Lower Dāntián and the False Lower Dāntián

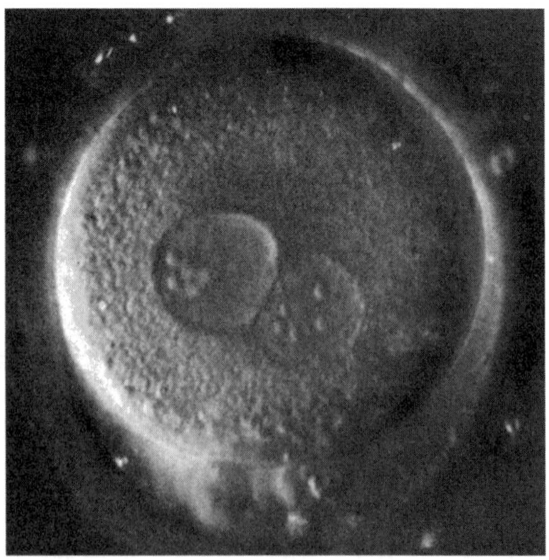

Figure 2-8. Original First Human Cell

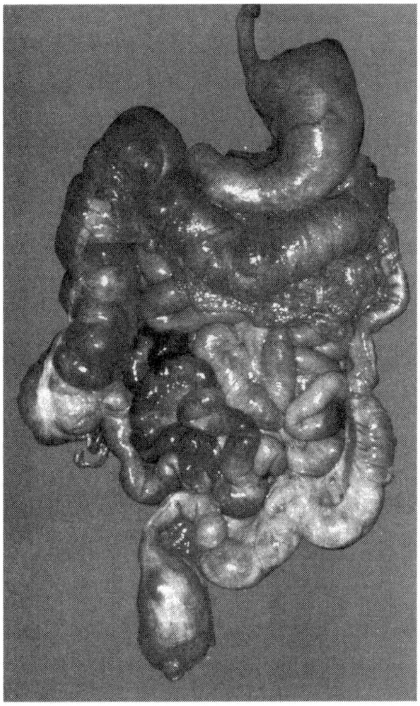

Figure 2-9. Anatomic Structure of the Real Lower Dāntián–The Second Brain

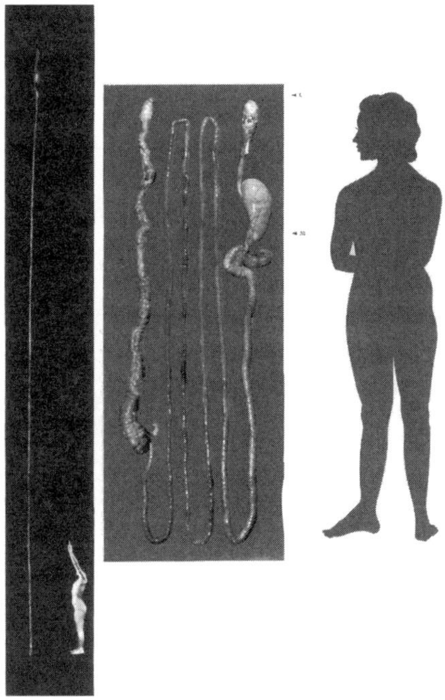

Figure 2-10. The Large and Small Intestines are About Six Times Your Height

The above argument adheres solely to the traditional point of view of the physical development of our body. Next, let us analyze this center from another point of view.

If we look at the physical center of gravity, we can see that the entire area is occupied by the Large and Small Intestines (Figure 2–9). We know that there are three kinds of muscles existing in our body, and we can examine them in ascending order of our ability to control them. The first kind includes the heart muscle, in which the electrical conductivity among muscular groups is the highest. The heart beats all the time, regardless of our attention, and through practice and discipline, we are only able to regulate its beating, not start and stop it. If we supply electricity to even a small piece of this muscle, it will pump like the heart. The second category of muscles are those which contract automatically, but over which we can exert significant control if we make the effort. The diaphragm (which controls breathing), our eyelids, and certain sexual responses are examples of this muscle type, and their electrical conductivity is lower than the first type. The third kind of muscles are those muscles which are directly controlled by our conscious mind. The electric conductivity of these muscles is the lowest of the three groups.

If you look at the structure of the Large and Small Intestines, the first thing you notice is that the total length of your Large and Small Intestines is approximately six times your body's height (Figure 2–10). With such long electrically conductive tissues

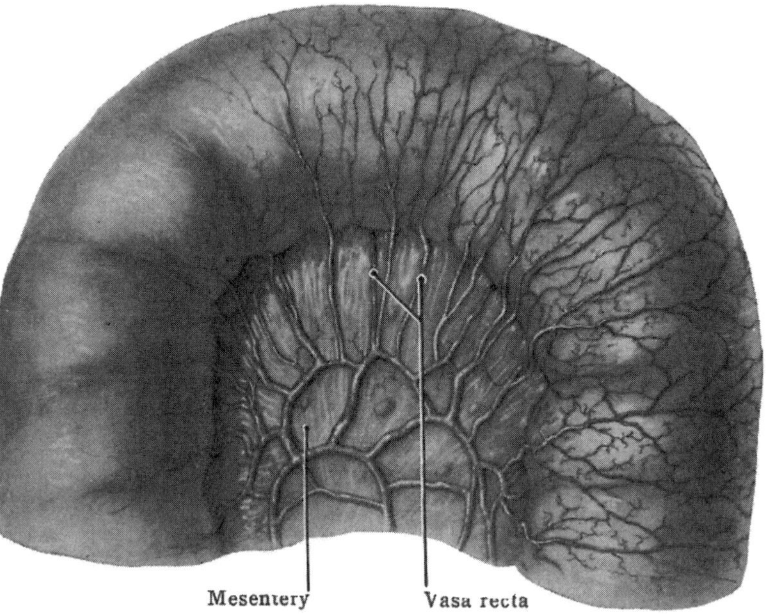

Figure 2-11. Low Electrically Conductive Material Such as Mesentery, Outer Casing, and Water in and Around the Intestines Makes the Entire Area Act Like a Battery
(Used with permission: James E. Anderson, M.D., Grant's Atlas of Anatomy, 7th ed., ©Williams and Wilkins)

sandwiched between all of the mesenteries, water, and linings (which it is reasonable to believe are poor electrical conductive tissues), the intestines act like a huge battery in our body (Figure 2–11).[16] From this, you can see that it makes sense both logically and scientifically that the center of gravity, rather than the false Dāntián, is the real battery in our body.

Furthermore, according to a 1996 article in *The New York Times*, a human being can be thought of as having two brains.[17,18] One brain is in the head, and the other is in the gut (i.e., the digestive system). Though these two brains are separated physically, through the connection of the spinal cord (highly electrically conductive tissue) (Thrusting Vessel, 衝脈), they actually function as one (Figure 2–12).

This article explains that the upper brain is able to think and has memory. It is able to store data, utilizing electrochemical charges. The lower brain has memory, but does not have the capability of thought. This discovery offers confirmation of the Chinese belief that the Real Lower Dāntián (Large and Small Intestines) is able to store Qì, while the Upper Dāntián governs thinking and directs the Qì. Theoretically speaking, if the upper brain is able to think, then it should be able to generate an EMF while the lower brain should have a large capacity for storing charge. In other words, the lower brain is the human battery in which the life force resides. Once the brain has generated an idea (EMF), the charge will immediately be directed from the lower brain, through the spinal cord and nervous system, to the desired area in order to activate the physical body for function.[18]

According to Ohm's Law in Physics,

$$V = I R$$

where V is potential difference or EMF, I is current, and R is resistance.[19]

From this formula, we can see that if R is a constant, then the higher the potential or EMF, the stronger will be the current that is generated. If we assume that the resistance of our body remains constant, then the more we are able to concentrate (higher EMF), the stronger the Qì flow will be. This parallels the Chinese Qìgōng concept that the more you concentrate, the higher your energy level. From Chinese Qìgōng, higher levels of concentration can be trained through still meditation. In addition, if we assume the EMF to be constant, that means the mind's concentration remains the same. Then, the lower the R (resistance), the higher the current flow will be. According to the past Qìgōng experience, the more relaxed you are, the more Qì (current) can flow.

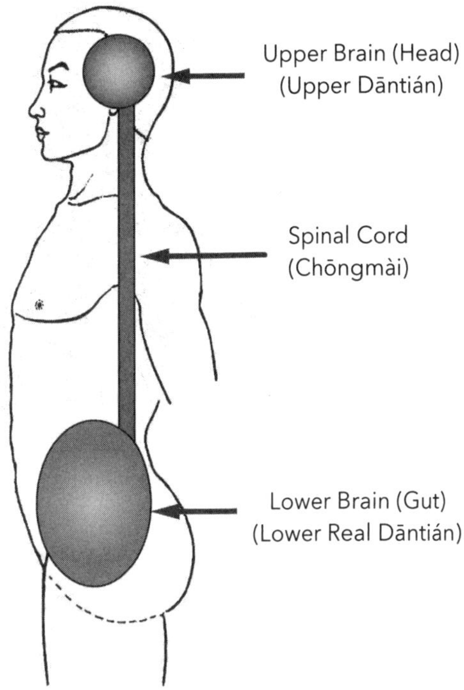

Figure 2-12. Two Polarities (Brains) of a Human Body

At this point you should also know that Qì can also be produced directly from food or herbs, and then stored at the Real Lower Dāntián. This means different food can produce different quantity and quality of Qì, which is why those herbs which can produce more Qì in the body were searched for and studied in Chinese herbalism in the past. For example, ginseng has been recognized as one of the many herbs able to produce more Qì when taken orally.

Cell Replacement. From the above discussion, you may have gained a better idea of how we can link ancient experience together with modern scientific understanding. In order to make the scientific concept of Qìgōng even clearer, let us look at Qìgōng from another scientific point of view, this time chemical.

If we examine how we breathe, we can see that we inhale to take in oxygen, and we exhale to expel carbon dioxide (Figure 2–13). Every minute we expel a great deal of carbon from our body through exhalation. Carbon is a material in physical form which can be seen. The question is, where in our body is the carbon coming from? Through breathing, how much carbon is actually removed?

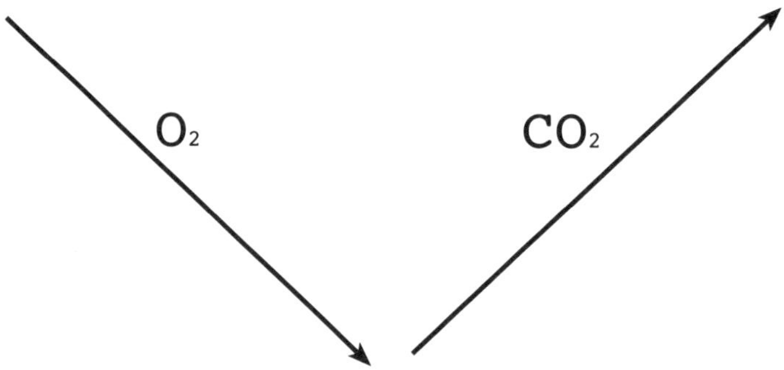

Figure 2-13. We Inhale to Absorb Oxygen and Exhale to Expel Carbon Dioxide

The first source of carbon is from the food (glucose) we eat. When this food is converted into energy through chemical reaction during our daily activities, carbon dioxide is produced.[20]

$$\text{glucose} + 6O_2 \longrightarrow 6CO_2 + 6H_2O$$
$$\Delta G^{o'} = -686 \text{ Kcal}$$

The second source of this carbon comes from the dead cells in our body. We already know that the majority (96%) of our body is constructed from the elements carbon, hydrogen, oxygen, and nitrogen, while other elements such as calcium (Ca), potassium (P), chloride (Cl), sulfur (S), potassium (K), sodium (Na), magnesium (Mg), iodine (I), and iron (Fe) comprise much less of our body weight. This means that the cells in our body contain a great amount of carbon.

In addition, consider that every cell in our body has a life span. As many as a trillion cells die in our body every twenty-four hours.[15] For example, we know that the life span of a skin cell is twenty-eight days. Naturally, living cells such as those of the bone, marrow, liver, etc., have their own individual life span. We rely on our respiration to bring the carbon (dead cells) out through exhalation, and to supply living cells with new oxygen through inhalation. We rely on food for new carbon, water, and other minerals. All this aids in the formation of new cells and the continuation of life.

From the foregoing, we can conclude that the cell replacement process (metabolism) is ongoing at all moments during our lifetime. Health depends on how smoothly and quickly this replacement process is carried out. If there are more new healthy cells to replacc the old cells, you live and grow. If the cells replaced are as healthy as the original cells, you remain young. However, if there are fewer cells produced, or if the new cells are not as healthy as the original cells, then you age. Now, let us analyze Qìgōng from the point of view of cell replacement.

Let us consider the materials needed to produce a healthy cell. From the structure of a cell, we know that we will need hydrogen, oxygen, carbon, nitrogen, and other minerals which we can absorb either from air or food. Therefore, air quality, water purity, and the choice of foods become critical factors for your health and longevity. Naturally, this has also been a major component of Qìgōng study.

However, we know that today's air and water have been contaminated by pollution, especially in big cities and in industrial areas. The quality of the food we eat depends on its source and processing methods. Naturally, it is not easy to find the same pristine environments as in ancient times. However, we must learn how to fit into our new environment and choose our way of life wisely.

Since carbon comprises such a major part of our body, how to absorb good quality carbon is an important issue in modern health. You may obtain carbon from animal products or from plants. Generally speaking, the carbon obtained from plants is more pure than that from animals.

According to past experience and analysis, red meat is generally more contaminated than white meat, and is able to disturb and stimulate your emotional mind and confuse your thinking. Fish are another animal source of carbon. Again, some kinds of fish are good, while others may be bad. For example, shrimp, though low in calories, has a high cholesterol content, which may increase the risk of high blood pressure.

Due to the impurities contained in most animal products, since ancient times Qìgōng practitioners learned how to absorb protein from plants, especially from peas or beans. Soybean is one of the best of these sources; it is both inexpensive and easy to grow. However, if you are not a vegetarian originally, then it can be difficult for your body to produce the enzymes to digest an all-vegetable diet immediately. Humans evolved as omnivores, and the craving for meat can be strong. Even today, we all still have canine teeth, which were used to tear off raw meat in ancient times. Therefore, the natural enzymes existing in our body are more tailored to digesting meat. In an experiment, if we place a piece of meat and some corn in human digestive enzymes, we will see that the meat will be dissolved in a matter of minutes, while the corn will take many hours. This means it is generally easier for a human to absorb meat rather than plants as a protein source.

However, the above discussion does not mean we absolutely cannot absorb plant protein efficiently. The key is that if it is present to begin with, the enzyme production can be increased within your body, but it will take time. For example, if you cannot drink milk due to insufficient lactose in your stomach, you may start by drinking a little bit of milk every day, and slowly increase it as days pass by. You will realize that you are able to absorb milk six months later. This means that if you wish to become a vegetarian, you must reduce the intake of meat products slowly and allow your body to adjust to it; otherwise you may experience protein deficiency.

Other than a protein source, you must also consider minerals. Although they do not comprise a large proportion of our body, their importance in some ways is more significant than carbon. We know that calcium is an important element for bones, and iron is crucial for blood cells. Therefore, when we eat we must consume a variety of foods instead of just a few. How to absorb nutrition from food has been an important part of Chinese Qìgōng study.

In order to produce healthy cells, other than the concerns of the material side, you must also consider energy. You should understand that when a person ages quickly, often it is not because he or she is malnourished, but instead is due to the weakening of their Qì storage and circulation. Without an abundant supply of Qì (bioelectricity), Qì circulation will not be regulated efficiently, and therefore your life force will weaken and the physical body will degenerate. In order to have abundant Qì storage, you must practice Qìgōng in order to build up the Qì in your eight vessels, and also to lead the Qì circulating in your body. This kind of Qìgōng training includes Wàidān (外丹) (External Elixir) and Nèidān (內丹) (Internal Elixir) practice.

Other than the concern for materials needed, and the Qì required for cell production and replacement, the next question is how this replacement process is carried out. The entire replacement process depends on the blood cells. From Western medicine, we know that a blood cell is the carrier of water, oxygen, and nutrients to everywhere in the body through the blood circulatory network. From arteries and capillaries, the components for new cells are brought to every tiny place in the body. The old cells then absorb everything required from the blood stream and divide to produce new cells. The dead cells are brought back through veins to the lungs. Through respiration, the dead cell materials are expelled as carbon dioxide.

However, there is something missing from the last process. This is the Qì or bioelectricity that is required for the biochemical process of cell division. It has been proven that every blood cell is actually like a dipole or a small battery, which is able to store bioelectricity and also to release it.[11] This means that each blood cell is actually a carrier of Qì. This is also understood in Chinese medicine. In Chinese medicine, the blood and the Qì are always together. Where there is blood, there is Qì, and vice versa. Therefore, the term "Qìxuě" (Qì-blood) (氣血) is often used in Chinese medicine.

If we look at our blood circulatory system, we can see that the arteries are located deep underneath the muscles, while the veins are situated near the skin's surface. The color of the blood is red in the arteries because of the presence of oxygen, and its color is darker red in the veins both because of the absence of this oxygen and the presence of carbon. This implies that cell replacement actually happens from inside of the body, moving outward. This can also offer us a hint that, if we are tense, the blood circulation will be more stagnant, and cell replacement will be slower. We can also conclude that most cell replacement occurs in the night, when we are at our most relaxed state during sleep. This can further lead one to conclude the importance of sleep.

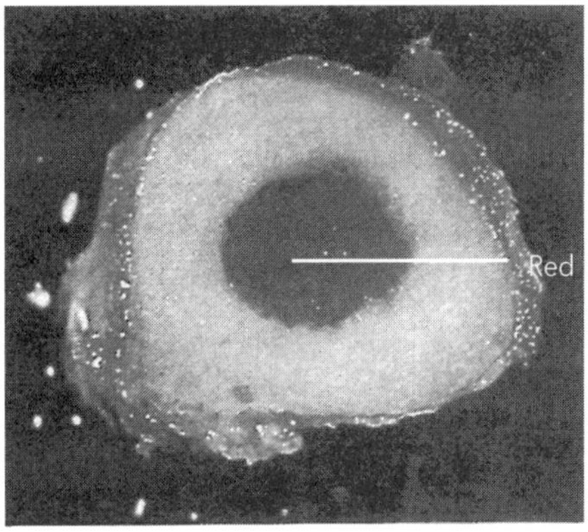

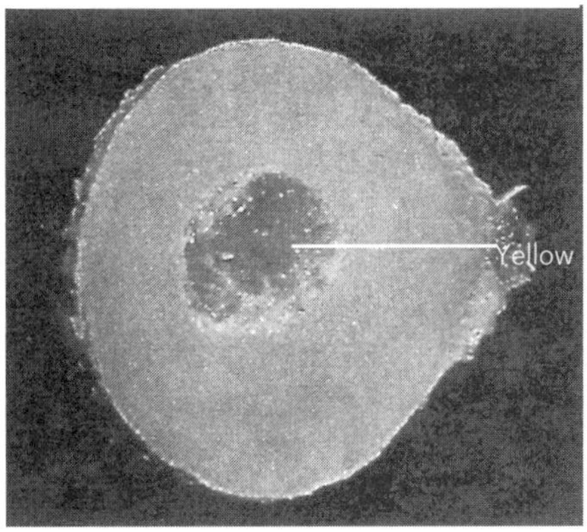

Figure 2-14. Structure of a Long Bone. Red Bone Marrow and Yellow Bone Marrow

If we accept that blood cells are the carriers of everything required for cell replacement, then we must also consider the healthy condition of our blood cells. If you have good health and a sufficient quantity of blood cells, then the nutrients and Qì can be carried to every part of the body efficiently. You will be healthy. However, if you do not have sufficient blood cells, or the quality of the cells is poor, then the entire cell replacement process will be stagnant. Naturally, you will degenerate swiftly.

According to modern medical science, blood cells also have a life span. When the old ones die, new ones must be produced from the bone marrow. Bone marrow is the major blood factory. From medical reports, we know that normally, after a person reaches thirty years of age, the marrow near the ends of the bone cavity turns yellow. This indicates that fat has accumulated there, which means that red blood cells are no longer being produced in the yellowed area (Figure 2-14).[21] Chinese Qìgōng practitioners believe that the degeneration of the bone marrow is due to insufficient Qì supply. Therefore, Bone Marrow Washing Qìgōng (Xǐsuǐgōng, 洗髓功) was developed. From experience, we know that, through Bone Marrow Washing Qìgōng practice, health can be improved and life can be extended significantly. If you are interested in this subject, please read *Qìgōng—The Secret of Youth*, published by YMAA Publication Center.

The next most important thing in human life is hormone production within your body. We already know from today's medical science that hormones act as a catalyst in the body. When hormone levels are high, we are more energized and cell replacement can happen faster and more smoothly. When hormone production diminishes, cell replacement will be slow and we will age quickly. It was only in the late 20th century that scientists discovered that, by increasing the hormone levels in the body, we may be able to extend our life significantly.[22]

Maintenance of hormone production in a healthy manner has also been a major concern in Chinese Qìgōng practice. Glands that produce hormones have been recognized by Chinese medicine since ancient times, even though hormones were not understood. Through thousands of years of practice and experience, the ancients understood that the essence of life is stored in the kidneys (Internal Kidneys) (Nèishèn, 內腎). Today, we know that this "essence" is actually the hormones produced by the adrenal glands on the top of the kidneys. The Chinese also believed that, through stimulation of the testicles and ovaries, the life force could be increased. Testicles and ovaries are considered "External Kidneys" (Wàishèn, 外腎) in Chinese Qìgōng and medical societies. In addition, from still meditation practice, they learned how to lead the Qì to the brain and raise up the "Spirit of Vitality." It has also been found that through practice, bioelectricity can be led to the pituitary gland to stimulate growth hormone production. All of these practices are believed to be effective paths to longevity.

From medical science, we know that our hormone levels are significantly reduced when the last pieces of our bones are completed between ages twenty-nine and thirty. Theoretically, when our body has completed constructing itself, it somehow triggers the reduction of our hormone levels. From this, you can see that maintaining the hormone levels in our body may be a key to longevity.

Finally, in order to prevent ourselves from becoming sick, we must also consider our immune system. According to Chinese medicine and Qìgōng, when Qì storage is abundant, you get sick less. If we take a careful look, we can see that every white blood cell is like a soldier who needs food to maintain his fighting strength. Likewise, if we do not have enough Qì to supply to the cell, its fighting capability will be low. When the Qì is strong, the immune system is strong. Therefore, the skin breathing technique was developed, which teaches a practitioner to lead the Qì to the surface of the skin in order to strengthen the "Guardian Qì" (Wèiqì, 衛氣), or an energetic component of the immune system near the skin surface.

From the foregoing, hopefully I have offered you a challenge for profound thought and further research. Although most of these conclusions are drawn from my personal research, further study and verification is still needed. I deeply believe that if we can all open our minds and share our opinions together, we will be able to make our lives more healthy and meaningful.

Breathing, Qìgōng, and Health (Hūxī, Qìgōng, Yǔ Jiànkāng, 呼吸、氣功、與健康). According to Chinese Qìgōng society, Qì can be distinguished as "Upper Level Qì" (Shàngcéngqì, 上層氣) or "External Qì" (Wàiqì, 外氣), and "Lower Level Qì" (Xiàcéngqì, 下層氣) or "Inner Qì" (Nèiqì, 內氣). These two levels of Qì are separated by the diaphragm. While the upper level manages the exchange of the external Qì, the lower level governs the production and storage of the inner Qì (Figure 2–15). The nose is the entrance and exit of the Upper Level Qì, the diaphragm is the pump, and the lungs manage and process this Qì. The abdomen and Huìyīn (Co-1) (會陰) are the pump and piston to produce and store the inner Qì at the Real Lower Dāntián (gut).

You may already have Figured out that the "External Qì" is actually air. Air is called "Kōngqì" (空氣) which means "the Qì in space." "Qì" here implies the energy existing in space. The bioelectricity which is stored at the Lower Dāntián and circulates in the body is called "Inner Qì" (Nèiqì, 內氣).[12]

From the scientific point of view, these two Qìs cannot be separated, though they are not directly related. You should understand that the entire body's inner Qì is produced from the biochemical reaction process.[20] The body's energy is metabolized from food. Remember the formula:

$$\text{glucose} + 6O_2 \longrightarrow 6CO_2 + 6H_2O$$
$$\Delta G^{o\prime} = -686 \text{ Kcal}$$

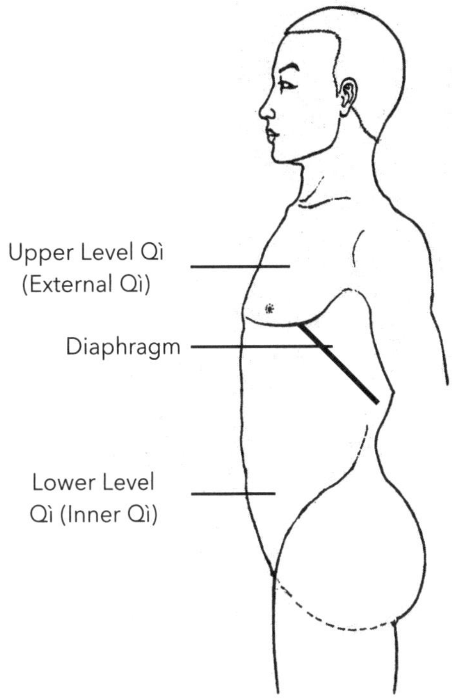

Figure 2-15. Upper Level Qì and Lower Level Qì

The energy produced is then converted into different forms of energy such as bioelectricity (Qì), heat, or light in the body. The quantity of oxygen is one of the most criticial factors in completing the transformation of glucose into energy. That is why whenever you need to manifest stronger force for exertion, such as lifting a heavy weight or pushing a car, you must first inhale deeply to take in more oxygen. Only then can the inner energy be manifested to a significant level.

In Daoist society, the space above the diaphragm (lungs) is considered the chamber where the external Qì is exchanged. The nose is the entrance and the exit, while the diaphragm is the piston or the pump of this chamber. The space below the diaphragm down to the groin area is considered the chamber (Real Lower Dāntián) of the inner Qì. Here, inner Qì can be built up and stored to an abundant level through the correct pumping movement of the abdominal area and the Huìyīn (Co-1) (會陰) cavity (perineum).

You can see the importance of breathing and how it can be so crucial in Qìgōng practice. If your breathing is shallow, the exchange of oxygen and carbon dioxide will not be completed and, naturally, cell replacement will not be fully accomplished. This is one of the major causes of sickness and aging.

2.3 Theoretical Foundations of Embryonic Breathing (Tāixí Zhī Lǐlùn Jīchǔ, 胎息之理論基礎)

From section 1–3, we have already grasped the idea of the Qì circulatory network in a human body. Here, I would like to summarize and review the concept of the eight vessels (Bāmài, 八脈). In order to comprehend the role which the eight vessels play in Qìgōng practice, you must have a clear concept of their function. This is especially true if you practice Nèidān (內丹) (Internal Elixir) Qìgōng.

Reviewing the Eight Vessels

1. The eight vessels include four Yīn Vessels and four Yáng Vessels, which balance each other. These eight vessels not only comprise the major framework of the body's Qì network, they function as Qì reservoirs that regulate the Qì status in the Twelve Primary Qì Channels (Shíèrjīng, 十二經).
2. The eight vessels are generally considered Qì reservoirs able to store Qì. However, much like the difference between Yáng and Yīn primary channels, the Yáng vessels are able to manifest the Qì while the Yīn vessels preserve it.
3. The Conception Vessel is classified as a Yīn vessel to balance the Governing Vessel, which is considered Yáng. The conception Vessel (Rènmài, 任脈) in the front is responsible for regulating the Qì status in the six Yīn primary channels (Qì rivers), while the Governing Vessel (Dūmài, 督脈) governs the Qì status of the six Yáng primary channels. Since the twelve primary Qì channels distribute Qì to the entire body, these two vessels play the controlling role in Qì distribution throughout the physical body.
4. The physical structure of the vessels is very likely constructed of various layers of tendons sandwiched between fasciae. Tendons are known to be better conductors than muscles, while fasciae are considered insulators (poor conductors). This structure comprises a sort of battery that is able to store the Qì to an abundant level. Naturally, Qì flows better in the tendons than in the muscles. For example, if you take a look at the structure of the Governing Vessel, you will see that various layers of tendons attached at the center line of the spine are sandwiched by fasciae (Figure 2–16).
5. The Girdle Vessel (Dàimài, 帶脈) is classified as an extreme Yáng vessel which counterbalances the Thrusting Vessel (Chōngmài, 衝脈) (Spinal Cord), which is considered an extreme Yīn vessel. The Girdle Vessel's Qì expands horizontally, which provides you with physical and mental balance, while the Thrusting Vessel keeps your physical body and mental body centered (Figure 2–17). These two vessels are the two most crucial vessels constituting the mainframe of the Qì network. When Qì expands in the Girdle Vessel, the Guardian Qì (Wèiqì, 衛氣) (Aura Energy) will be strongly manifested, and

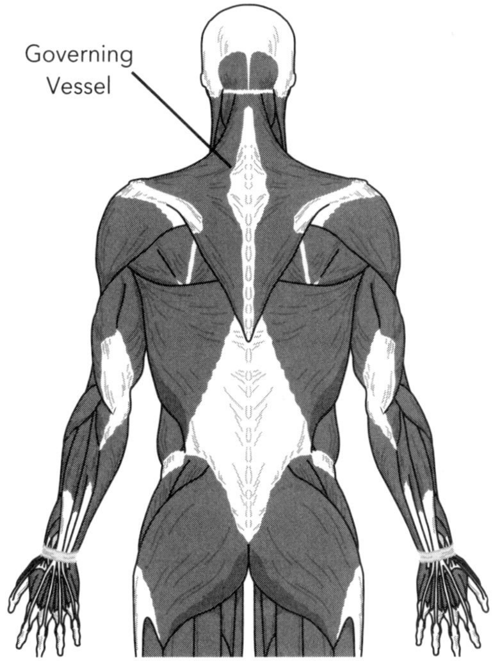

Figure 2-16. Anatomic Structure of the Governing Vessel

the functioning of the immune system will be robust. When the Qì stored in the Thrusting Vessel is abundant, the central energy line will be strong. Consequently, the Shén can be raised to a high level, and the glands located along the central energy line (such as the pineal, pituitary, adrenals, and testicles or ovaries) will also be nourished and produce hormones. In addition, the Marrow Qì can also be abundantly stored, so healthy blood cells can be produced. We will discuss this in more detail in the book: *Qigōng—Grand Circulation for Spiritual Enlightenment*.

6. Once you wake in the morning, you naturally start to use your physical body. Your exhalation is longer than your inhalation, since your mind is now being directed out of your body to your surroundings. The Qì is led outward for manifestation through the Twelve Primary Channels, whose Qì circulation is regulated by the Conception and Governing Vessels, and therefore the Qì is strongly and aggressively circulated in the Conception and Governing Vessels (i.e., the Small Cyclic Circulation). However, when night comes, you fall asleep. Your entire body is relaxed and your inhalation is longer than your exhalation. Consequently, the Qì is led inward to the central energy line, and the Guardian Qì shrinks. When this happens, hormones are produced by the pineal, pituitary, adrenal, and testicular or ovarian glands. The brain obtains Qì nourishment. This may be the reason for dreaming, as the brain cells readjust their energy storage status.

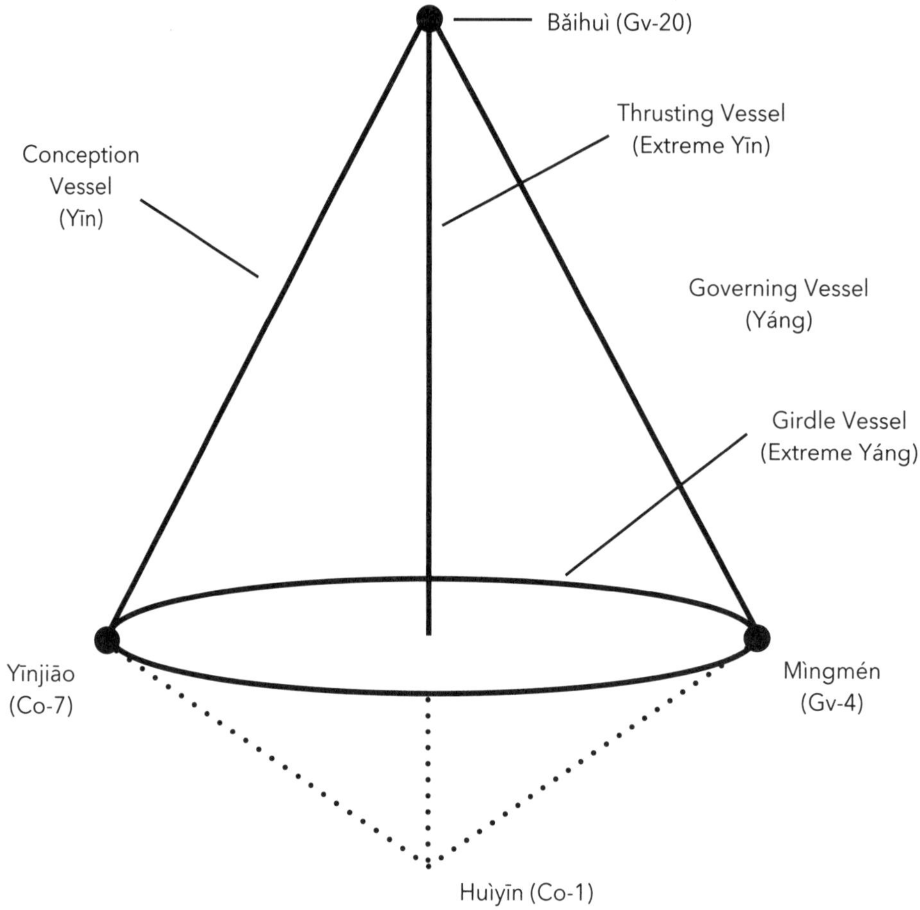

Figure 2-17. Thrusting Vessel and Governing Vessel

This is no different from the Qì cycle of a fish. During the daytime, Qì circulates strongly along the upper and lower contours of the fish. Thus, the fins and tail are moving aggressively. However, when night comes, this Qì circulation weakens and the Qì will be focused at the center line. Electromagnetic waves are emitted from the fish's Third Eye, enabling it to swim around without colliding with obstacles or other fish. (Figure 2–18).[23]

Similarly, in the daytime, a tree's energy emerges upward and outward from the root (i.e., the tree's biobattery) to be exchanged with the energy from the sun. At night, the tree's Qì will return to its center and down to the root (Figure 2–19). Remember, all living things are part of the Dào. Thus, the Dào remains the same through nature. If you are able to comprehend one clearly, you are able to interpret others easily.

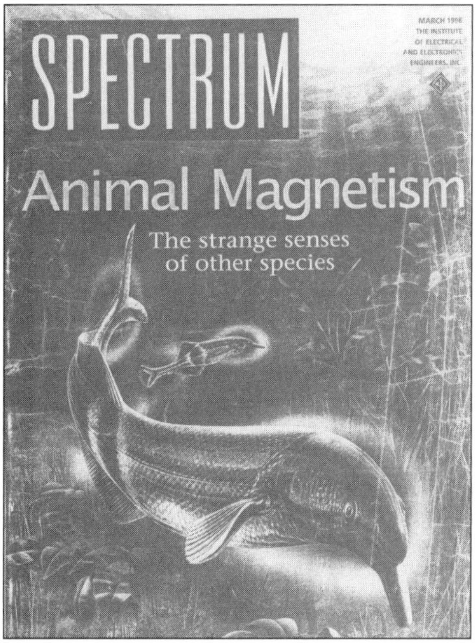

Figure 2-18. How Fish See Things in the Dark

7. The other four vessels exist in pairs. They are the Yīn Heel Vessel (Yīnqiāomài, 陰蹺脈), Yīn Linking Vessel (Yīnwéimài, 陰維脈), Yáng Heel Vessel (Yángqiāomài, 陽蹺脈), and Yáng Linking Vessel (Yángwéimài, 陽維脈). The two Yīn vessels connect at the Huìyīn (Co-1) (會陰) cavity (i.e., the perineum) and meet the other two Yīn vessels, the Conception and Thrusting Vessels. That is why the perineum is named "Huìyīn," which means "meet Yīn." From this, we can see that the Huìyīn is the gate connecting all four Yīn vessels in the body. When this gate opens, the Qì is manifested, and when this gate is closed the Qì is preserved. For example, when you are happy and excited,

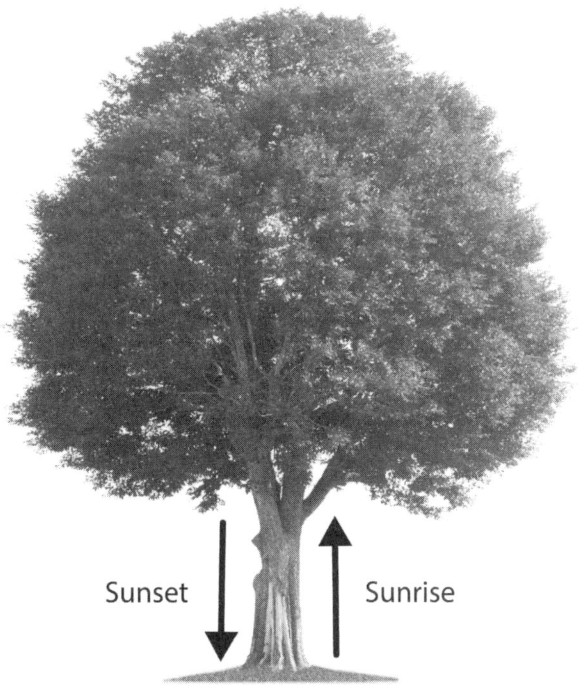

Figure 2-19. The Tree's Energy Moves Upward and Outward in the Daytime, and Moves Downward and Inward at Nighttime

(Photo by Shutterstock)

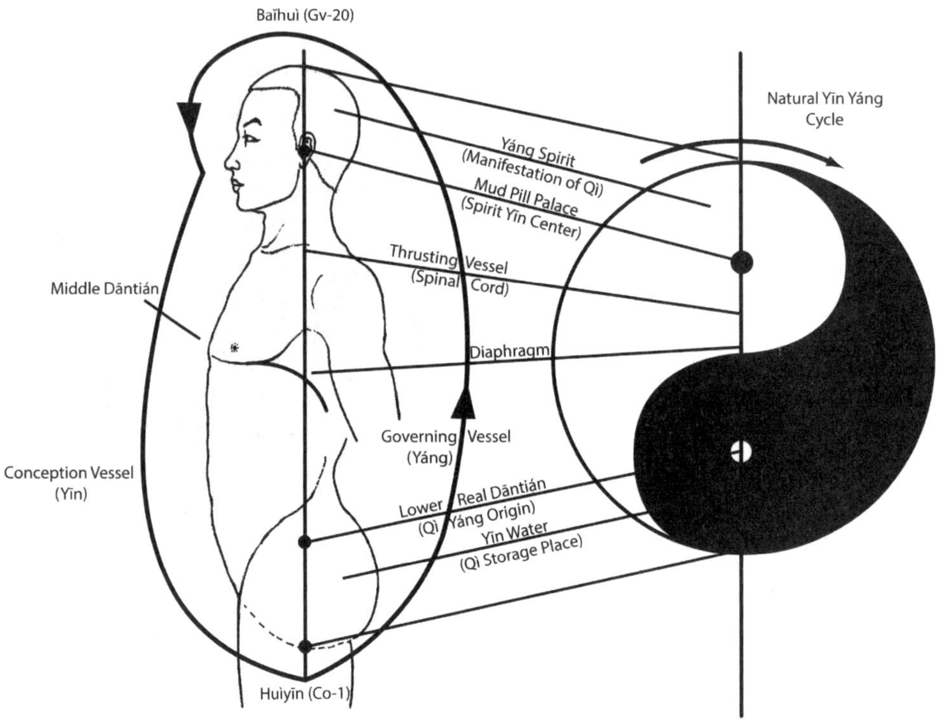

Figure 2-20. The Body's Yīn and Yáng, and the Two Polarity Centers

your exhalation is longer than your inhalation, and the body turns Yáng. This may lead to excess Yáng in the internal organs (especially the heart). When this happens, you will naturally make a sound of "Hā" (哈) while pushing the perineum out (i.e., opening the gate) without thinking. On the contrary, when you are sad or scared, your inhalation is longer than your exhalation and you feel chilly. In order to preserve the Qì in the body, you will hold up the perineum (i.e., close the gate) automatically. In fact, using the perineum to control the Qì status in the body is a crucial hidden key in ancient Qìgōng practice.

Illustration of the Body's Yīn and Yáng Poles. In this subsection, I would like to compare the natural Tàijí Yīn-Yáng symbol with the body's Yīn and Yáng energy structure. From this comparison, you can easily see through many things which may inspire your Qìgōng pondering and practice. Remember, this is only my personal conclusion. You should keep your mind open and see if you are able to discover more links between the human body and the Yīn-Yáng cycle. Since a human body is a part of nature, Qì manifestation in this body should be able to be interpreted by the natural Yīn-Yáng symbol (Figure 2–20).

1. The Qì circulation along the Conception and Governing Vessels (Rènmài, Dūmài; 任脈・督脈) is reversed from the natural Yīn-Yáng cycle so the Yīn and Yáng in the body can be balanced from natural Yīn and Yáng. We will discuss this more in the book: *Qìgōng Meditation Small Circulation*.
2. Shén is generally thought of as Yáng. That is why the term "Yángshén" (陽神) (Yáng Spirit) is commonly used in Chinese Qìgōng documents. Shén is the general who controls the manifestation of the Qì. When Shén is high, the Qì can be controlled and manifested efficiently and effectively. That means once you are able to raise your Shén to a higher level, your vital force will be enhanced. Normally, the raising of the Shén takes place through the Bǎihuì (Gv-20) (百會), located at the top of the Yīn-Yáng symbol, the place of extreme Yáng. "Bǎihuì" means "hundred meetings" and implies the meeting place of the entire body's Qì. That means it is the pivotal controlling point of the entire body's energy. Bǎihuì is considered the most Yáng place of the entire human body.
3. Huìyīn (Co-1) (會陰) is considered as the most Yīn place in a human body. Huìyīn is also commonly called "Hǎidǐ" (海底), meaning "sea bottom." This is because Qì is analogous to water, with the Large and Small Intestines (Qì residence) as the ocean which is able to store the water (Qì). When the Qì stays at its residence, the physical body will be calm and peaceful. However, when the Qì is led away from its residence for manifestation, then the mind and body will be excited, and the Shén will be divergent. In this way the Qì is consumed. The way of maintaining calmness of the mind (and Shén) and of the physical body is to lead the Qì downward. For example, when you are excited, your breathing is shallow and fast, and your body is tensed. In this case, if you are able to calm your mind, inhale deeply, and use your mind to lead the Qì down to the abdominal area, and then exhale while relaxing your mind and physical body, the body's mental and physical tension will disappear gradually. This is one of the crucial keys to lowering high blood pressure in Qìgōng practice. On the contrary, if you lead the Qì upward to the brain, you will become still more excited and tense, and the blood pressure can also be raised.
4. The body's two Poles, Yīn and Yáng, are connected by the Thrusting Vessel (Chōngmài, 衝脈) (Spinal Cord). The top "Spirit Yīn Center," located at the Mud Pill Palace (Níwángōng, 泥丸宮) (the site of the pineal and pituitary glands) in the Yáng Spirit (Yángshén, (陽神) (the brain or Upper Dāntián), controls and restrains the Yángshén's manifestation. This Spirit Yīn Center is like a steering wheel that can govern the status of the Shén's actions. If the Shén can stay at this center, then it can be focused. If the

Shén is away from this center, even if it is high, it is scattered. In order to bring the Shén to this Yīn center, your mind must first be calmed. To keep your mind calm, you must avoid any emotional disturbance and desires. This is one of the main focal points in Qìgōng Embryonic Breathing.
The site of the lower of the two Poles is the Real Lower Dāntián, located at the center of the Large and Small Intestines (Second Brain). This area acts as a bio-battery to store the Qì (bioelectricity). It is in this area that the food essence is absorbed and converted into energy (Qì). In order to keep the Qì at its residence, you must also learn how to keep your mind at the Qì Yáng Origin (Real Lower Dāntián or Center of Gravity). Here the Qì can be preserved and stored to an abundant level (Yáng).

5. The Real Lower Dāntián produces and stores the Qì, and is thus able to increase the quantity of the Qì supplied to the body and brain for them to function. However, the quality of the Qì manifestation is controlled by the Upper Dāntián center (Spirit Yīn Center) (Figure 2–20). With the Girdle Vessel (Extreme Yáng Vessel) and Thrusting Vessel (Extreme Yīn Vessel), it forms a "spiritual cultivation triangle" (Figure 2–21). The more abundant the storage of Qì (strong Guardian Qì), the higher the Shén can be raised. The base of the triangle represents physical life, while the height of the center line represents spiritual life.

Interaction of Yīn and Yáng (Intercourse of Dragon and Tiger) (Lónghǔ Jiāogòu, 龍虎交媾). Once you are able to keep your Shén and Qì at their residences (centers), then you have reached the first goal of "Embracing Singularity" (Bàoyī, 抱一). Remember, these two centers are the two Poles of the same thing: life. They synchronize and correspond with each other. Physically, they are in two places, but in function they must be treated as one. They cannot separate from each other. One is for physical life and the other is for spiritual life.

It was mentioned in Chapter 1 that, according to the available documents, there are two definitions of Embryonic Breathing. The first one is to unite the Shén and the Qì at the Real Lower Dāntián; that is, to return our being to the very beginning of life. Remember, it is from this Real Lower Dāntián that a human life is initiated and developed. Therefore, to many Daoists, the first goal of Embryonic Breathing is to find this center so the Shén and Qì (son and mother) can be united there (Figure 2–22). Since the goal of this breathing practice is to return our beings to their Wújí center (center of gravity), I call this Embryonic Breathing "Wújí Breathing" (Wújíxí, 無極息).

The second definition of Embryonic Breathing is to conceive a "Spiritual Embryo" (Shéntāi, 神胎) at the Huángtíng (黄庭) cavity located between the Middle and Real Lower Dāntiáns. In order to reach this goal, you must learn how to use

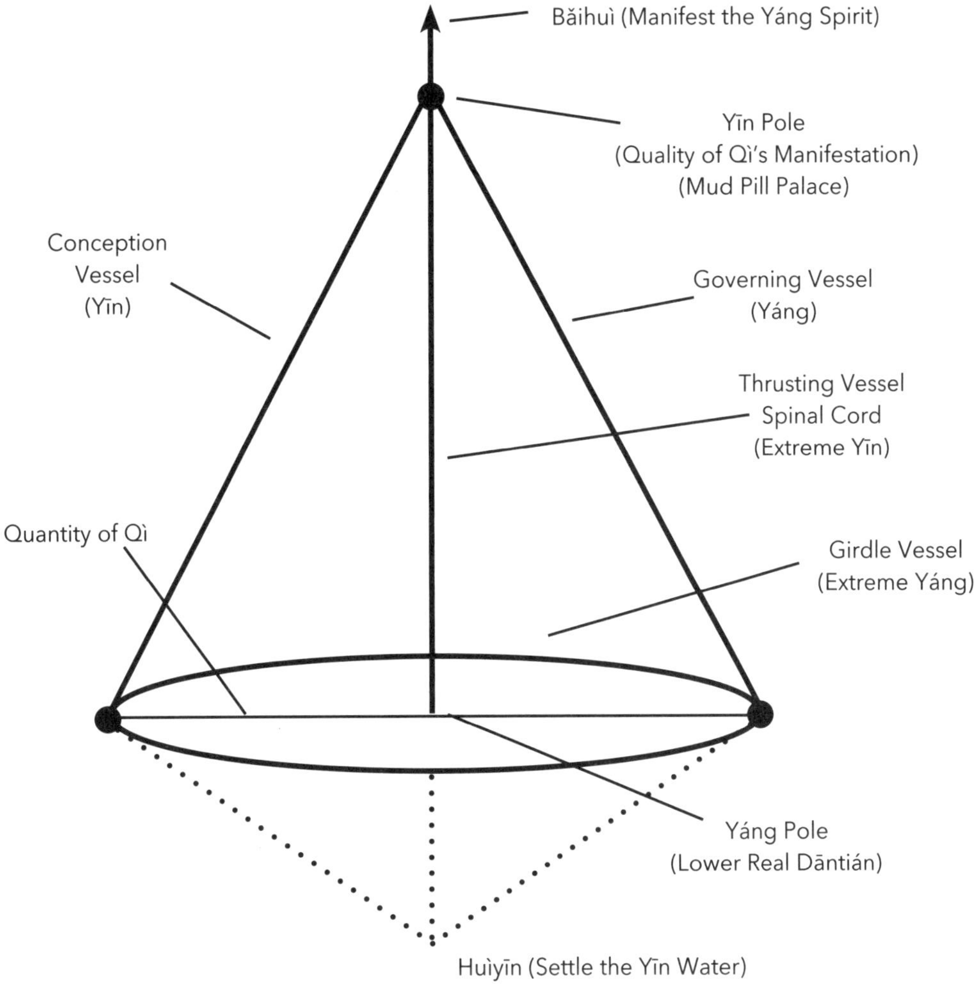

Figure 2-21. Spiritual Triangle

your concentrated Wisdom Mind (Yì, 意) to lead the Fire Qì (Huǒqì, 火氣) (Post-Birth Qì) down from the Middle Dāntián and the Water Qì (Shuǐqì, 水氣) (Pre-Birth Qì) up from the Real Lower Dāntián, and allow them to meet at the Huángtíng cavity (Figure 2-23). This process is called "the Intercourse of Dragon and Tiger" (Lónghǔ Jiāogòu, 龍虎交媾), which refers to the interaction of Yīn and Yáng, and is also called Kǎn-Lí (離) (water-fire). Having done this, you will lead the Shén down from the Upper Dāntián to unite with this Qì so the Spiritual Embryo can be conceived.

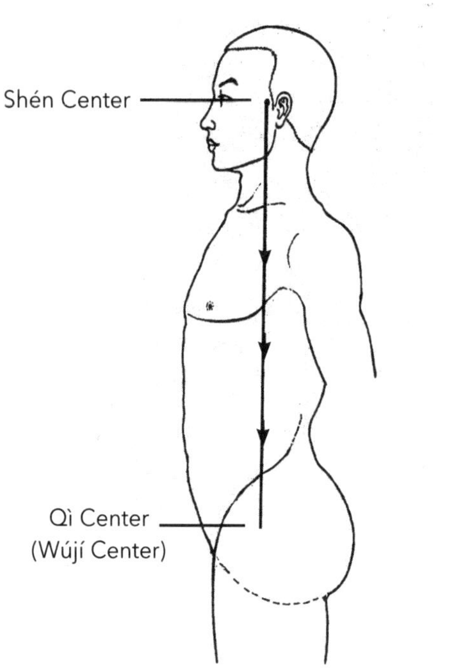

Figure 2-22. Unification of Shén and Qì at the Wújí Center

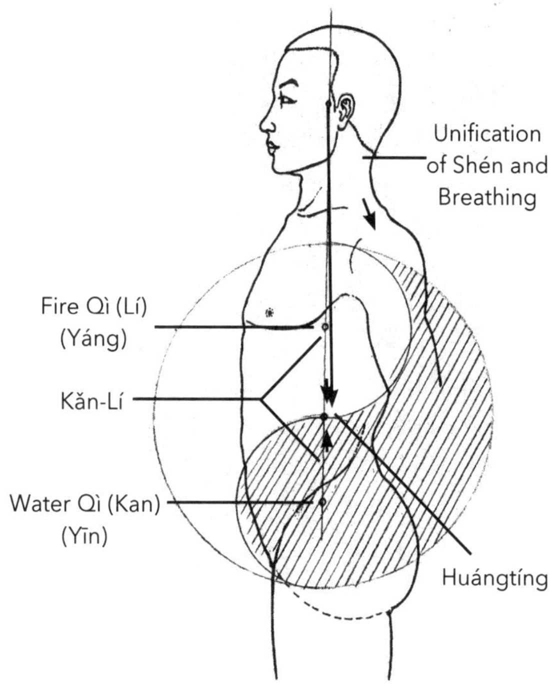

Figure 2-23. Conceiving the Spiritual Embryo

Summaries

1. Within the Daoist document *The Complete Book of Principal Contents of Human Life and Temperament* (*Xìngmìng Guīzhǐ Quánshū*, 性命圭旨全書), the section "About Large and Small Tripod and Furnace" ("Dàxiǎo Dǐnglú Shuō," 大小鼎爐說) says: "Huángtíng (黃庭) is the tripod, Qìxuè (氣穴) (Qì cavity) is the furnace. Huángtíng is just on the top of the Qìxuè, mutually connected with numerous Luò (絡) (secondary Qì channels), and is the meeting place of hundreds of Qì vessels (and channels) in a human body. The Original Qì (Yuánqì, 元氣) is dense between these two cavities (between Huángtíng and Qìxuè) and is called 'Small Tripod Furnace' (Xiǎodǐnglú, 小鼎爐). If 'the position of Qián (乾) (the brain or head) is the tripod and the position of the Kūn (坤) (the abdomen) is the furnace,' then it means that the Níwán (泥丸) (Upper Dāntián or brain) is the tripod and the Lower Dāntián is the furnace. This is called 'Big Tripod Furnace' (Dàdǐnglú, 大鼎爐)."[24] This document has offered you an idea of major sites explained in the large Yīn-Yáng and Small Yīn-Yáng symbols and how they relate to a human body (Figures 2–24 and 2–25). Please read Chapter 3 for a detailed explanation of the tripod (Dǐng, 鼎) and furnace (Lú, 爐).

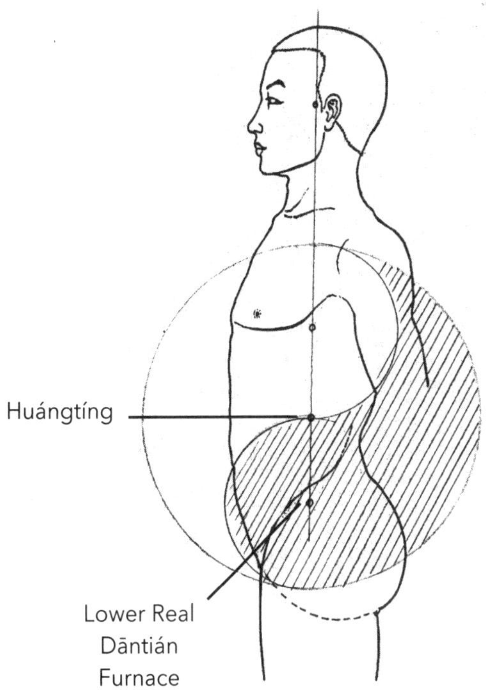

Figure 2-24. Small Tripod and Furnace

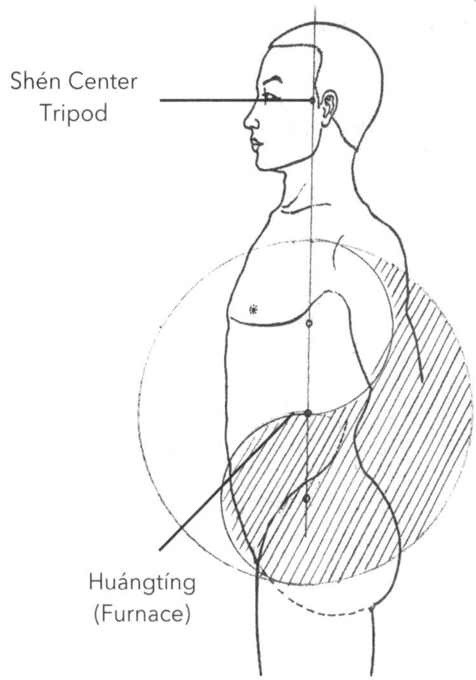

Figure 2-25. Large Tripod and Furnace

2. In the "Small Tripod Furnace" (Xiǎodǐnglú, 小鼎爐), first you are searching for the Wújí state of Kǎn (坎) (Water Qì) and Lí (離) (Fire Qì). That means bringing the Fire Qì and Water Qì to the Huángtíng (Qì cavity) and allowing them to meet and interact there. This is the process of Yīn-Yáng interaction or Dragon-Tiger intercourse. In order to conceive a Spiritual Embryo at Huángtíng, the Shén must be brought down to Huángtíng and unified with the Qì. This is called "the unification of the Shén and the Qì" (Shénqì Xiànghé, 神氣相合). When this happens, the "Spiritual Embryo" (Shéntāi, 神胎) can be conceived. Later, when the Spiritual Embryo is matured, then it can be led upward for the cultivation of spiritual enlightenment (i.e., to reopen the Third Eye).
3. In the "Big Tripod Furnace" (Dàdǐnglú, 大鼎爐), you are looking for the Wújí (無極) (No Extremity or No Discrimination) state of your original being; that is, returning your life to the very beginning. Therefore, after you have located the two Poles of the body, you will bring your Shén downward to the Real Lower Dāntián to unite with the Qì. This is the process of returning the life to its origin.

2.4 Meanings and Purposes of Meditation (Jìngzuò Zhī Yìyì Yǔ Mùdì, 靜坐之意義與目的)

If we look carefully, we can see that meditation practice has existed in almost every culture in the world, especially in religious societies. There are many ways of meditation, and, depending on one's purpose, the training methods are also different. In this section, I would like to explain the possible meaning and the purposes of meditation. Then, I will summarize those meditation practices from Chinese Qìgōng society.

General Meanings and Purposes of Meditation

1. **Searching for a Peaceful Mind.** The first and the most common purpose of meditation is probably the search for a relaxed, peaceful, and harmonious mind. Generally, our mind is emotionally agitated by the surrounding environment. When this happens, the mind becomes scattered, confused, and excited, and it consequently leads us to a state of emotional disturbance. Through meditation with deep, profound breathing, we are able to calm down and make our mind clear.

   Measurements with an EEG (electroencephalogram) machine show four groups of different brain waves (oscillating electrical currents), which research has associated with different activities. Normally, brain waves are classified according to frequency bands in cycles per second (Hz). These four categories are (Figure 2–26):[26]

   1. Beta activity (above 13 Hz): Occurs in bursts in the anterior part of the brain and is associated with mental activity.
   2. Alpha activity (8–13 Hz): Relaxation; is abolished by attention
   3. Theta activity (4 to less than 8 Hz): Drowsy and asleep
   4. Delta activity (below 4 Hz): Deep sleep and coma

   From these classifications, we can see that when we are awake and involved in heavy thinking (Beta), the activity is busy and the signals are weak (i.e., the amplitude is low). We can see that on average, there are thirteen or more thoughts per second passing through our brain. Once we are relaxed (Alpha), the number of oscillations is significantly reduced. Furthermore, the amplitude is increased, though still weak. This means that when you are relaxed, your mind is more clear, calm, and peaceful. This implies that concentration is increased. When you are in a drowsy or sleeping state, the number of oscillations is also reduced, but the thoughts are more irregular (Theta). Once you are in a deep, sound sleep (Delta), the number of oscillations is reduced to only a few and the oscillation amplitude is also significantly increased. From the fundamental principles of physics, we know that the power of oscillation is:[27]

$$P = \text{Frequency}^2 \times \text{Amplitude}^2$$

This implies that when you are in a deep sleeping state, although your conscious mind is not heavily involved in thought (frequency reduced), the brain cells are obtaining a strong supply of nutrition, oxygen and Qì nourishment. In this calm state, there is less distortion or disturbance in the brain. Under these extremely calm and relaxed conditions, if you are nevertheless able to maintain consciousness, you can build up a better sensitivity for energy correspondence with the outside world. This is one of the desired states in meditation practice; there are also other states that correspond to different meditation goals.

In meditation, you are trying to reach the state in which the brain waves are between Theta and Delta. This means that you seem to be sleeping, yet your conscious mind is still governing your being. According to Chinese meditation theory, this is the state of semi-sleeping, or a self-hypnotic state. In this state, the brain's sensitivity to or energy correspondence with natural vibrations, including other brain waves, reaches a peak. It is in this stage that a meditator seeks for the connection between his spiritual being and the spirit of nature.

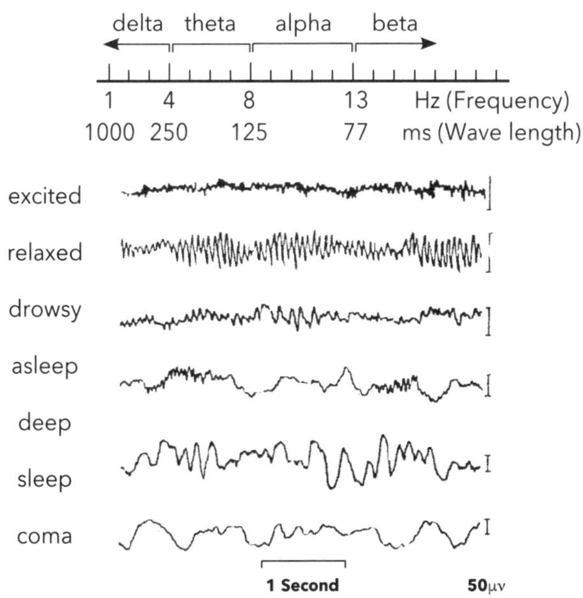

Figure 2-26. Typical Brain Wave Patterns From a State of Excitement to One of Deep Coma

2. **Healing and Improving Health.** When the mind is relaxed and calm, the physical body will also be relaxed and calm. From past experience, we know that the more profound the meditative state the mind reach, the deeper the body is able to relax. When both the mental and physical body are relaxed, the Qì will be able to circulate in the body smoothly and naturally. In this case, irregular Qì circulation due to illness or any other reason can be regulated to a harmonious healthy state. According to Chinese medical science, this is the primary method of maintaining health and healing. In addition, during the deep meditative and relaxed state, the mind-body communication will be efficient and effectively carried out. When this happens, you will be able to use your mind to lead the Qì and regulate it to a healthy state. With the mind's concentration, the Qì circulation will be stronger and, consequently, the healing process will be faster.
   In addition, during deep meditation the breathing will be deep, soft, and slender. When this happens, you are able to more efficiently absorb oxygen and expel carbon dioxide. From Western science, we already know that each brain cell consumes at least twelve times more oxygen than other cells. This implies that the oxygen supply is a crucial factor in maintaining healthy brain function. Not only that, through deep exhalation of carbon dioxide, waste in the deep places of the body can be brought out. This is the important key for the process of cellular replacement in our body to be successful.

3. **Finding the Center of Self-Being.** Normally, when you calm down, your mind will become clear and its thinking can be logical. Naturally, you must also stop yourself from indulging in fantasy. Whenever your imagination begins to take you away from reality, you must continue to lead the thought back to reality. Otherwise, you may enter into deep fantasy, which is called "entering the devil" (Rùmó, 入魔) in Chinese meditation. The best way to stop it is to pay attention to the breathing and keep the mind straight and truthful.
   In Buddhist and Daoist religion, normally there are four steps involved in the process of cultivating meditation to reach spiritual freedom. The first step is "self-recognition" (Zìshì, 自識). In this first step, the mask on your face starts to drop off, which allows you to see your spiritual being more clearly. Mistakes and lies you have committed and hidden in your subconscious mind will gradually appear in your conscious mind. In Chinese Qìgōng society, it is believed that your subconscious mind is always truthful and is associated with the spiritual being. Once your mask drops off, you must face your real self. You must face the past and analyze it. Not only that, in order to gain permanent emotional

balance, you must search for ways to let go of the feeling of guilt hidden deep inside you. This process will make you humbleand better able to understand yourself, and will finally help you find the center of your being.

The second step is "self-awareness" (Zìjué, 自覺). In this step, if you pay attention, you will be aware of your spiritual being and the problems existing within yourself. Not only that, you will start to recognize the existence of other spiritual beings. You will slowly and gradually pay more attention to your thinking and behavior, and that of others as well. From this awareness, you will be able to understand your existence, your problems, and the role you should play in this society. Through this "self-awareness" meditation process, you will establish a calm and peaceful mind that allows you to harmonize with others and with nature.

4. **Seeking and Understanding the Meaning of our Lives.** From awareness, you gradually enter the third stage of cultivation, that of "self-awakening" (Zìxǐng, Zìwù; 自醒・自悟). From self-awareness, you have paid attention, collected information, and understood yourself and your environment. Now you gradually start to wake up and see things differently. Many people, after awakening, have seen how ugly human spiritual beings are, and decided to become hermits or monks and keep away from lay society. Many others, after awakening, change their thinking about the meaning of life. Still others are able to build their confidence and make their lives more meaningful.

5. **Searching for Spiritual Freedom.** Many people, once having awakened, start to realize how we have been abused by political and spiritual leaders, both spiritually and physically. They start to search for ways to achieve "freedom from spiritual bondage" (Jiětuō, 解脫) or "spiritual independence." When you have reached this stage, your spiritual being does not have to rely on someone else. Naturally, in this case, you will not easily be abused.

6. **Comprehending the Meaning of this Universe.** Even many non-religious people in China, through meditation, are trying to comprehend the meaning, the root, or the origin of nature. In other words, they are searching for the truth of the Dào. To reach this goal, the first step is to search for the root of our lives (Shēngmìng Zhīběn，生命之本). Since we are a part of nature, by understanding the root of our lives, we are able to comprehend the meaning of nature. The search for this root is called "Embracing the Origin" (Bàoyuán, 抱元) or "Embracing Singularity" (Bàoyī, 抱一).

"Embracing" here means to keep, to maintain, to enfold, and to cherish. To find the origin of our spiritual and physical lives, Chinese Qìgōng practitioners pay attention to the "Three Origins" (Sānyuán, 三元) of our lives: Original Essence (Yuánjīng, 元精), Original Qì (Yuánqì, 元氣), and Original Spirit (Yuánshén, 元神). It is believed that by understanding and cultivating these three origins, we will be able to find the truth of our lives. It is also thought that the Original Spirit is the origin of the other two, since it existed even before physical life. Therefore, searching for the spiritual root has become the most important cultivation in all Chinese societies. The Daoist family says: "Cultivate the Xīn (emotional mind) to cultivate the human temperament. Keep the center and Embrace the Singularity (very origin)."[28] The Scholar family says: "Exist the Xīn (pay attention to the Xīn) to cultivate the human temperament. Maintain the center, thread together (i.e., comprehend completely) the one (origin)."[29] The Buddhist family says: "To brighten (understand clearly) the Xīn to meet the human temperament. Millions of methods return to one."[30] The Medical family says: "Void Xīn (humble mind) to stabilize the human temperament, embrace the origin and keep singularity (origin)."[31] It is explained in a classic, *Classic of Great Peace* (*Tàipíngjīng*, 太平經), about the "one." It is said: "Ponder to keep singleness, why? What is singleness? The beginning of the counting number; what is the one, the Dào of begetting; what is one, the beginning of the raising Qì; what is one, the principle of the heaven and the earth (universe)."[32] From this, you can see that "the one" means the very origin of every thing, or even of energy. According to the *Book of Changes* (*Yìjīng*, 易經), this "one" refers to the state of Wújí (無極) (No Extremity). What is meant by the Scholar's family that says "to go through the one?" It is explained in a Daoist book, *The Complete Book of Principal Contents of Human Life and Temperament* (*Xìngmìng Guīzhǐ Quánshū*, 性命圭旨全書): "What the scholar means by 'to go through the one' is to use the original body to thread together (understand) (human nature)."[33] It is also said in the Daoist family that: "Dào, (use) the one to thread (understand thoroughly)."[34]

In China, meditation has existed in almost every level of society. In Chinese medical and scholar societies, meditation is commonly called "Jìngzuò" (靜坐) which means "sit quietly." In these societies, meditation is used to search for ways to bring the mind to a peaceful, neutral, and calm state. It is believed that many illnesses and human mental pain are generated from the mind's emotional disturbance. If we are able to neutralize the imbalance of the emotional mind, we will remove the cause of sickness and emotional pain. Therefore, this kind of meditation has also commonly been considered as meditation for the layperson. Naturally, it remains at the level of regulating the mind, and the level of regulating the spirit is not actively pursued.

However, meditation in Chinese martial society focuses not only on regulating the emotional mind, but also on pursuing the meaning of life and the way to raise the Shén. When the Shén is raised, the Qì can be effectively led to the physical body for power manifestation (Yáng manifestation). When the meaning of life is pondered and comprehended during meditation, a peaceful mind can be achieved (Yīn calmness). From this Yīn and Yáng balance, a person will be able to reach deep martial skill as well as profound understanding of harmony and peace. Here, I would like to point out an important fact: since most of the well-known Chinese martial styles—Shàolín (少林), Tàijí (太極), Wǔdāng (武當), Éméi (峨嵋), Tiānshān (天山), Qīngchéng (青城), Kūnlún (崑崙), Kōngdòng (崆峒), etc.—were developed in religious monasteries, all of the meditation methods and purposes in these styles are heavily influenced by religious meditation. In many ways, they cannot even be separated.

Finally, religious meditation is called "Zuòchán" (坐禪) (meaning "sit for Chán") by Buddhists, and "Dǎzuò" (打坐) ("engaged sitting") by Daoists. Chán (禪) means to relate or to associate with Buddhism, which includes to cultivate, to refine, and to pursue Buddhahood. In the Buddhist classic *Āhánjīng* (阿含經) it says: "Sitting for Chán and ponder for the origin, do not be neglectful and lazy."[25] That means through Chán meditation, you are searching for the origin of spiritual life.

The final goal of religious meditation is enlightenment (Daoism) or Buddhahood (Buddhism). Religious meditation has been recognized as the highest level of meditation in Chinese society. The monks are not only searching for the peaceful and harmonious mind by neutralizing their emotional mind, but also aiming for the unification of the human spirit and the nature spirit (Tiānrén Héyī, 天人合一). In order to reach this goal, the Qì storage in the Real Lower Dāntián must be abundant. The abundant Qì can then serve two purposes: to strengthen the physical body, and to nourish the brain to an enlightened state. When the body is strong, physical life will be long, allowing you a longer time for spiritual cultivation. When the brain is nourished to a high level, the Third Eye can be re-opened. Then our spirit and the natural spirit will be reunited, and the meaning of life will be understood.

From the above, you can see that different societies aim for different purposes. When you train meditation, first ask yourself: What are the purposes of my meditation training—a peaceful mind? Martial arts? Enlightenment? Second, you must ask: how do I reach the goal? Do I know the way? How do I find the correct way? Do I have enough patience, perseverance, and commitment to pursue my goal?

If you are interested in spiritual cultivation through Internal Elixir (Nèidān, 內丹) Qìgōng practice, the first step is learning Embryonic Breathing (Tāixí, 胎息). Through correct Embryonic Breathing, you will be able to find your spiritual center and Qì center. Later, you will unify the spirit and the Qì at the Real Lower Dāntián and reach the state of "Embracing Singularity" (Bàoyī, 抱一). This is the state of "Wújí" (無極), the state of returning life to its origin. In addition, through Embryonic Breathing the Qì can be built up to an abundant level and stored at the Lower Dāntián. This is the crucial key to Muscle/Tendon Changing and Marrow/Brain Washing Qìgōng practice.

To reach the goal of Muscle/Tendon Changing, you must learn "Small Cyclic Heaven" (Xiǎozhōutiān, 小周天) (Small Circulation) meditation. The purpose of the Small Circulation is for the mind to lead the Qì to circulate smoothly and abundantly in the Conception and Governing Vessels (Rènmài, Dūmài; 任脈・督脈). Then the Qì in the twelve primary Qì channels will also be smooth and abundant, and your physical body will become conditioned and healthy.

To reach the goal of spiritual enlightenment, you must learn Brain Washing Grand Circulation. This is to lead the Qì from the Real Lower Dāntián through the Thrusting Vessel (Chōngmài, 衝脈) to the brain to activate more brain cells and energize them to a higher vital state. When this happens, the Third Eye can be re-opened. This is the state of "enlightenment."

Embryonic Breathing is only the first step toward reaching any of these goals. Its practice is crucial to achieve longevity or spiritual enlightenment. Therefore, you must read this book carefully, ponder it, and then practice what you have learned. Once you have established a habit for your meditation, soon you will realize that you are dancing in a spiritual garden which is hard to describe to other people.

References

1. 《易》曰：〝一陰一陽之謂道。〞
2. 《道德經・四十二章》：〝道生一，一生二，二生三，三生萬物。〞
3. 《道德經・二十五章》：〝有物混成，先天地生。寂兮寥兮，獨立而不改，周行而不殆，可以為天下母。吾不知其名，強字之曰道。〞
4. 《道德經・一章》：〝玄之又玄，眾妙之門。〞
5. 《道德經・五十一章》：〝道生之，德畜之，物形之，勢成之。〞指萬物變化。
6. 《道德經・二十五章》：〝人法地，地法天，天法道，道法自然。〞指以自然為法。
7. 《淮南子・天文訓》：〝道始于一，一而不生，故分為陰陽，陰陽和合而萬物生。〞
8. 《道德經・一章》：〝無，名先天之始；有，名萬物之母。常無，欲以觀其妙；常有，欲以觀其徼。〞指事物正在變化之中。
9. 指事物一分為二，合二而一的對立統一規律。
10. 《朱子語類》：〝謂之太極者，所以指天地萬物之根。〞
11. "Life's Invisible Current," by Albert L. Huebner, *East West Journal*, June 1986.
12. *The Body Electric*, by Robert O. Becker, M.D. and Gary Selden, Quill, William Morrow, New York, 1985.

13. "Healing with Nature's Energy," by Richard Leviton, *East West Journal*, June 1986.

14. *A Child is Born, by Lennart Nilsson*, A DTP/Seymour Lawrence Book, 1990.

15. *A Study of Anatomic Physiology* (解剖生理學)，李文森編著。華杏出版股份有限公司。 Lǐ, Wén-Sēn, Táipěi, 1986.

16. *Grant's Atlas of Anatomy*, James E. Anderson, 7th Edition, Williams & Wilkins Co., 9–92, 1978.

17. *Complex and Hidden Brain in the Gut Makes Stomachaches and Butterflies*, by Sandra Blakeslee, The New York Times, Science, January 23, 1996.

18. *The Second Brain: The Scientific Basis of Gut Instinct and a Groundbreaking New Understanding of Nervous Disorders of the Stomach and Intestine*, Michael D. Gershon, New York: Harper Collins Publications, 1998.

19. *Fundamentals of Physics*, Holliday and Resnick, pp. 512–514. John Wiley & Sons, Inc. 1972.

20. *Bioenergetics*, by Albert L. Lehninger, pp. 5–6, W. A, Benjamin, Inc. Menlo Park, California, 1971.

21. *Photographic Anatomy of the Human Body*, by J. W. Rohen, 邯鄲出版社， Táipěi, Táiwān, 1984.

22. "Restoring Ebbing Hormones May Slow Aging," by Jane E. Brody, *The New York Times*, July 18, 1995.

23. "Animal Magnetism, The Strange Senses of Other Species," p. 32, *IEEE Spectrum*, March, 1996.

24. 《性命圭旨全書 》（大小鼎爐說）：〝黃庭為鼎，氣穴為爐。黃庭正在氣穴上，縷絡相連，乃人身百脈交會之處。〞元氣氤氳二穴之間，謂之〝小鼎爐。〞〝乾位為鼎，坤位為爐。〞即泥丸宮為鼎，下丹田為爐，謂之〝大鼎爐。〞

25. 《阿含經》：〝坐禪思惟，莫有懈怠。〞

26. *The New Encyclopedia Britannica*, Vol. 4, Encyclopedia Britannica Inc., 1993.

27. *Fundamentals of Physics*, David Holliday and Robert Resnick, p. 308, John Wiley & Sons, Inc. New York, NY, 1970.

28. 道家：修心養性，守中抱一。

29. 儒家：存心養性，執中貫一。

30. 佛家：明心見性，萬法歸一。

31. 醫家：虛心定性，抱元守一。

32. 《太平經》：〝以思守一，何也？一者，數之始也；一者，生之道也；一者，元氣所起也；一者，天地之綱紀也。〞

33. 《性命圭旨全書．大道說》：〝儒之一貫者，以此本體之一而貫之也。〞

34. 道，一以貫之。

PART II

Translations and Commentaries of Ancient Documents Related to Embryonic Breathing

CHAPTER 3

Translations and Commentaries of Ancient Documents

3.1 Introduction (Jièshào, 介紹)

More than 150 documents related to Embryonic Breathing practice, written throughout nearly four thousand years of Chinese Qìgōng history, are now available. Many of these documents focus on theory, while others emphasize the general concept of the practice. Naturally, the contents of many of these documents are redundant or repetitious. I have read and filtered them, studied and experimented with them, and searched for possible explanations written in each document. With all of these efforts, I still believe that there are many more related documents that I have not yet discovered. However, through the available documents, I am able to conclude and formalize a clear idea of what Embryonic Breathing is, the theory behind it, and its practice methods.

From these ancient documents, we are able to see the verification and achievement of this spiritual practice. This provides us with encouragement, confidence, and inspiration to pursue our final goal of spiritual enlightenment. In order to benefit from these documents, we should have a correct attitude when we study them. We should remain humble, feel deep appreciation, and establish our confidence. We should be open-minded, yet we should not hesitate to challenge the statements in the documents, to test them, and to verify them. We should try to judge the entire practice from a logical and scientific point of view. Study these documents repeatedly and ponder them carefully. This will lead us to the path of profound internal feeling.

Such an internal sensitivity will enable us to find our true natural identity and the real meaning of our lives. It will also lead us to appreciate the greatness of the natural universe. We can free ourselves from the matrix of spiritual bondage that has been formalized over the course of human history. Only if we are able to liberate ourselves from this human spiritual matrix, can we expect to have a neutral mind to further develop our spiritual science. We must recognize that all religions created in the past are spiritual matrices which act against the true science which continues to pursue the truth of nature.

Most of these documents originated in Daoist and Buddhist society, with a few coming from Scholarly and Medical societies. Documents produced by martial arts society are very scarce. Even though there are some, their discussion and practice remains superficial.

The majority of the documents translated and commented upon in this book are from the following sources, 1–7:

1. *Dào Dé Jīng and Qìgōng* (道德經與氣功), by Dīng, Xīn-Bǎi (丁辛百) and Pān, Míng-Huán (潘明環), 安徽科學技術出版社, Ānhuī, China 1996.
2. *Chinese Qìgōng Dictionary* (中國氣功辭典), by Lǚ, Guāng-Róng (呂光榮), 人民衛生出版社, Běijīng, China, 1988.
3. *The Great Completion of Chinese Qìgōng* (中國氣功大成), by Fāng, Chūn-Yáng (方春陽), 吉林科學技術出版社, Jílín, China, 1989.
4. *The Study of Practical Chinese Medical Qìgōng* (實用中醫氣功學), by Mǎ, Jì-Rén (馬濟人), 上海科學技術出版社, Shànghǎi, China, 1992.
5. *The Complete Book of Nourishing the Life in Chinese Daoist Qìgōng* (中國道教氣功養生大全), by Lǐ, Yuǎn-Guó (李遠國), 四川辭書出版社, Chéngdū, Sìchuān, China, 1991.
6. *The Great Completion of Chinese Life Nourishing* (中國養生大成), by Fāng, Chūn-Yáng (方春陽), 吉林科學技術出版社, Jílín, China, 1992.
7. *Important Collection of Concealed Daoist Qìgōng* (道藏氣功要集), by Hóng, Pī-Mó (洪丕謨), 上海書店, Shànghǎi, China, 1991.

Before you read the next section, you should understand that it is very difficult to translate ancient Chinese writings. Because of the cultural differences, many expressions would not make sense to the Westerner if translated literally. Often, knowledge of the historical context is necessary. Furthermore, since in Chinese every sound has several possible meanings, when anyone tries to understand a poem or write it down, he has to choose from among these meanings. For this reason, many of the poems or articles have several variations. The same problem occurs when the poems or articles are read. Many Chinese characters also have several possible meanings, so reading involves interpretation of the text, even for the Chinese reader. Also, the meaning of many words has changed over the course of time. When you add to this the grammatical differences (generally no tenses, articles, singular or plural, or differentiation between parts of speech) you find that it is almost impossible to translate Chinese literally into English. In addition to all this, the translator must have much the same experience and understanding, as well as similar intuitive feelings as the original author, in order to convey the correct meaning.

With these difficulties in mind, I have attempted to convey as much of the original meaning of the Chinese as possible based on my own Qìgōng experience and understanding. Although it is impossible to fully translate the original meaning, I feel I have managed to express the majority of the important points. The translation has been made as close to the original Chinese as possible, including such things as double negatives, and at times, idiosyncratic sentence structure. Words that are implied but not actually written in the Chinese text have been included in parentheses. Also, some Chinese words are followed by the English in parentheses, for example Shén (Spirit).

In order to assist your understanding, I have included commentaries from my personal understanding of the documents. Again, it is not easy to offer you a perfect commentary with 100% accuracy. Many specialized Qìgōng terminologies were used in the past, and these terms can have different meanings depending on when, how, where, and by whom they were used. For example, the crown of the head is called "Bǎihuì" (Gv-20) (百會) (Hundred Meetings) by medical society, "Tiānlínggài" (天靈蓋) (Cover of Natural Spiritual Divine) or "Níwángōng" (泥丸宮) (Mud Pill Palace) by Daoists. In order to translate these terms correctly, I have consulted many Qìgōng dictionaries and documents and searched for the best answer. Often, it does not make sense when you read the translation; however, after you read and understand the commentaries, the documents can be understood.

To make it easier for you, I have tried to classify these documents according to their main focus. Through this effort, I hope you can establish a structural sense from the beginning. In section 3-2, I have included those documents which talk about the general concept of Embryonic Breathing. Next, I have gathered those which talk about the Dāntián in section 3-3. Then, I have classified those related to the concept of regulating the breathing, the mind, and the spirit in section 3-4, 3-5, and 3-6, respectively. As to the training methods, I have included them in section 3-7. Finally, the last section includes a few documents that do not belong to any of the above categories.

3.2 General Concepts (Yībān Gàiniàn, 一般概念)

1. Dào Dé Jīng (Chapter 10)[1]

《道德經・十章》

When bearing and managing the Pò (Vital Spirit) and embracing (maintaining) it to a singularity (simplicity), can it be not separating? When concentrating the Qì to reach its softness, can it be as (soft as) a baby? When cleansing the thought to reach its purity, can it be flawless? When loving the people and ruling the country, can it be no ruling? The opening and closing of the Heaven Gate, can it be (calm and tender) as a female? To comprehend (nature) and reach the four directions (everywhere), can it be known without knowing? When bearing and raising, (if one can) bear without keeping it to self, raising without being meritorious, leading without controlling, then this is the way of "profound natural virtue."

載營魄抱一，能無離乎？專氣致柔，能如嬰兒乎？滌除玄鑒，能無疵乎？愛民治國，能無為乎？天門開闔，能為雌乎？明白四達，能無知乎？生之畜之，生而不有，為而不恃，長而不宰，是謂玄德。

The book commonly known as *Dào Dé Jīng* (道德經), also called *Lǎozi* (老子), was written by Lǎozi (604–531 BCE) during the Chinese Zhōu Dynasty (周朝) (1122–255 BCE). Lǎozi was also named Lǐěr (李耳) or Lǎodān (老聃), and nicknamed Bóyáng (伯陽). Scholarly Daoism originated from Lǎozi's philosophy. Later, during the Chinese Eastern Hàn Dynasty (Dōnghàn) (東漢) (25–220 CE), Zhāng, Dào-Líng (張道陵) combined Daoist and Buddhist philosophies and created a religious Daoism, called "Dàojiào" (道教).

In *Dào Dé Jīng*, there are many sayings related to Qìgōng practice, especially Embryonic Breathing and spiritual cultivation. Unfortunately, almost all of the interpretations of *Dào Dé Jīng* were done by Chinese scholars instead of Qìgōng experts, so there are very few Chinese books or English translations available that show the relationship of the *Dào Dé Jīng* to Qìgōng practice. This chapter is one of few which talk about the cultivation of spiritual life and Qì, as well as the purification of human nature and personality.

In the first sentence, you must first understand the meaning of Pò (魄). Pò is the vital spirit which is supported by vital energy (Qì) when a person is alive. When a person is dead, the Pò becomes Hún (魂) (Soul), which means the spirit after death. When we were born, the spirit incarnated into our physical body and, with Qì nourishment, became Pò. Pò enables us to manage our lives vigorously. However, in the process, we must keep our spirit in its spiritual center, and not allow it to be confused and influenced by the surrounding environment. This spiritual training, keeping the spirit in its original simplicity, is called "Bàoyī" (抱一), meaning "Embracing Singularity" or "Embracing Simplicity." Therefore, the first sentence asks: when handling our spirit, can we keep it simple (pure) and maintain it at its residence without distraction?

Not only that, Qì is the inner energy that supports our physical life and continues to nourish our spirit. Can the Qì circulation be as soft as a baby? Since the air (Kōngqì, 空氣) (External Qì) is related to the inner Qì, it is also commonly believed that when this chapter mentions Qì, it is referring to the breath. We know that the body's inner energy is generated by metabolism, the conversion of glucose into bio-energy. During this process, an abundant oxygen supply is necessary. The greater the oxygen supply, the more energy can be produced. That is why when we lift weights or push a car, we must first inhale deeply in order to generate more power.

The third important point raised in this chapter is about the mind. It asks: can we keep our mind simple and pure, so there is no disturbance or confusion about life? In a common Qìgōng analogy, the Mind is the king of a country, the Body is the country, and Qì is the populace. Therefore, the sentence means that when you use the mind to love and lead the Qì, and use it to nourish the physical body, you can reach the stage of "regulating without regulating."

Tiānmén (天門) means "Heaven Gate" and refers to the "Third Eye" that allows you to communicate with nature. The Third Eye is also called "Yìntáng" (印堂) in Chinese medicine and Qìgōng society. You should never forget that this place is the residence of the spirit (Shén, 神), the origin of life. In order to reopen the Third Eye, you must be soft and tender. Once you have reopened the Third Eye, you are considered enlightened, since you will comprehend everything around you without any intention of knowing it, and will be able to communicate with nature. In addition, once you have reached the Dào of enlightenment, you will educate others and help them to grow their spirits. You should not control their spirit or abuse them, but teach them to be spiritually independent, so they will no longer be abused either physically or spiritually. When this happens, everything has become natural. This is the way of "Dào" (道) or "Xuándé" (玄德) (profound natural virtue).

The Complete Book of Principal Contents of Human Life and Temperament (*Xìngmìng Guīzhǐ Quánshū*, 性命圭旨全書) said: "If (you are able to) concentrate the training of Qì to reach its softness, the spirit will stay (in its residence) for a long time. To and fro, the real breathing will become natural and smooth. Softly and continuously to lead the Qì to its origin. (In this case), the spiritual spring will always emerge automatically without pumping."[8] This saying implies that in order to keep the spirit at its residence for a long time (longevity), you must first learn how to breathe softly, so you can build up the Qì storage to a higher level, and then circulate it in the entire body smoothly and continuously. Through this practice, the Original Qì (Yuánqì, 元氣) can be maintained at its residence. When this Original Qì is used to nourish the Original Spirit (Yuánshén, 元神), your spirit can be raised to a high level of longevity and spiritual enlightenment. In Qìgōng breathing practice, "uttering must be slender and receiving must be soft."[9] You must practice regulating the breathing until no regulating is necessary. In order to reach this stage, at the beginning, you must learn how to "condense (your) spirit in regulating breathing which can be reached only through peaceful Xīn and harmonious Qì."[10] *The Complete Book of Principal Contents of Human Life and Temperament* (*Xìngmìng Guīzhǐ Quánshū*, 性命圭旨全書) said: "When regulating the breathing, it must be regulated until the regulating has ceased. When you train the spirit, you must train it until no spirit is necessary."[11] This implies that at the end, all of the training and cultivation have become natural and no more training is necessary. When this happens, you are training always and everywhere.

Scientifically, it is known that we have two brains that constitute two inner energy poles of the body (Yīn and Yáng), which are connected via the spinal cord.[12,13] Qì (bio-electricity) is constantly circulating in our body in order to maintain our lives. The upper pole regulates our spiritual life while the lower pole manages our physical life. These two poles synchronize, coordinate, and harmonize with each other.

2. Dào Dé Jīng

(Chapter 16) [1]

《道德經・十六章》

Approach (Follow) the nothingness (emptiness) to its extremity and maintain calmness with sincerity. Millions of objects (lives) are in action which allows us to observe their cyclic repetitions. Though there are so many objects, each individual must repeatedly return to its root (origin). When it returns to the root, it means 'calmness.' When it is calmed, then it means 'repetition of a life.' When the life repeats, it means 'constant natural routine.' If (one) knows this constant natural routine, then (his mind) is clear (enlightened). If (one) does not know this constant natural routine, then various unfortunate dangers could occur. If (one) knows this constant natural routine, then (life) is permitted. When life is permitted, then it is impartial. If it is impartial, then it can be completed. When it is completed, then it is heaven (nature). When it is heaven, it is the Dào. If it is the Dào, then it can be long and the death of the body will not be near.

致虛極，守靜篤；萬物并作，吾以觀其復。夫物芸芸，各復歸其根。歸根曰靜，靜曰復命。復命曰常，知常曰明。不知常，妄作凶。知常容，容乃公，公乃全，全乃天。天乃道，道乃久，歿身不殆。

All lives originated from nothingness. Therefore, in order to see the repetition of lives, we must first reach this nothingness. This nothingness is called the state of Wújí (無極) (No Extremity), where there is no discrimination of Yīn (陰) and Yáng (陽). It is a neutral state of everything. Therefore, "nothingness" here means the emptiness of the emotional mind and material world. In order to reach this state, the first step is to maintain extreme calmness of both mental and physical bodies. Then you will be able to see the actions of all lives and understand their repetitions. Even though there are millions of various living objects, each individual, at the end, must return to its origin (root). It is from this origin that the initiation of life begins again. When one has returned to this origin, it is calm, quiet, and peaceful. When new life is initiated again, the natural constant routine (Cháng, 常) will be repeated. If you know this constant natural routine, then there is no doubt about life—you will have understood its meaning and become enlightened. If you are able to follow the natural routine and the way of natural rules, then your life will be long and healthy. This is what the "Dào" means. If you do not know this routine, then you rub against nature, and consequently various disasters may occur.

Embryonic Breathing is to keep the mind at the Wújí (無極) state. In order to trace back to our origin, we must first know how to keep our mind at the center, meaning the center of the Qì (氣) (Real Lower Dāntián, 真下丹田), and the center of the spiritual being (Upper Dāntián, 上丹田). As mentioned earlier, one of these two Poles is Yīn and the other Yáng. The Real Lower Dāntián provides the quantity of Qì that allows the physical body to perform its life with vigor and strength. The Upper Dāntián (spiritual center) governs the usage of the Qì and improves the quality of the Qì manifestation. These Two Poles are connected through the spinal cord (Chōngmài, 衝脈). Physically, there are Two Poles, but in function, they are one, and cannot be separated. When your mind is able to remain in these Two Poles as one (Embracing Singularity) (Bàoyī, 抱一), then you are able to conserve and govern your Qì effectively and efficiently. This is the key to longevity and maintaining health.

3. The Song of Great Dao

(Eight Notes of Life Abidance; The Marvellous Theory of Abidance for Pure Cultivation) [2] (Gāo, Lián; Míng Dynasty)
《大道歌》
《遵生八箋・清修妙論箋》
(明・高濂撰)

The Great Dào (Dàdào) is not far (away), but inside the body. Ten thousand objects are empty, but the human temperament is not empty. If the human temperament cannot be empty and stay together with the Qì harmoniously, (how can) Qì return to its original ocean (i.e., Real Lower Dāntián) and (expect) unlimited longevity. If (you) wish to keep the spirit in the body, (then) do not leave (even) an object in Lingtai (i.e., spiritual platform). (If) any object (i.e., thought) stays in the heart (i.e., mind), the spirit will not be clear. (This) will waste the real essence and damage the tendons and bones (i.e., physical body). The spirit directs the Qì and from Qì the shape remains (healthy). (In this case, you) will live for a long time without needing herbs. The techniques are easy; however, the secrets are hard to meet (i.e., obtain). (The correct ways) have always been changed (into wrong ones) and separated from the expert path. Therefore, even though a thousand people or ten thousand people have learned (about this), after all, there is not even one who has accomplished (i.e., few have succeeded). (Whenever) the spirit has exited (from the physical body), immediately bring it back. When the spirit has returned to the physical body, the Qì will also return automatically. As such, practice every morning and evening, the Spiritual Embryo will be conceived and born naturally.

> 大道不遠在身中，萬物皆空性不空。性若不空和氣住，氣歸元海壽無窮。欲得身中神不出，莫向靈台留一物。物在心中神不清，耗散真精損筋骨。神御氣兮氣留形，不須藥物自長生。術則易知訣難遇，總然易了不專行。所以千人萬人學，畢竟終無一個存。神若出兮便收來，神返身中氣自回。如此朝朝並暮暮，自然赤子產靈胎。

In this song, it states that the Great Dào (Dàdào, 大道) of longevity and enlightenment is in our bodies. As long as we cultivate it, we will be able to reach this Dào. The mind should not stay on the objects around us. All of these objects, after all, are empty. What the Daoists and Buddhists train is to keep away from the influence of the objects generated from earth, fire, water, and air. Since your spiritual body originated from physical and emotional nothingness, in this training, you are returning to nothingness. The Buddhists call this "Sìdà Jiēkōng" (四大皆空), or "Four Large Are Empty." You should cultivate your human nature and temperament and raise your spirit to a higher stage. Once you have reached a high spiritual level and are able to harmonize with the Qì, then it can be kept at the Real Lower Dāntián. Then, through the conservation of Qì and the high governing power of your spirit, you will live for a long time. Língtái (靈臺) means the spiritual platform, the residence of the spirit (Shénshì, 神室) which is located at the center of the brain. This residence is also commonly called "Níwángōng" (泥丸宮), or "Mud Pill Palace."

In order to keep Qì at the Real Lower Dāntián, first you must have a simple and pure mind which is free from the temptation of the objects around you and from emotional bondage. If so, your spirit will be able to stay in its spiritual center, but once your mind strays from this center, it will naturally lead the Qì away from its residence and waste it. Therefore, when the spirit is firmly kept inside of the body, the Qì will also stay. When the Qì is abundant and able to stay in the body, the physical body (shape) will be strong and healthy. This is the key to longevity. The crucial key to producing the Spiritual Embryo is to keep the spirit inside the body all the time.

From this song, you can see that in order to produce the Spiritual Embryo (Shéntāi, 神胎), you must cultivate your spirit. In order to raise your spirit to a higher level, you must first have abundant Qì stored in the Real Lower Dāntián. When this Qì is led upward to nourish the brain, the spirit can be raised. However, during this period of training, if your mind has been tempted and influenced by external attractions both physical and mental, you will not be able to store the Qì to a higher level to generate a Spiritual Embryo. In conclusion, this is the stage of cultivating your human nature or temperament so you can be free from physical and emotional bondage (human desires).

4. Jade Pendant Inscription of Transporting Qì [2,5]

《行氣玉佩銘》

When transporting Qì, (if) deep, then accumulate. If (Qì is) accumulated, then can be extended. When it is extended, it can be sunken downward. If sunken downward, then steady. If steady, then firm. If firm, then able to germinate. Having germinated, then grow. When grow, then retreat. When retreat, then (return to) the heaven. The foundation of the heaven is at the top (i.e., brain or Upper Dāntián) and the foundation of the earth is at the bottom (i.e., Real Lower Dāntián). If following (these rules), then live; if adverse, then die.

行氣，深則蓄，蓄則伸，伸則下，下則定，定則固，固則萌，萌則長，長則退，退則天。天几舂在上，地几舂在下，順則生，逆則死。

When you circulate the Qì in the body, if your breathing is deep, then the body is relaxed and the mind is calm. When this happens, the Qì circulation can also be deep, and the Qì storage can reach an abundant level. Only if you have an abundant store of Qì can this Qì be strong enough to extend and be distributed everywhere in the body. It is said: "Transport Qì as though through a pearl with a 'nine-curved hole,' not even the tiniest place won't be reached."[14] When this happens, the body's metabolism will be smooth and natural, and you will be healthy. Not only that, if you have abundant Qì, it can be led downward and stored in the Real Lower Dāntián. Then life can be stabilized and firm.

Leading the Qì and storing it in the Real Lower Dāntián is the process of Embryonic Breathing (Tāixí, 胎息), the process of returning the mental and physical life to its origin (Wújí state). Once the Wújí state is reached, new life can be germinated and grown strong again. After you have fulfilled the purpose and completed the Qì manifestation, retreat and return the Qì to its origin, the Real Lower Dāntián. This process is the way of the heavenly cycle (Dào, 道). You must know how to return the Qì to store it at the Real Lower Dāntián and how to conserve it, then you will be able to manifest it efficiently for your life. How to manifest the usage of the Qì to its highest efficiency depends on how much you are able to purify your spirit and raise it to a higher level. This spirit will then be able to govern the Qì circulation smoothly. In Chinese Qìgōng, the head is considered the heaven (Tiān, 天) while the abdomen area is considered the earth (Dì, 地). The Upper Dāntián is located at the heaven and is the residence of the spirit, while the Lower Dāntián is situated at the abdominal area, the residence of Qì. If you know how to store the Qì at the Real Lower Dāntián and keep your spirit focused and high at the Upper Dāntián, you will achieve longevity.

5. Stele with One Hundred Words

(Lǚ, Yán)[2]
《百字碑》
(吕岩作)

When cultivating Qì, do not just constantly talk about how to keep (i.e., protect) it. When descending the mind (i.e., calming the mind), it should be doing without doing. If (you) know the origins (i.e., causes) of movement (Yáng) and stillness (i.e., Yīn), then there is nothing (i.e., no reason) for (you to) ask anyone else. To face the real reality, (you) must deal with daily affairs. However, when (you) deal with these daily affairs, (you) should not be infatuated by them. If (you are) not infatuated, then (your) temperament can be steady (i.e., self-controlled). When the temperament is steady, the Qì will naturally return (i.e., be preserved). If the Qì can be returned, the elixir (i.e., Baby Embryo) can be conceived, consequently, Kǎn and Lí can coordinate with each other within the kettle (i.e., under control). When there is Yīn-Yáng (interaction), the repeated cycle will be initiated, this will bring (you) a natural derivation (of new life) like thunder (i.e., enlightened). White clouds are moving upward, and sweet dew is sprinkling Xūmí (i.e., completeness of human virtue). I will drink the wine of longevity by myself, how can others know how free and unfettered I am? (I) sit down to listen to the songs (generated from the instrument) without strings, I comprehend clearly the pivotal function of natural creation. In total, these are twelve sentences which offer (you) the ladder to ascend to Heaven (i.e., enlightenment).

養氣忘言守，降心為不為。動靜知宗祖，無事更尋誰？真常須應物，應物要不迷。不迷性自住，性住氣自回。氣回丹自結，壺中配坎離。陰陽生反復，普化一聲雷。白雲朝頂上，甘露洒須彌。自飲長生酒，逍遙誰得知？坐聽無弦曲，明通造化機。都來十二句，端的上天梯。

Cultivating Qì is not just learning how to maintain it. The most important thing of all is learning to regulate your Xīn (emotional mind). This mind must be regulated until no more regulation is necessary, and it becomes natural. When this happens, your mind will be clear and your judgments will be neutral and accurate. Then, whether you are active or still, you know where the origins are. If you know clearly what is happening, why do you need to ask anyone else? In order to live in this world of human society, you must deal with many necessary affairs. However, when you are handling them, you should not be lured by money, glory, dignity, pride, jealousy, power, or other human desires and emotions. If your mind is separated from these temptations, then it can be calm and steady. Then Qì will naturally return to its origin (Real Lower Dāntián). This will result in the formation of the elixir (Spiritual Embryo). Then you are able to control your life easily through the adjustment of Kǎn (坎) (Water) and Lí (離) (Fire). Through the Kǎn and Lí, the Yīn and Yáng status of your spiritual and physical bodies can be regulated as you wish. Kǎn and Lí are the methods which change the body's Yīn and Yáng. Through the cultivation of the Yīn and Yáng of your spiritual and physical body, when the time is ripe, you can reopen your third eye for enlightenment suddenly, like a clap of thunder. When this happens, you have no doubt about your life. Your life will be just like the pure white clouds floating in the sky, or like the sweet dew upon Xūmí (須彌). Xūmí is the Daoist term for the human spiritual being in the fullness of human virtue. In this case, you will be able to live long and enjoy life to the fullest. Not only that, you will be able to communicate with nature like listening to songs without sound and also understanding the pivotal functions of nature.

6. Classic of Embryonic Breathing [2,3,5]

《胎息經》

The embryo is conceived from the concealed Qì. Qì is developed through the (regulated) breath of the embryo. When Qì is present, the body may live; when spirit (Shén) abandons the body and the shape (i.e., embryo) disperses, death will follow. Knowing (how to cultivate) the spirit and Qì makes long life possible. Firmly protect the insubstantial emptiness (i.e., Spiritual Embryo at the Real Lower Dāntián) so as to cultivate spirit and Qì. When spirit moves, the Qì moves; where spirit stops, the Qì stops. If you wish to have a long life, spirit and Qì must harmoniously coordinate (with each other). When the Xīn (heart-mind) is not infatuated by thoughts coming or going, then (spirit and Qì) will not exit and enter, and thus will always stay naturally. To practice intelligently is the true way (of success).

胎從伏氣中結，氣從有胎中息。氣入身來為之生，神去離形為之死。知神氣可以長生，固守虛無以養神氣。神行則氣行，神住則氣住。若欲長生，神氣相住。心不動念，無來無去，不出不入，自然常住。勤而行之，是真道路。

Nobody knows when or by whom this classic was written. However, it has been passed down for generations and considered as one of the most important documents about Embryonic Breathing.

Basically it says that the Holy Embryo (Shèngtāi, 聖胎) (Shéntāi, 神胎) is conceived from Qì concealed at the Real Lower Dāntián. In order to reveal this concealed Qì, you must practice Embryonic Breathing. Once you have stored this Qì to an abundant level, your life force will be strong, bringing you good health and longevity. However, in order to manifest this Qì into physical life force, you must have a strong spirit to focus the circulation and manifestation of Qì. Once you have lost this living spirit, you will lose your health and die. Therefore, he who knows how to cultivate his spirit and develop his Qì will live a long and healthy life. This first part of the classic explains how to regulate the relationship between physical life, Qì, and spirit.

In order to reach this goal, first you must firm your mind and keep it at the Real Lower Dāntián. The Real Lower Dāntián is called "Xūwú" (虛無) and means "nothingness." When your mind remains at the Real Lower Dāntián, it is the state of Wújí (無極) (No Extremity) and the state of "no discrimination"—in other words, the state of nothingness. To reach this, you must clear out emotional thoughts and desires. Only when your mind is in this state can you really be in the neutral state of your mental being. This is the state described in *Dào Dé Jīng*, "Approach the nothingness (emptiness) to its extremity, and maintain calmness with sincerity." You should know that "the mind leads the Qì." When your mind is actively thinking, you are leading the Qì away from its residence, the Real Lower Dāntián, and consuming it. In order to store your Qì to an abundant level, you must know how to conserve, protect, and build it. These are three important things always emphasized in Internal Elixir Qìgōng (Nèidān Qìgōng, 內丹氣功) practice.

In order to build up the Qì to an abundant level, you must not only keep your mind at the Real Lower Dāntián, but also know the techniques of Embryonic Breathing. In order to manifest your Qì efficiently in your daily life, you must have a strong and highly controlled spirit. Then Qì consumption will be limited and performance efficiency will be high. Therefore, the key to longevity is to keep the spirit and Qì in mutual coordination and harmonization. To keep the spirit a pure and at a high level, your Xīn (emotional mind) must be calm. Xīn is compared to a monkey, while the Yì (Wisdom Mind) is compared to a horse (Xīnyuán Yìmǎ, 心猿意馬). In order to keep the monkey steady, you must restrain it in its cage, the Wújí state. This is the crucial key to success.

7. Embracing Simplicity; Explain Stagnation[2]

《抱朴子・釋滯》

> *Those who have obtained (the capability) of Embryonic Breathing are able to breathe without using the nose and mouth, like (the breathing of) a fetus in the womb.*
>
> 得胎息者，能不以鼻口噓息，如人在胞胎之中。

This document describes that one who has really reached the Dào of Embryonic Breathing is able to stop the breathing for a while just like a fetus in the womb who does not use the nose or mouth to breathe. In order to extend your breathing to a longer time, your physical body must reach a higher level of relaxation and your mind must achieve a profoundly calm meditative state. When this happens, your heartbeat will slow down and the oxygen consumption in your body will decrease to its minimum. In this case, your breathing will be long, quiet, slender, soft, calm, smooth, and continuous, as if you were not breathing at all.

Technically, in Embryonic Breathing, in order to lead the Qì to the center (Real Lower Dāntián) and store it there efficiently, you must first inhale deeply, and then hold your breath until the Qì reaches this center. This is the Kǎn (坎) (Water) of the Qìgōng practice. The longer you are able to hold it without sacrificing the relaxation of your physical body, the faster the Qì can be led to the Real Lower Dāntián. If you tense while doing so, the consumption of oxygen will increase and the breathing will become urgent and short once more. This kind of holding of the breath is the crucial key to leading the Qì to the center. By the same token, in order to lead the Qì outward and manifest it into physical power, we often hold the breath until the exhalation has reached its maximum. For example, when you push a car or lift a heavy weight, often you inhale deeply first to take in oxygen sufficiently. In this case, the biochemical reaction process can reach its highest efficiency, and Qì can be produced more abundantly for the physical body's action. Then, you exhale and lead the Qì to the physical body for action. At the end of your exhalation, you often hold your breath to allow the Qì to reach its maximum performance level. This is the Lí (離) (Fire) of the Qìgōng practice.

8. Língjiànzi's Dǎoyǐn Zǐwǔ Recording[2]
《靈劍子導引子午記注》

What is Embryonic Breathing? It is a method of Embracing (i.e., maintaining) Singularity (i.e., simplicity, Wújí center) and keeping it in the neutral state. An embryo in the womb takes air through the umbilical cord. After ten months (of pregnancy), (it) becomes a newborn. Then (the baby) will take the air from the head (Shénlú). A truthful person (i.e., person who has reached the Dào) breathes deeply but not from the nose. Embryonic Breathing is what Lǎozi said about returning to the baby state (of breathing). This is Embryonic Breathing.

胎息者，抱一守中之法也。嬰兒在腹中，取氣于臍管，十月脫胎，即取氣于神爐。真人鼻無出入，其息深深。老子所謂復歸于嬰兒者，胎息之謂也。

"Dǎoyǐn" (導引) is one of the ancient terms in Qìgōng which means "to guide and to lead." "Zǐwǔ" (子午) means "midnight and noon" and implies the timing of the cultivation. Língjiànzi (靈劍子) is the name of the Daoist who wrote this classic. In the Chinese calendar each month has only 28 days, since it follows the lunar cycle. Therefore, ten months is 280 days and approximately the same as the Western concept of nine months of pregnancy. "Shénlú" (神爐) means "the spiritual residence," namely the head. Finally, "Zhēnrén" (真人) means "the truthful person" and refers to those Daoists who have reopened the Third Eye and reached the Dào. The reason for this is simply that in order to reopen the Third Eye, a person must be truthful. As long as a person is not truthful and continues lying, then the Third Eye cannot be reopened since he will be afraid others will see through to his original intention.

This simple document clearly points out that the key to Embryonic Breathing is to keep the mind at its spiritual center, and also to preserve the Qì and allow it to stay in the Qì residence (Real Lower Dāntián). As mentioned earlier, there are two energy Poles in our body, one in our head and the other in our abdomen. The upper pole is the residence of the spirit (Shén) and the lower pole is the residence of the Qì. Western science has recognized the upper pole as the brain in the head, while the lower pole (abdomen) is the "second brain."[12,13] These two brains are connected through the spinal cord, which is highly electrically conductive fiber. Since there is nearly no resistance to Qì circulation in the spinal cord, it implies that though there are two brains physically, they actually function as one. It is the Yīn and Yáng side of the same thing. The spirit in the upper brain controls the quality of the Qì manifestation, while the lower brain builds up and stores the quantity of Qì. Therefore, when the document mentions "the one" (simplicity) or the neutral state, it means to keep the mind and Qì at these two centers, respectively. When this happens, the mind will be centered and the Qì can be preserved. This is the crucial key to Embryonic Breathing.

9. The Classic of Tàishàng's Embryonic Breathing for Life Nourishment 2

《太上養生胎息氣經》

> *Concerning the method of breathing, (you) must have a Xīn (i.e., emotional mind) like an embryo in the mother's womb. After ten months (of pregnancy) it matures, tendons and bones are harmonious and soft. Use the Míngxīn (i.e., Yīn mind) to cease thoughts, (then) the harmonious Qì will arrive automatically.*
>
> 凡服氣法，存心如嬰兒在母胎，十月成就，筋骨和柔，以冥心息念，和氣自至。

"Tàishàng" (太上) means "Grand Uppermost" and is an abbreviation of "Tàishàng Lǎojūn" (太上老君) which means "Grand Uppermost Old Gentleman." In Chinese culture, to be called "old" is a sign of respect, rather than an insult as in the Western world. Traditionally in China, the older you are, the more respected you are by people around you. "Tàishàng Lǎojūn" is a respected name of Lǎozi (老子) given by Daoists.

Again, Xīn (心) is the emotional mind developed after birth. Míng (冥) means the Yīn world. According to Chinese tradition and belief, there are two worlds (or spaces) coexisting in this universe. One is the "Yáng world" (Yángjiān, 陽間), the material world in which we live. The other is the "Yīn world" (Yīnjiān, 陰間), the spiritual world where we go after death. Yáng is the manifestation and is active, while Yīn is calm and conceals energy. Míngxīn therefore means the mind of the Yīn world. When your mind is in this world, all material attractions will disappear, since substance has no meaning in the spiritual world. If you are able to keep your mind in this state, your thoughts and physical activities will cease. This will lead you to the source of life (Wújí state).

At this time, you are pure and without emotional disturbance, and the harmonious Qì will be generated in the Real Lower Dāntián. This harmonious Qì is the origin of the spiritual baby embryo (Shéntāi, 神胎).

10. The Complete Book of Principal Contents of Human Life and Temperament

(Zhāng, Jǐng-Hé's Secret of Embryonic Breathing)[2]

《性命圭旨全書》
(張景和胎息訣)

Real Xuán and real Pìn, inhale and exhale by itself automatically. It is just like the pond fish swimming in the spring time, like torpidity of hundreds of insects, the Qì contained inside is joyful and harmonious, and the spiritual wind blows constantly, neither dirty nor clean, not from the mouth nor from the nose, going nowhere and coming from nowhere, no exit and no entrance. (Everything has) returned to its root and origin. This is the real Embryonic Breathing.

真玄真牝，自呼自吸，似春沼魚，如百蟲蟄，灝氣融融，靈風習習。不濁不清，非口非鼻，無去無來，無出無入。返本返原，是真胎息。

To understand this document, first you must know what Xuán (玄) and Pìn (牝) mean in Daoist terminology. In the ancient document The Interpretation of Embryonic Breathing Classic (Tāixíjīng Zhù, 胎息經注) it says: "Three inches under the navel is Qìhǎi (氣海), also called Lower Dāntián (Xiàdāntián, 下丹田), or Xuánpìn (玄牝). What is Xuán? It means water; what is Pìn, it means mother... Those who cultivate the Dào, always conceal their Qì under the navel, keep their spirit (Shén, 神) inside the body. From the mutual harmonization of the spirit and Qì, the 'Marvellous Embryo' (Xuántāi, 玄胎) will be formed. Once this miracle is formed, it will grow and survive. This is the Internal Elixir (Nèidān, 內丹)."[15] This document points out that the Lower Dāntián or Real Lower Dāntián is the place of conception of the Spiritual Embryo. The way of doing so is to keep the Qì there and maintain the spirit and mind at their centers. When this happens, the spirit and Qì will harmonize with each other and the Spiritual Embryo will be formed.

Another document, Concealed Secret of Féng's Family (Féngshì Jǐnnáng, 馮氏錦囊) says: "There is a crux in the body which is named 'Xuánpìn' (玄牝). This place is how life can be alive. In fact, this place is the residence of spirit. It is the place where the

Three Origins (Sānyuán, 三元) (Jīng, Qì, and Shén; 精・氣・神) (Essence, Qì, and Spirit) gather. The cavities where the essence (Jīng, 精), spirit (Shén, 神), soul (Hún, 魂), and vigor (Pò, 魄) meet. It is the root where the Golden Elixir (Jīndān, 金丹) (Qì) returns and the place where the immortals conceive their Holy Embryo."[16] Also, *Dào Dé Jīng* (道德經) (Chapter 6) said: "(If) the Valley Spirit does not die, it is called 'Xuánpìn.' The gate of the Xuánpìn is the root of heaven and earth. It exists softly and continuously. When you use it, it will not be exhausted."[17] This document clearly points out that "Xuánpìn" is the place where the spirit resides (Shénfǔ, 神府). This place is at the middle of the brain and is commonly called "Spiritual Valley" (Shéngǔ, 神谷) or "Mud Pill Palace" (Níwángōng, 泥丸宮). It is called "valley" because physically the brain is constructed of two hemispheres, and a valley is formed between them which can generate resonance to correspond with energy outside the body (Figure 3–1). The spirit which resides in this valley is called "Valley Spirit" (Gǔshén, 谷神). The center of this valley is actually where the pineal and pituitary glands are located (Figure 3–2). In spiritual cultivation, Daoists believe that through cultivation of essence (Jīng, 精), Qì (氣), and spirit (Shén, 神), and gathering them at the spiritual center, the Spiritual Embryo can be grown, which will result in the birth of the spiritual baby (i.e, the reopening of the Third Eye) (Kāitiānyǎn, 開天眼). When this happens, enlightenment can be achieved.

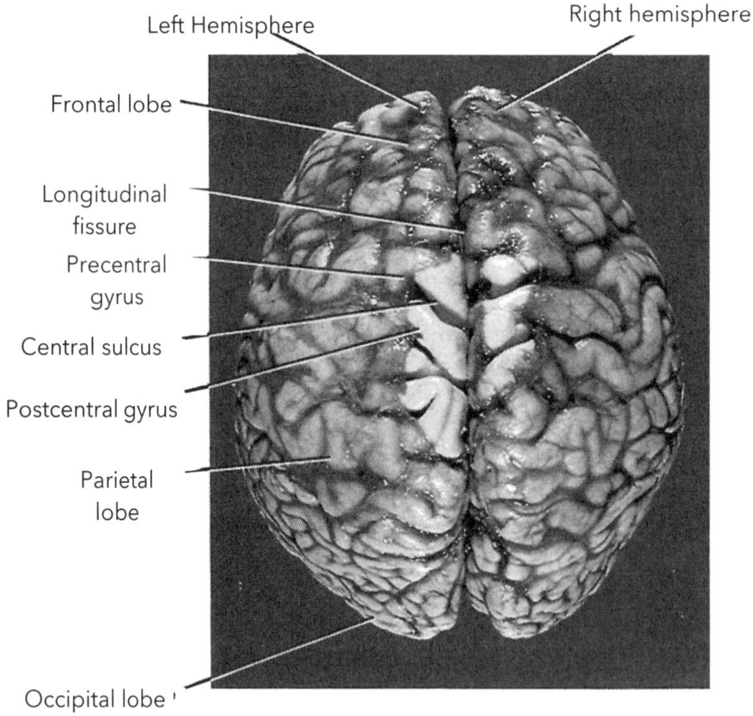

Figure 3-1. The Brain Encompasses Two Hemispheres

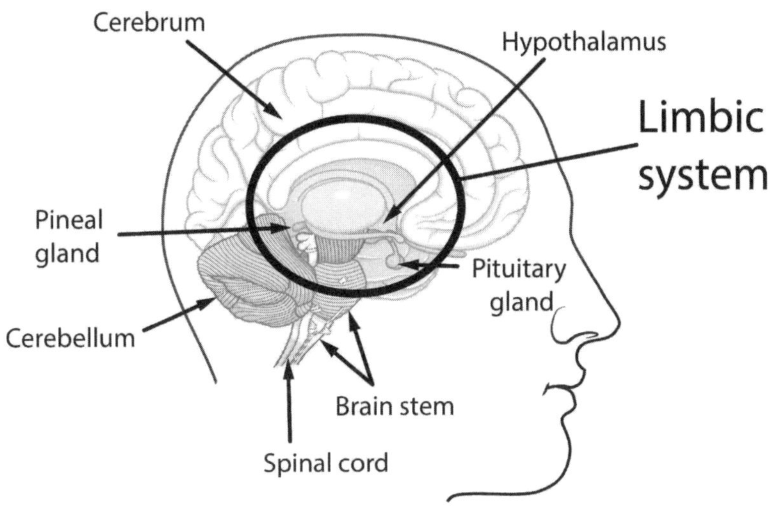

Figure 3-2. The Pituitary and Pineal Glands (Mud Pill Palace) in the Spiritual Valley

Scientifically, when you condense your spirit at this center, your mind is leading the stored Qì from the Real Lower Dāntián (bio-battery) upward through the spinal cord (Thrusting Vessel) (Chōngmài, 衝脈) to this center, and stimulating hormone production. Hormones act as catalysts in the body's biochemical metabolic process. When the hormone content is high, the vital force is strong and longevity can be reached.

From this, we can see that in Embryonic Breathing we are, in fact, aiming for Spiritual Breathing at the Upper Dāntián (Shàngdāntián, 上丹田) and Qì Breathing at the Real Lower Dāntián (Zhēn Xiàdāntián, 真下丹田). As mentioned earlier, these Two Poles are the Yīn and Yáng aspects of the same thing. Therefore, while it seems there are two places, nevertheless they function as one. Spiritual Wind (Língfēng, 靈風) implies the flow of spiritual energy that passes through your body.

11. The Thesis of Retaining the Shén and Firming the Qì[2]
《存神固氣論》

In addition, according to the theory of bearing and variation, those (who carry) only Yáng will not bear (the offspring) and those (who carry) only Yīn will not grow. Those Perfect Men (Zhìrén) (i.e., those who have reached the Dào) talk about nourishing the Holy Embryo, and searching for the exit way (of death) know that

> *Kǎn or Lí, lead or mercury, cannot be left alone. If it is not from the intercourse of the Dragon and Tiger (i.e., Yīn and Yáng) and from establishing the key axis at the marvellous extremity (i.e., Lower Rear Dāntián), who is able to stabilize the original harmonization (of spirit and Qì) and breathe as an embryo?*
>
> 且生化之理，獨陽不生，孤陰不長。至人謂養聖胎，求出路，坎離鉛汞不相孤。苟非龍虎交媾，立關軸于玄極，誰能住元和而息胎呼？

"Kǎn" (坎) means "water" and "Lí" (離) means "fire." Lead (Qiān, 鉛) and mercury (Gǒng, 汞) are terms commonly used in Daoist society. Lead and mercury were used in Daoist alchemy to adjust the Yīn and Yáng of the elixir. Dragon (Lóng, 龍) and Tiger (Hǔ, 虎) are commonly used to represent Yīn and Yáng. Kǎn and Lí are the methods which could result in a change of Yīn and Yáng.

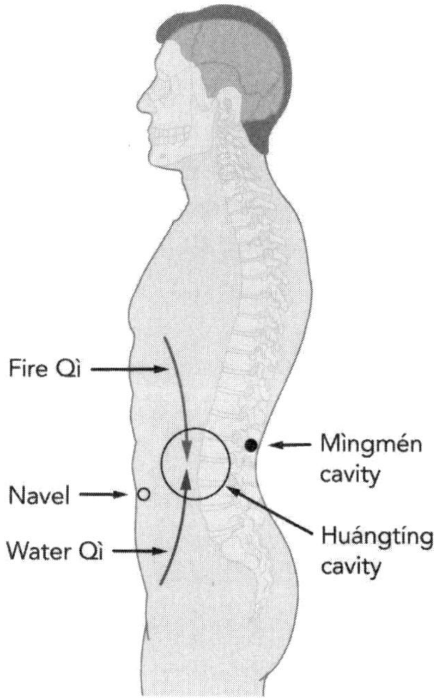

Figure 3-3. Interaction of the Yīn (Water) and Yáng (Fire) Qì in the Huángtíng Cavity

This article emphasizes that in order to have a congelation of a Spiritual Embryo, you must first know how to create the harmonious interaction of Yīn and Yáng. Yīn or Yáng alone will not generate life. In order to have a harmonious interaction of Yīn and Yáng, you must know the crucial keys of Kǎn and Lí. For example, exhale is Lí while inhale is Kǎn; the mind is Yáng when it is excited and Yīn when it is calm. Also, when the Qì stays in its residence it is Yīn, and when led away from its residence it is Yáng. Not only that, it is believed that the Fire Qì (Yáng Qì) generated from the Post-Birth essence (air and food) resides at the Middle Dāntián (Zhōngdāntián, 中丹田) (area near lower section of sternum) while the water Qì (Yīn Qì) produced from the Original Essence (Yuánjīng, 元精) resides at the Real Lower Dāntián. When you lead the Fire Qì downward and water Qì upward to interact with each other at Huángtíng (黃庭), it is called "Kǎn-Lí" (坎離) (Figure 3–3).

12. Refined Thesis of Embryonic Breathing[3,7]

《胎息精微論》

Lǎozi said: "Those who know the Dào (natural way), Heaven will not kill, and those who have contained the Dé (natural virtue), Heaven will not harm. Dào and Dé embrace each other mutually." If (you) do not wish to be weak and old, the most important key is to absorb the internal grand harmonious Original Qì (Yuánqì). Train yourself to (keep the mind) clear and pure, to keep the body relaxed and natural, do not hold onto thoughts of the ego, maintain the internal organs in their peaceful and steady healthy state, comprehend the grand harmony (of nature) profoundly, ponder the theory of longevity deeply, conceal the Qì (at the Real Lower Dāntián) without moving it away, the Yì (i.e., Wisdom Mind or logical thinking) is like a stream flowing (i.e., without disturbance). (If you are able) to train this without ceasing (i.e., continuously), then (you) have really gained the Dào.

老君曰：〝知道者，天不殺。含德者，天不害。道德相抱。〞身不衰老。內食太和元氣為首。清淨自練，委身放體，志無念慮，安定臟腑，洞極太和，長生久視，潛氣不動，意如流水，行之不休，得道真矣。

It is very difficult to explain the real meaning of "Dào." In *Dào Dé Jīng* (道德經), Chapter 1, it is said: "Dào, if it can be talked about, then it is not the real Dào." In Chapter 25, again, it said: "There is something formed (in nature), which existed before heaven and earth (i.e., nature); quiet and rare, independent and unchanging, it continues cycling and does not rest; it can be the mother of the heaven and the earth. I don't know its name and named it 'Dào.' It can be called 'Dà' (大) (Grand)."[19] From this, you can see that once we start to talk about the great nature, we are using our limited knowledge, influenced by emotion, to make an interpretation of the Dào. This has already led the real meaning of the Dào away from the truth. This is because humans are not truthful. We lie and play tricks on each other, so we all have a serious mask on our faces. Not only that, we have created an emotional matrix through our limited thinking and beliefs, and become trapped in this emotional bondage. Therefore, the closest way to describe the Dào is "The Natural Way." "Dé" (德) is the manifestation of the Dào or the activities of nature.

Whoever follows nature will live a long and healthy life. Dào and Dé must match and be harmonious with each other. To keep the body from getting withered, weak and old, you must practice a few things. These are: 1. Cultivate the internal Original Qì (Yuánqì, 元氣), and conserve it; 2. Keep the mind clear and pure (calm and peaceful). Do not have an ego which makes you worry and disturbs your emotional mind. Keep the Wisdom Mind active. When this happens, the spirit can be maintained at a high level; 3. Maintain the body's strength (Yáng) and keep the physical and mental bodies relaxed and comfortable (Yīn). Then the circulation of the entire internal Qì will be harmonious, consequently, the internal organs will be healthy and harmonious. This is stage of "Tàihé" (太和) and means "Grand Harmonization." Naturally, the key to reaching this harmonious stage is constant practice.

> *Go into a quiet room every day and protect (i.e., preserve) the Xuányuánqì. (Xuányuán means to stay at the two Xuán gates, keeping the mind in the Real Lower Dāntián which is connected with them). If there is Xuán (i.e., Qì) in the Xuán (i.e., insubstantial center, namely Real Lower Dāntián), then I have my life. If there is an alive (Qì) in life, then I have a shape (i.e., physical body). When there is a shape in the shape (i.e., healthy physical body), then I have the (Original) Essence. When there is a (refined Original) Essence in the Essence, then I have an (abundant) Qì. When there is an (abundant Qì) in (my) Qì (circulation), then I have a (strong) spirit. When there is a (highly cultivated) spirit in my spirit, then I will become natural (i.e., unification of human spirit with the natural spirit). Dé (i.e., natural virtue) uses the shape (i.e., physical body) as a carriage and Dào (i.e., natural way) uses the Qì as the horse. Hún (i.e., soul) uses the Essence as its root and Pò (i.e., vigorous spirit) uses the eyes as the doors. When the shape is fatigued, then the Dé is dispersed. When Qì is derailed, then the Dào revolts. When the Essence is over-consumed, then the Hún is damaged. When the eyes are touched (i.e., attracted), the Pò is weakened.*
>
> 每日入靜室，守玄元氣。〔玄元謂存玄門。〕玄中有玄是我命，命中有命是我形，形中有形是我精，精中有精是我氣，氣中有氣是我神，神中有神，是我自然。德以形為車，道以氣為馬，魂以精為根，魄以目為戶。形勞則德散，氣越則道叛。精銷魂損，目動魄微。

Literally, "Xuán" (玄) means "marvellous" or "incredible," and when this word is used in Daoist documents, it means "mysterious." "Xuányuán" (玄元) means the "mysterious origin" and implies the Dāntiáns (丹田). Normally, it means the Upper Dāntián and/or Real Lower Dāntián (or Lower Dāntián). Since the Lower Dāntián generates and stores the Water Qì (Shuǐqì, 水氣), Xuán sometimes implies water. Therefore, in this document, "Xuányuán" means the "Real Lower Dāntián." If you are able to keep your mind at the Real Lower Dāntián, then there is a marvellous Qì at the Dāntián, which is the root of your life. If you are able to manifest this marvellous Qì into living form, then you will have a strong and healthy physical life and your shape will be complete. When you have a complete and healthy physical body, then the physical essence (hormones) can be produced and preserved efficiently. Once you have this abundant essence, then you can convert it into Qì and make the Qì circulation and storage abundant. When my Qì is abundant, you can lead it upward to nourish your spirit so as to raise your vitality. Finally, if you can keep this spirit high and in its residence, then you will be able to connect your spirit with the spirit of nature. This is the stage of the "Unification of Heaven and Human." (Tiānrén Héyī, 天人合一).

Dé (德) is the natural manifestation of the Dào (道) in the shape of a human. When this Dé is in action, it is like a carriage in motion. Dào is the natural way. Qì is the crucial energy for the Dào to be manifested. Therefore, it is like a horse (Mǎ, 馬), meaning the forerunner or the entire derivation of the Dào. The Dào (道) is "the way" where the horse runs.

When your essence is pure and abundant, the soul can be powerful. Therefore, the essence is the root of the soul (Hún, 魂). The strength of Pò (魄) (vigorous spirit) can be seen from the expression of the eyes and therefore, the eyes are the doors of the soul. The eyes manifest the deep and profound subconscious mind and thinking, which is connected to the soul.

In order to maintain a healthy life, you should not allow your physical body to be fatigued. Fatigue can be caused from too much working, lack of rest, or too many worries. When this happens, the manifestation of the Dào will be incomplete, and the Dé dispersed. In addition, you should not manifest your Qì to an excessive level. Too much Qì manifestation will exhaust the Qì stored in your body, and make the physical body too Yáng. In this case, you are away from the Dào. Naturally, you will have a short life. Furthermore, you must learn how to protect or conserve your Original Essence. For male practitioners, the first step is to regulate your sexual activities. Too much sex will exhaust your essence, and your physical spiritual bodies will be weakened.

> *Therefore, (you) should keep the shape (i.e., physical body) calm and safeguard (your) Qì. Protect (your) essence and treasure (your) spirit. Dào and Dé should be kept condensed and closed (i.e., maintained in the right path closely) and the Hún and Pò should be safeguarded firmly. This is what is meant by: containing the Dào without speech, gaining the real Qì, muscles and skin are moist and glossy, obtaining the root of the Dào, hands and feet sweat, the essence (Qì) is abundant, (not hungry and thirsty as a) turtle or dragon's Embryonic Breathing, soft and slender existing for a long time. When used, it is not exhausted. Drink in the marvellous spring, ascend the spirit to the ultimate purity, returning the years back to the infant, and the Dào is kept natural. The ultimate Dào is not far but close to your own body. If (you) study and practice diligently and carefully, life can exist forever.*
>
> 是以靜形愛氣，全精寶神。道德凝密，魂魄固守。所謂含道不言，得氣之真，肌膚潤澤，得道之根，手足流汗，精〔氣〕之充溢，〔不飢不渴，〕龜龍胎息，綿綿長存，用之不竭。飲于玄泉，登于太清，還年反嬰，道之自然。至道不遠，近在己身，用心精微，命乃永存。

This paragraph concludes that in order to have a healthy life, you must protect and safeguard four things in your body. These are your physical body (Xíng, 形), Qì (氣), essence (Jīng, 精), and spirit (Shén, 神). In order to protect them, you must follow the rules of nature (Dào, 道) and the ways of its manifestation (Dé, 德). In this case, your spirit, soul, and vigorous energy can be firmed and protected. Once you have comprehended these theories, you simply have to practice it constantly. Just talking about it will not lead you to the goal of practice. Those who comprehend the Dào and also know how to practice it diligently will verify its truth. The verifications of this practice are: a healthy physical body, strong Qì circulation, without becoming fatigued easily; and breathing smoothly, softly, and slenderly. In this case, you have learned how to follow the Dào and the Dé.

Those who cultivate the Dào today, absorb the Qì either from the Five Elements (Wǔyá), Eight Directions (Bāfāng) (ether), Four Timings (Sìshí) (Four Seasons), Sun and Moon (Rìyuè), or stars, and mistakenly think (the Qì) can be taken from the crown and nose. Though all of these methods were recorded in ancient classics, however, it is rare to see one who has accomplished (the goal of this cultivation). This (goal) also cannot be reached by those who rely on food (and herbs). Therefore, all of those who cultivate the Qì cannot obtain its secret and waste the essence (i.e., effort) frequently. Even if (you) have obtained the entrance (i.e., the keys of training), you must also comprehend this secret and practice it diligently and delicately without slackness and laziness. [Those who wish to absorb the Qì through Embryonic Breathing, must absorb the internal Qì by seven gulps after midnight. Whenever a gulp is completed, then regulate the Qì for six or seven breaths, and then again gulp. When gulp, it is like the water passing (the throat) with the sound of Kǎn. This means the Qì is transportable. (Lead the Qì) straight downward to the Qìhǎi (i.e., Lower Dāntián) and condense it there until (the Qì) is full at the abdomen as if there were an embryo inside.]

今之修道者，或服五牙、八方、四時、日月、星辰等氣，並誤但思自頂鼻而入，雖古經所載，為之少見成遂，亦非食穀者所能行致爾。是以修氣者，皆不得其訣，虛精勤矣。既得其門，復悟其訣，要在精勤無退懈耳。〔凡胎息服氣，從夜半後服內氣七咽，每一咽既，調氣六、七息，即更咽之。每咽如水流過坎聲，是氣通也。直下氣海中凝結，腹中充滿，如含胎之狀。〕

"Wǔyá" (五牙) means the "alive Qì of the Five Elements" (Wǔxíng, 五行): metal, wood, water, fire, and earth.[20] These five Qìs correspond with the five Qìs in five internal organs: lungs, liver, kidneys, heart, and spleen. Bāfāng (八方) means "eight directions" and implies the space or air around us. Sìshí (四時) refers to nature's four seasons.

This paragraph explains that there are many Daoist practitioners who have learned to absorb Qì from the Five Elements, the ether, the four seasons, or the sun, moon, and stars through Bǎihuì (百會) (crown) and nose (breathing). However, it is rare to see that the result of longevity practice is significant. The results are the same for those who attempt to accomplish longevity by diet and taking herbs. If you cannot comprehend the secret, and practice diligently, then you are wasting your time and effort.

This paragraph follows with a practice method in parentheses. It says, in order to reach the goal of maintaining health and extending life, you must learn two things: one is Embryonic Breathing and the other is the correct way of generating saliva and swallowing it. According to medical Qìgōng, swallowing the saliva (Yàn, 咽) is considered one of the crucial keys of maintaining health. It is believed that the saliva is able to balance the body's Yáng and bring the Fire Qì down. Then we can be calm and peaceful both mentally and physically. A well-known Chinese medical Qìgōng, The Eight Pieces of Brocade (Bāduànjǐn, 八段錦), teaches how to use the method of circling the tongue in the mouth to produce saliva and then swallowing it. When you swallow it, make a sound "Ń" (嗯) and at the same time use the mind to lead the Qì downward to the Lower Dāntián (or Real Lower Dāntián). In this article, it says that you should do this after midnight and repeat seven times. Between each swallowing, you should maintain your Embryonic Breathing for at least six or seven respirations. If you are interested in the The Eight Pieces of Brocade, please refer to the book: *Eight Simple Qìgōng Exercises for Health*, published by YMAA Publication Center.

> *Embryo is formed from the (concealed) Qì and the Qì is initiated from the embryo; consequently, the embryo is completed due to (the supply of) Qì. Once the embryo has been formed and completed, millions of illnesses will automatically be repelled and the spirit will therefore reside (at its residence). Keep the three (i.e., Essence, Qì, and Shén) united as one and maintain them at the center (i.e., Upper Dāntián), the corpse worms (Shīchóng, causes of death) will be falling and this will gradually lead (you) to immortality. Today's learners, either learning from ancient methods or instructed by those who do not know the Dào, all close the mouth and seal the nose (i.e., hold the breath) and emphasize holding the breath long. They do not know that this will cause the obstruction and stagnation (of the Qì) in the five internal organs, thus harming the righteous Qì (Zhèngqì). This is not the way of natural breathing. This will make the shape (i.e., physical body) and spirit become fatigued constantly, therefore useless.[When absorbing the Qì (i.e., training or cultivating the Qì), the joints must be transportable (i.e., loose and moveable), stomach ocean (i.e., stomach area) must be opened (i.e., loose), then receiving the original air essence (i.e., inhaling) and firming the Qì (at the Qì center). When the receiving has been completed, then return the joints into the closed condition while gradually allowing the external Qì (i.e., air) to exit through the nose. In this case, the internal and external will not be separated automatically. The Qì concealed in the embryo will be retained. However, (you) should bend (your) fingers and count the number of breathings in (your) mind, from ten to one hundred, from one to two, to three hundred. This is called "Little Smoothness" (Xiǎotōng). This will result in the sharpness of the ears (i.e., listening) and eyes (i.e., seeing), hundred illnesses can be healed.]*

凡胎從氣中結，氣從胎中生，胎因氣中成。結成即萬病自遣，神靈居之。三一守中，尸蟲亡墜，即漸通仙靈矣。今之學者，或傳古方，或受非道，皆閉口收縮鼻，貴其氣長，而不知五臟壅閉，畜損正氣，殊非自然之息，此繫勞形神，無所益也。〔凡服氣之時，即須關節通，胃海開，納元氣固，納畢，即關節還閉，徐徐鼻出納外氣，自然內外不離，胎中氣亦不出。但潛屈指數息，從十至百數，從一百至二百、三百，此為小通，即耳目聰明，百病皆愈。〕

"Shīchóng" (尸蟲) means "corpse worms" and implies "three emotional worms" which are able to agitate your emotions and lead you to the path of death. These three worms are: 1. Desires at the Upper Dāntián; 2. Seven emotional attachments at the Middle Dāntián; and 3. Desires for alcohol and sex. As long as you have these three worms, your Righteous Qì (Zhèngqì, 正氣) will be affected and harmed. This will lead you to sickness and finally, death. "Xiǎotōng" (小通) means "little smoothness" and means the smooth circulation of the Qì.

In order to achieve longevity, you must first form a "Holy Embryo" (Shèngtāi, 聖胎) in your Real Lower Dāntián through correct Embryonic Breathing. Once this Holy Embryo is formed, then you can be healthy and live long.

However, in order to reach enlightenment, you must also learn how to lead Qì upward to the Upper Dāntián (Spiritual Residence) so the Three Origins (Sānyuán, 三元) (essence, Qì, and spirit) can be united there.

The correct way of Embryonic Breathing is to first keep your mind at the Real Lower Dāntián, and also to know the correct way of breathing. If you simply hold the breath without knowing the methods, you can only cause more problems internally. Then, in the parentheses of the original text, the method for correct breathing is explained. First, you inhale deeply and lead the Qì to the Real Lower Dāntián while relaxing all the joints of your entire body and stomach area. Then, immediately restrain the Qì at the joints while allowing the air to be released slowly and gradually. In this case, the Qì generated can be maintained internally. You should begin your practice with ten respirations first, and gradually increase the number without any uncomfortable and tightened feeling. If you are able to do it for a few hundred times, then you have accomplished the small achievement.

The Dào (i.e., Daoist documents) says: "If (you) restrain and stuff the nose and mouth in the practice of the Embryonic Breathing, then this theory is unreasonable. Since the mouth and the nose are not transportable, then (the Qì) will be stagnant at the lungs and damage them. How can it be beneficial?" Those who absorb (i.e., train) the internal Qì, though the effort is very little, the result can be seen quickly. The accomplishment of this all depends on the peaceful spirit and calm mind, no vexation and no disturbance. This means the Qì paths are opened for smooth circulation. There is an original internal harmony which stays the whole day without dispersion. The flesh and skin are moist and shining, the hands and feet sweat (healthily). This is the secret of the Dào for longevity. [After midnight, swallow seven times and then immediately hold the Qì. Keep this internal Qì (internally) and do not release it, while using the nose and mouth to inhale and exhale external Qì (i.e., air) gradually and slowly without any mixture with the internal Qì. Before dawn swallow seven times and after dawn again swallow seven times. Total there are twenty-one swallows, then stop. Those whose body is large, then it should not be limited by this number. Whenever there is an empty stomach, immediately swallow internal Qì. When the internal Qì is full, there is no hunger.] At the beginning, it will have a little difficulty. After practicing for a long time, it becomes marvellous. The hairs are black, the teeth are strong, the eyes are sharp and shining, tendons and bones are all solid (i.e., firmed), brave with embryonic spirit, the face is lustrous, walking light, the mind without desires, the spirit not greedy (i.e., longing for glory), profound father (i.e., an understanding father) with a newborn baby, and there is no boundary which cannot be reached. Keep the Hún (i.e., soul) and Pò (i.e., vitality) firmly at their origins, the three (i.e., Essence, Qì, and Shén) will automatically and truly be unified into one. Forever conserve Dào, keep the spirit peaceful and calm, the spirit will naturally and automatically be connected to the supernatural divine. This is called "Yǒngbǎo" (i.e., a lasting treasure) in Dào and is the accomplishment of Embryonic Breathing (through cultivating) Original Qì. This is also the final marvelousness of Zhēnrén's (i.e., truthful persons who have reached the Dào) Embryonic Breathing.

道曰：〝若抑塞鼻口，擬習胎息，殊無此理。口鼻氣既不通，則畜損肺臟，有何益哉！” 餌內氣者，用力雖微，而速見功成。全在安神靜慮，不煩不擾。即氣道疏暢，關節開通，內含元和，終日不散。肌膚潤澤，手足流汗，長生之道，訣在此矣。〔從夜半后服七咽，即閉氣，但內氣不出，鼻口常徐徐出納外氣，內氣都不相雜，至五更又服七咽，平旦又服七咽，都在二十一咽止。若體糧者，即不限此數，肚空即咽內氣。〕內氣滿，無饑渴。初習即小難，久久甚妙。髮黑齒堅，眼瞳英明，筋骨全實，壯勇胎神，面貌光澤，行步舉輕，心自無欲，神不貪榮，玄父赤子，固際無傾。魂魄守元，三一自真，永寶其道，靜安其神，神自通靈，道曰永寶，胎息元氣克成。自為真人胎息之妙窮于此也。

This last paragraph emphasizes that when you practice Embryonic Breathing, you should not hold your breath, which causes internal stagnation of the Qì circulation. The key to Embryonic Breathing is keeping the breathing deep and long while the body is relaxed and the mind calm. Scientifically, in order to keep the breathing long, you must keep the oxygen consumption to its minimum. For this, you must have a calm and meditative mind, centered at the Real Lower Dāntián (Qì residence), combined with an extremely relaxed physical body.

In the document, the practice method is inserted in parentheses. It says that, right after midnight, you need to swallow saliva seven times. Naturally, as explained earlier, you must also repeat Embryonic Breathing six or seven times, inhaling deeply into relaxed joints (relaxed physical body) with a calm mind. Then slowly and gradually release the air without feeling uncomfortable. You should repeat the same practice between 3–5 a.m. and also at dawn, making a total of twenty-one swallowings. However, you should not be limited to this number. The more you practice, the more benefit you will receive. "Yǒngbǎo" (永寶) means the treasure that you are able to keep forever. "Zhēnrén" (真人) means "truthful person," referring to those who have achieved the Dào.

13. A Brief Classic about Embryonic Breathing

(Wáng, Wén-Lù's Embryonic Breathing Method)[2]

《胎息經疏略》

(王文祿胎息法)

In the Tàixū (i.e., Great Emptiness or Universe), the spirit is harmonious and prosperous. There is a Qì (i.e., energy) through which the spirit is able to exist. Consequently, (the spirit) is conceived and the embryo is formed. Once the embryo is formed, it begins to breathe. The beginning of an embryo is just like a flower and the navel is like the footstalk, where the stem (i.e., the umbilical cord) connects to the embryo. When the mother exhales, (the embryo) also exhales and when the mother inhales, (the embryo) also inhales. This respiration is called "Xí" (i.e., breathing). When it (i.e., breathing) has reached its extreme calmness, the pure Yáng will grow daily. When the embryo is matured, the shape is completed and (the baby) is born. This is the first original shape (i.e., physical body) to show the world. (This is) the breathing training which (you) should focus on so as to reach its softest as a baby.

太虛氤氳，一氣孔神，伏始結胎，胎結乃息。胎初入花，臍如蒂，蒂帶連胞，母呼亦呼，母吸亦吸，呼吸為息，靜極純陽日長，彌月形全誕生，此原始以示人，欲專氣致柔如嬰兒也。

"Tàixū" (太虛) means "Grand Emptiness" and implies the great nature of the universe. It is believed that there are many forms of Qì (energies) filling up this universe. Through these energies, the spirit is able to exist and grow. From the existence of the spirit and the Qì, the embryos of various life forms can be conceived and formed. Once the embryo is formed as an independent life, it can breathe by itself. This embryonic respiration is called "Xí" (息). At the beginning of this respiration, the embryo is connected with the mother through the umbilical cord and breathes in unison with her. During this growing stage, the body is in an extremely calm and relaxed state. The breathing is soft and slender, and the mind is in a neutral and extremely peaceful state, without emotional disturbances. From this extremely calm (Yīn) state, the Yáng physical body begins to grow. When the manifestation of Yīn has matured, the baby is completed, then born. This tells us clearly that in order to return to the beginning of our life, we must return our breathing to our baby stage. When this happens, we can expect to have a long, peaceful life.

14. Important Fundamental Secrets of Embryonic Breathing[3]

《胎息根旨要訣》

All of the writings written by those who cultivated Embryonic Breathing in ancient times did not reach the marvellous key door (of the training). According to the explanation in words, all of them either have lost or gained (only) in some special areas. Some may say: "If there is no breathing, then there is an embryo. When the breathing is restrained without panting, then it is breathing." All of them have their own individual sayings and have not gained the real content of the subject, thus have misled those who learn later. It makes (you) doubt whether these writings are still beneficial and useful. However, those who cultivated the life have already (wasted the time and) reached the end of their lives. It is really sad! That (i.e., the secret) which I have obtained is actually very simple and easy. Those who wish to learn in the future should keep it preciously. To receive the Qì (i.e., cultivate the Qì) is the marvellous application of the Embryonic Breathing. This must be done through analyzing the internal and external Qì, and also the Qì of the internal organs and bowels. This is all related (to the Qì) generated in the body, therefore, they must be understood.

古修胎息者，尋其所著，皆未達于玄門，據其文字所陳，悉皆互有得失。或云：'無氣是胎，閉氣不喘是息。' 各執一門，未有所趣，迷誤后學，疑或益滋，而修生之人，性命已殆，足可悲哉！余今所得，實為簡易，將來學人，保而深惜。夫云服氣，即胎息之妙用也。切在分析內、外氣，及在臟腑之氣，統一身之所生，不可得而知也。

This first paragraph mentions the importance of obtaining the true and correct way of cultivating the Qì through Embryonic Breathing. Even though there are many documents in existence today, most of them cover only one or two of the possible aspects of the training. Therefore, they are not complete. In order to obtain the real secret of the training, you must have an open mind which allows you to see the different aspects of the same thing. You should not be stubborn in keeping only one belief. Only after you have collected and studied all of the existing documents, through logical pondering and practice, will you understand the correct way of practice.

For example, most documents do not discuss the relationship between Embryonic Breathing and the internal organs. In fact, the external Qì (Wàiqì, 外氣) (Guardian Qì, Wèiqì, 衛氣) and internal Qì (Nèiqì, 內氣) (Managing Qì, Yíngqì, 營氣) are both manifestations of the Qì from the Real Lower Dāntián. In order to have a strong Guardian Qì for your immune system and Managing Qì for the healthy functioning of the organs, you must first have abundant Qì stored in the Real Lower Dāntián. The keys to reaching this goal are through correct Embryonic Breathing and knowing the way of making the Qì manifest more efficiently, both internally and externally.

"External Qì" (Wàiqì, 外氣) here does not mean "air" as explained earlier but the "Guardian Qì" on the skin and its surface. The Internal Qì (Nèiqì, 內氣) also does not mean the Qì (bioelectricity) circulating in the whole body, but refers specifically to the Managing Qì of the internal organs.

> *This Qì must be produced daily. The coarse Qì manifested at the surface for guarding (i.e., protection, Guardian Qì) is the Qì generated from (the breathing of) panting with sounds. If the Qì is originally coarse, then the life is short. If the Qì is slender, then the life is long. Those Qìs concealed in the internal organs and bowels are the Qìs of function (i.e., Managing Qì). These two Qìs do not originate from cultivation and receiving. The Embryonic Breathing aims for the two Yīn and Yáng Qìs from the heaven and the earth. It is the Qì that is used to congeal the essence (Jīng) at the beginning (i.e., Original Qì). When this Qì is congealed, the shape (i.e., physical body) is formed. Once the shape is established, then this essence Qì first congeals and produces two eyes. These two eyes are the essence Qì of the father. It is called the "essence of pure Yáng," thus millions of objects can be seen and inspected. In addition, from receiving mother's Yīnqì, Xuánpìn (i.e., heaven and earth of the body) is constructed and this is the mouth and the nose. Therefore, it is known that the shape is the origin of Qì's receiving while the Qì is the root of the shape. In this case, these two Qìs are the root and stalk of the shape. Once these root and stalk have been established, then (the embryo) is able to breathe softly by following the mother's (breathing). After ten moons (i.e., months), the body of the baby is completed. This is how those cultivators use it as a model. It is said that (this) is for returning to the root. This is why the Embryonic Breathing is so important.*
>
> 此氣須日日生之。凡粗氣在榮衛之中，為喘鳴之氣。氣本粗者命促，氣本細者命長。眾氣在臟腑之內，為運動之氣。此兩者並非修服之氣。其胎息者，是天地陰陽二氣，初結精之氣，氣結而為形，形既成立，則精氣先凝為雙瞳子。雙瞳子者，即父之精氣，號為純陽之精，故能鑒視視萬物。又受母之陰氣，而成玄牝者，即口鼻也。是知形為受氣之本，氣為成形之根，則此二氣為形之根蒂也。根蒂既成，則能隨母呼吸綿綿，十月胎體成而生，故修養者效之。夫云復其根本，此胎息之要也。

We know that the body's metabolism is completed through biochemical reaction in the body. During this reaction process, oxygen is one of the most essential ingredients for the new cells' construction and also for the production of energy. The quantity of oxygen is important and directly influences the production of Qì. For example, when you push a car or lift up a heavy object, before you tighten your muscles, you will inhale deeply first and then manifest the power. If the inhalation is shallow, the power manifested will be weak.

This translation distinguishes the Managing Qì (Yíngqì, 營氣) from the Guardian Qì (Wèiqì, 衛氣). Managing Qì is used to maintain the organ functions and to regulate the production of Qì through biochemical reaction. Here, it is pointed out that these two Qìs are obtained by breathing through the nose. It is different from the Qì produced through Embryonic Breathing. The Qì produced from nose breathing is for maintaining life and not for forming new life. New life is formed through Embryonic Breathing, which allows you to convert the Original Essence (Yuánjīng, 元精) into Qì. This Qì can then be used to conceive the Spiritual Embryo. In order to reach this goal, breathing through the nose must be slow, soft, quiet, and slender. When this happens, the Qì produced from the respiration will only be used to maintain physical activity instead of making it excited. In this case, through the calm meditative mind and abdominal exercises, we will be able to convert the Original Essence into Original Qì (Yuánqì, 元氣) and then lead it inward to store it at the Real Lower Dāntián (Zhēn Xiàdāntián, 真下丹田). In this case, physical activity ceases, and through the mind's concentration in the Wújí state (無極), we will be able to store the Qì at the Real Lower Dāntián. This is the key to Embryonic Breathing.

> *Ancient people all said: "Qìhǎi is the root and origin of the Qì." This saying is not true. This is because they did not know how (the Qì) ceases (i.e., returns to its origin), and therefore it is useless if repeated (i.e., re-initiate the Qì circulation). Ancient immortals all passed down the teaching orally and did not write it down in words. This is because they only wanted to share (the secret) with those who had the same aspiration. What is called the "root" is opposite to the navel on the number 19 of the vertebrae. This is the space between two spine muscles and under the bladder (external kidneys) which is called "Mìngdì" (i.e., Life Stalk), also called "Mìngmén" (i.e., Life Door), "Mìnggēn" (i.e., Life Root), or "Jīngshì" (i.e., Semen Residence). It is the place where the male conceals the sperm, and female preserves vaginal secretion. This is the root of producing the Qì for longevity. This is the root which (we should) recover today and cultivate (i.e., increase) its production. This is just like mother and son in shape (i.e., apparent), why do (we) keep it. Qì is considered as mother while the spirit is considered as son, and this Qì is the origin of the essence. Qì does not have shape, is not a substance, it follows the essence up and down. First it establishes the shape, and due to the existence of the shape, the Qì is able to reside. (The spirit) relies on the mother (i.e., Qì) and does not abandon the mother, thus lives with mother. Thus the spirit and the Qì can reside in the shape firmly, therefore longevity can be expected. Therefore, all of those who cultivate their lives always keep the spirit and the Qì unified (i.e., in harmony with each other), the son and the mother mutually stay with each other. In this case, there is no breathing from the mouth and the nose naturally. Zhuāngzhōu (i.e., Zhuāngzi) said: "Those truthful persons (i.e., those who have obtained the Dào) breathe with soles." This*

means the breathing is very deep. Lǎozi in his classic said: "Keep the root deep, and firm the stalk, means to repeat life." This means the most fundamental crucial key is maintaining the Qì in Mìngmén (i.e., Life Door). Therefore, in the future, those gentlemen should not let out (the semen) easily.

古皆云：'氣海者，為氣之根本。' 此說非也。為不知其所止，是以復之無益。古仙皆口口相授，非著于文字之中，蓋欲胎其同志。所謂根本者，正對臍第十九椎，兩脊相夾脊中空處，膀胱下近脊是也，名曰命蒂，亦曰命門，亦曰命根，亦曰精室，男子以藏精，女子以月水，此則長生氣之根本也。今之所復其根本，修其所生，斯則形中母子，何不守之。夫氣為母而神為子，氣則精液也。氣無形質，隨精液以上下，但先立形，則因形而住氣，為其母而不舍母，則依母而住，神氣住形中，故能住世長生久視。故修生之人，常令神與氣合，子母相守，自然玄牝無出入息也。莊周云：真人息以踵。言其息深深也。老子經云：深根固蒂，是為復命。此乃命門元氣根本之旨也。將來君子，勿得輕泄耳。

The author of this article believed that Qìhǎi (Co-6) (氣海) is not really the main concern in protecting the Qì. It is true that Qìhǎi is the place where the Original Qì is produced from the conversion of Original Essence. However, more important than producing Qì is to keep it without losing it. Therefore, he specified that the most important place you should protect and cultivate is the place under the bladder (external kidneys, which means testicles or ovaries) where the semen is produced. He called this place "Mìngdì" (命蒂) (Life Stalk), "Mìngmén" (命門) (Life Door), "Mìnggēn" (命根) (Life Root), or "Jīngshì" (精室) (Semen Residence). The reason for this is if this place is not firmed, then even if you have built up an abundance of Qì at the Real Lower Dāntián, eventually you will lose it. For example, sexual activities for a male practitioner will make him lose this semen, the root of life. Therefore, cultivation is useless. Here, I would like to point out that there is a place between L2 and L3 of the vertebrae also called "Mìngmén" (Gv-4) (命門) by Chinese medicine. You should not be confused by this.

In this document, the author also pointed out that in order to establish a Spiritual Embryo, you must know how to unify your spirit and Qì. Spirit and Qì are just like son and mother which cannot be separated. This training is called "Shénqì Xiànghé" (神氣相合) and means the unification of the spirit and Qì.

In summary, in order to conceive a Spiritual Embryo through Embryonic Breathing, you must know how to produce Qì at the Qìhǎi (Qì furnace), lead it inward to store it at the Real Lower Dāntián, protect it from loss, and unify the spirit and Qì.

15. Marvellous Applications of Inner Truth[3,7]

內真妙用訣》

Frank Discussion of the Correct Theory of Becoming Heavenly Immortal, Commented by Wǔ, Shǒu-Yáng, Míng Dynasty; Frank Discussion of Embryonic Breathing, #9: Chōngxūzi said: "Ancient Embryonic Breathing document said: 'Embryo is conceived from the concealed Qì and Qì is initiated from the breathing of embryo.' These sayings are the important methods of becoming deities and immortals in the past and future. Again, I would like to comment on it in detail and discuss it frankly."

《天仙正理直論・明伍守陽撰注・胎息直論第九》：沖虛子曰："古胎息云：'胎從伏氣中結，氣從有胎中息。' 斯言為過去未來諸神仙天仙之要法也。予愿再詳譯而直論之。"

Wǔ, Shǒu-Yáng (伍守陽) (1552–1640 CE) was a Daoist Qìgōng practitioner and scholar during the Chinese Míng Dynasty (明朝). Chōngxūzi (沖虛子), or Wǔchòngzi (伍沖子) are the Daoist names of Wǔ, Shǒu-Yáng. In the first paragraph, he explains the purpose of this document.

When a human has just been conceived, the two Qìs (i.e., Yīn Qì and Yáng Qì) are combined as one. This is only the Qì of the emptiness (i.e., no shape). There is neither embryo nor breathing. From mother's breathing, the embryo grows into a fetus. The fetus grows due to the inner breathing (i.e., Xí). When the fetus has formed its structure, it is marvellous that it can be breathing by following (its) mother's breathing. Therefore, it will not feel suffocating and stuffy in its breathing whole day. At this time, it does not breathe through the mouth and nose. There is only a connection with the mother through the umbilical cord. Consequently, he can be (alive) even though there is no breathing. This is the scenery of the real Embryonic Breathing. Once the baby has separated (from the mother), this (inner breathing) is broken. There is no more umbilical cord connection between the mother and the baby. Therefore, there is no choice but relying on self, breathing through mouth and nose. Though this serves the same purpose (in absorbing the air) as when he was still a fetus, the difference is that the knack of (receiving) is different. If (we) wish to reverse the situation and return ourselves to youth, how can we not change our current breathing into the breathing as we were as a fetus?

> 夫人身初時，只二氣合一，為虛空中之氣而已。無胎也，亦無息也。因母呼吸而長為胎，因胎而長為息，及至胎全，妙在隨母呼吸而為呼吸，所以終日呼吸而不逼悶。此緣不由口鼻呼吸，只臍相通，故能似無氣息一般，此正真胎息景也。離胎而息即斷，無母臍與子臍相通，不得不向自身口鼻起呼吸，即與胎中呼吸同，而暫異其竅耳。逆修返還之理，安得不以我今呼吸之息，而返還為胎中息耶？

It is believed that an embryo is formed due to the interaction of the father's and mother's Qì. The father's Qì is considered to be Yáng while the mother's is considered Yīn. Since these two Qìs are only inner energy, they are empty without any physical shape. At this time, there is no embryo formed yet, and naturally there is no Embryonic Breathing. When these two Qìs congeal and form into an embryo, then the embryo will do its own breathing. Even though the embryo absorbs oxygen and nutrients through the umbilical cord from the mother, the mother does not have the capability to push the oxygen and nutrition into the embryo. The mother is simply a supplier. The embryo has to absorb the oxygen and nutrition through the up-and-down movements of his abdomen. These up-and-down movements pump and suck in the supplies from the mother's body. Therefore, the first step in learning Embryonic Breathing is Abdominal Breathing. The Abdominal Breathing is also called "Back to Childhood Breathing" (Fǎntóng Hūxī, 返童呼吸). Theoretically, through these up-and-down abdominal movements, you will be able to convert the food essence, or fat, stored at the abdominal area into Qì through biochemical reactions.

In addition, to reach the goal of Embryonic Breathing, you must also know how to minimize the consumption of oxygen which is taken in from the nose or mouth. In order to do so, your physical body must be extremely relaxed and your mind extremely calm and neutral. When this happens, you will be able to keep your mind at the Real Lower Dāntián and thus lead Qì there for storage. These are the crucial keys to Embryonic Breathing.

> *Whenever (you) return (your) breathing (to the Embryonic Breathing) by using the nose and mouth, (you) are returning (yourself) to the place where the Embryonic Breathing originally was. It is as if (you) have returned to the time of Embryonic Breathing. Practice gradually until reaching the stage that Embryonic Breathing is "as if there and as if not there." What does the "as if there and as if not there" mean? It means (as if) the breathing has reached the end of the breathing. It is just like before birth returning to the stage of no breathing and no embryo, or Wújí state. This is the path which has neither life nor death. It can be done so is not because suddenly there is nothing (for you) to rely on or to coordinate with so (you) are able to return the breathing to its center for Embryonic Breathing. This is what is called "single Yīn will not be completed." This is also one of the reasons. It must be done when the Pre-Heaven Qì (i.e., Original Qì) has just started to generate,*

there is also a unique feeling, (i.e., existence) of the Original Spirit. In addition to the coordination of the breathing, these three treasures are gathered. The great herb (i.e., Qì) can be refined and completed (i.e., gathered). This great herb can then be led in the correct timing to the Huángtíng, the place where the embryo is formed.

凡返還呼吸時，以口鼻呼吸之氣，而復歸于胎息之所，如處胎息之時，漸漸煉至胎息亦真無。真無者，滅息盡之義也。方是未生時，而返還于未有息、未有胎已（以）前之境界，不落生死之途者矣。所以得如此者，亦非驀然無所憑依配合，便以呼吸歸中而可胎息者。所謂孤陰不成者，此亦其一也。必要有先天氣機發動之時，又有元靈獨覺，及呼吸相依，三寶會合，已先煉成大藥者，而轉歸黃庭結胎之所，于此之時。

When you start the practice Embryonic Breathing, you are using the nose and mouth for your respiration while keeping your spirit at the Upper Dāntián (Yīn pole center) and mind at the Real Lower Dāntián for the Qì's storage (Yáng pole center). Once you have reached an extremely calm and relaxed state, the mind or the spirit will not be led away from its center and the Qì consumption will reach its minimum level. When this happens, the breathing will slow down and reach the stage where it seems as if it is there and as if it is not there. Then, you can unify and harmonize the spirit and the Qì (Shénqì Xiànghé, 神氣相合), and return to the Wújí state of life before the embryo was formed. This is the stage of nothingness and insubstantiality, therefore, there is no meaning to life or death.

In order to reach this stage, you cannot just rely on the breathing and return the Qì to its residence. Without the unification of the spirit, this single pole will not accomplish anything. In order to reach this goal, you must have three things: to cultivate the Original Qì (Yuánqì, 元氣) and store it at the Real Lower Dāntián; to reach a high level of cultivation of your Original Spirit (Yuánshén, 元神); and finally, correctly harmonize your breathing. Only then will the condensed Qì, or great herb, be formed. When this Qì is led to Huángtíng (黃庭), then the Spiritual Embryo can be formed. Huángtíng is the space behind the navel. *Yellow Yard Classic* (Huángtíngjīng, 黃庭經) said: "Yellow is the earth color and the earth (in Five Elements) represents the center. Yard is the empty space in front of the house. It is named Huángtíng and means the empty space in the center." It also said: "The empty space behind the navel is Huángtíng."[21] In fact, Huángtíng is the inner space between abdomen and diaphragm.

As mentioned in Chapter 1, there are four stages of cultivation for spiritual enlightenment in Daoist society:

A. Refining the Original Essence and Converting it into Qì (Liànjīng Huàqì, 煉精化氣)—One Hundred days of Building the Foundation (Bǎirì Zhújī, 百日築基)

B. Purifying Qì and Converting it into Spirit (Liànqì Huàshén, 煉氣化神)—Ten Months of Pregnancy (Shíyuè Huáitāi, 十月懷胎)

C. Refining Spirit and Returning it to Nothingness (Liànshén Fǎnxū, 煉神返虛)—Three Years of Nursing (Sānnián Bǔrǔ, 三年哺乳)

D. Crushing the Nothingness (Fěnsuì Xūkōng, 粉碎虛空)—Nine Years of Facing the Wall (Jiǔnián Miànbì, 九年面壁)

From this, you can see that this paragraph is talking about the first stage of cultivation.

Thereafter, use the Embryonic Breathing to nourish, (i.e., conceive) the spiritual embryo. The spirit and Qì (i.e., son and mother), when united at the (Huángtíng) center, with the assistance (i.e., coordination) of Embryonic Breathing, then it is the beginning of conceiving the embryo. This is just what was stated in the document, Entering the Herbal Mirror, that "the forming of the (spiritual) embryo at the beginning depends on (the cultivation) of the original (physical) life (i.e., respiration). Though it seems there is a fine slender breathing existing, as if at the navel and as if not at the navel but in the emptiness, (i.e., Huángtíng)." It's just like the (Buddhist) document, Classic of Releasing Human Purgatory said: "The very original beginning, (it is) as if there is a suspended precious pearl apart from the ground for 50 feet; as if it has appeared right in front of the Buddha, as if there is a precious pagoda emerged from the ground, as if it exists in the empty insubstantiality." All of these are (the verification) of the result. All of these are accomplished by applying and transporting the Real Breathing (i.e., Embryonic Breathing) in the cultivation and gradually forming the embryo until it is matured. Though it seems suddenly there is no breathing from the mouth and nose, there is some respiration. It is just like when the embryo (is in the womb). It seems there is the respiration at the beginning and eventually it ends with nothingness. This is what the real Embryonic Breathing is. It is from this real Embryonic Breathing that the Yáng Spirit (Yángshén) can be established.

而后以胎息養胎神，得神氣乘胎息之氣，在中一定，即是結胎之始，正《入藥鏡》所謂初結胎看本命而得者。雖似有微微呼吸，若在臍輪而若不在臍輪在虛空。正《度人經》所謂元始懸一粒寶珠，去地五丈，如世尊之前，地湧之寶塔，在虛空中等語，皆是也。皆用運旋真息，以漸至成胎，頓然絕離口鼻，不存呼吸，滅卻有作，恰然處胎相似，而胎中之息，始雖似有而終絕無，即是真胎息，所以成陽神者。

Once you are able to unify and harmonize your Shén and Qì at the Huángtíng, then you will gradually form the Spiritual Embryo. The forming and growth of this embryo must rely on Embryonic Breathing at the Huángtíng area. When the embryo begins to form, it is very small like a precious pearl suspended in empty space. Right in front of it is the future of Buddhahood. This must be done continuously through Real Breathing, (Zhēnxí, 真息) (Embryonic Breathing) until the embryo has matured. This is the second stage of spiritual cultivation, Purifying Qì and Converting it into Spirit (Liànqì Huàshén, 煉氣化神) (Ten Months of Pregnancy) (Shíyuè Huáitāi, 十月懷胎).

"Zhàng" (丈) is a Chinese unit of length which is a little bit longer than 10 feet (3 meters). "Shìzūn" (世尊) is a respectful name for Buddha (Fó, 佛) (Sakyamuni). A human's central energy body is constructed of Two Poles connected by the Thrusting Vessel, (Chōngmài, 衝脈) (spinal cord). The Yīn pole at the Upper Dāntián where the spirit resides, controls the quality of the Qì manifestation, while the Real Lower Dāntián, or second brain, is considered as the Yáng pole which stores the Qì. When the Yīn spirit unites with the Qì at the Huángtíng, a new Yáng spirit (Yángshén, 陽神) will emerge and thus form a new life.

Practice this for a long time without breaking, very soft and dense, not even a second (that you are) not in the scene of no breathing as in the embryo. Train until it has reached the verification of the great firmness of the Yáng Spirit (Yángshén), (where) there is absolutely no movement or stillness, no initiation or termination (of the mind). This is the roundness of the embryo. Then, (you) will still aim to return to the beginning of the embryo's formation in (your) mother's womb, when the sole Qì (i.e., the interaction of Yáng and Yīn Qì) has not formed you (i.e., embryo) yet. This is the time when there is no discrimination of essence, Qì, and spirit yet. It is just what the (Buddhist document), Classic of Releasing Human Purgatory called: "the final stage of disembodying and observing the four directions to accomplish (immortality)." This is the final disembodying or returning the spirit through Embryonic Breathing. This is (also) the final stage of ten months (of carrying the Spiritual Embryo) so as to verify the immortality.

如是而久久無間斷，綿綿密密，無時無刻而不是在胎中無息之景，直証陽神大定，絕無動靜起滅，即是胎圓，乃返還到母胎初結，一氣未成我，而未分精、氣與神之時，正《入藥鏡》所謂終脫胎看四正而得者。胎息還神，固曰畢矣，畢其十月中關之事，神仙之証也。

After you have practiced for a long time, the embryo matures and becomes a spiritual baby. This is the completeness of the second stage of cultivation, Ten Months of Pregnancy (Shíyuè Huáitāi, 十月懷胎).

Then in the next stage, you lead the baby spirit upward to the Upper Dāntián for the birth of the spiritual baby. To enable the birth of the spiritual baby, you must have reached the Wújí state, which is even before the existence of the essence, Qì, and spirit. This will lead you to the third stage of spiritual cultivation, Refining Spirit and Returning it to Nothingness (Liànshén Fǎnxū, 煉神返虛)—Three Years of Nursing (Sānnián Bǔrǔ, 三年哺乳). The birth of the Spiritual Embryo means The Third Eye's opening so the new spirit is able to exit and enter from this eye or gate. When this stage has been reached, it means you are able to disembody and become a human immortal (Tuōtāi

Huàngǔ, 脫胎換骨). This spirit has its own life and is able to travel anywhere in heaven and earth (i.e., nature). Nature, or the universe, (i.e., heaven and earth) is called "Sìzhèng" (四正) which means "four directions" (east, west, south, and north).

> *Furthermore, there is further (training) which is to refine the spirit and return it to the empty insubstantiality at the Upper Dāntián so as to verify the cultivation of divine immortality (Tiānxiān). Therefore, (you) must move the (embryonic) spirit upward to the Upper Dāntián and exit through the Heaven Gate (Tiānmén), (i.e., Third Eye) through the manifestation of the Yáng Spirit (Yángshén). (This spirit) is able to exit hastily and enter suddenly. Why can it be done so? When it (i.e., the embryo) was still under the ten month (pregnancy), the spirit may have exited (the Heaven Gate). However, this is the exit which should not be. This is because the exit (of the spirit) was caused due to the six roots of desires (Liu Gen) which were attracted by the devil. Once it has exited, the spirit will be seized and enters the devil territory. (When this happens), the respiration will be again carried out through the mouth and nose. (When this happens, you) should immediately bring (your mind) in, and follow the (embryonic) breathing again and return the embryo to its residence. When the Spiritual Embryo is matured, then it should exit. Whenever there is a thought of exiting, the Yáng Spirit will exit from Heaven Gate. However, if it is parted (from the mother body) too long, it can be lost. In this case, immediately return to the (Upper Dāntián) and again enter the insubstantial steadiness, (i.e., emptiness). This is because when the spirit is born (i.e., exits the Heaven Gate), it is just like a newborn human baby, which needs three years of nursing.*
>
> 猶有向上田煉神還虛，而証天仙者，在所必當知。故遷神于上丹田而出天門，以陽神之顯見者，倏出而倏入，何也？當前之十月之內，而或有出者，是不宜出之出也，由六根之為魔而妄出。妄出則神走而著魔境，而息亦走著于口鼻，必急入則依于息而歸胎。此時之出，是當出而出也。故起一出念，而出陽神于天門，若出之久，恐神迷失而錯念，故即入丹田，而依于虛無之定。所以神既出胎，喻同人生之幼小，須三年哺乳者，以定為哺乳也。

There are two definitions of immortality. One is called "Rénxiān" (人仙) which means "Human Immortality." If you have reached the stage of human immortality, your physical life will continue for a long time. That means you have completed the second stage of establishing a Spiritual Embryo at the Huángtíng. However, in order to have spiritual immortality and avoid reincarnation of human life, you must establish an independent spiritual life. That means the spiritual baby is able to exit through the Heaven Gate (Tiānmén, 天門) or Heaven Eye (Tiānyǎn, 天眼) (Third Eye). Heaven Gate means the forehead area where the Heaven Eye (Third Eye) is located. Often, either one of them can be used to represent the Third Eye on the central lower part of the forehead. If you are able to grow an independent spiritual life, then your spirit will last forever, and you achieve eternal spiritual life. This is the third stage of cultivation, Refining Spirit and Returning it to Nothingness (Liànshén Fǎnxū, 煉神返虛)—Three Years of Nursing (Sānnián Bǔrǔ, 三年哺乳). This is the beginning stage of reaching "Heaven Immortality" (Tiānxiān, 天仙) which means the eternity of spirit. Six Roots (Liùgēn, 六根) means the eyes, ears, nose, tongue, body, and Yì (mind), the six roots which can generate emotions and desires.

It is also said that surely it will need nine years and three years (of cultivation) is talking about at the beginning of the (spiritual) exiting, (you) should occasionally enter (the body) for (spiritual) steadiness. This is to complete the stage of returning insubstantiality for heaven immortality (i.e., spiritual eternity). When (you) have (reached and) verified the stage of extreme insubstantiality and nothingness, then (you) have verified, (i.e., accomplished), the stage of Heavenly Immortality. In this case, the steadiness is more for entrance and less for exiting. It is also appropriate that (the spirit) should be able to be active when exited and reach high level of steadiness when entered. Therefore, I say: "The beginning of the exiting from the steadiness is actually the beginning of the entering steadiness." Though the heaven immortality has been verified, however, there is no limitation of timing. Therefore, Buddha also said: "When (you) have reached the end of insubstantial and empty world (i.e., Wújí world), my cultivation will not be ended after all." It is for this reason, (the spiritual life) will (only) be ended after the Heaven and the Earth, (i.e., nature), so I can avoid ill fortune (i.e., reincarnation). This achievement will again not be restricted by the timing. (In this case, you) have reached the marvellous world of immortality or Buddhahood. This is the ultimate goal of the heavenly immortal Buddhahood. Those who cultivate (this) holy truthful training should know all of these trainings and verify this result.

又言九載三年一定者，言出定之初，時而入定，以完成還虛之天仙也。証到至虛至無，即証天仙矣。然是定也，入定時多而出定時少，又宜出之動而入之遠也。我故曰：〝出定之初，即為入定之始也。〞雖天仙已証，亦無不定之時也。故世尊亦曰：〝虛空界盡，我此修行，終無有盡。〞正如此也。至于終天地之后，超過劫運，亦無不定之時也。此猶仙佛以上無仙無佛之妙境，而天仙佛之至者也。后來聖真，共知之，共証之。

After three years of nursing, the spiritual baby has become stronger and more independent. It will become very active due to the new discovery of the new world (i.e., enlightenment). Even though this has happened, you must occasionally return your spirit to its center and keep it firm and steady. This center remains the residence and the root of spiritual growth. Once you have reached this stage, your spirit will be able to reach spiritual eternity and escape from the natural destiny of reincarnation or rebirth.

However, the last stage of spiritual cultivation will not be ended here. In order to complete the final cultivation of heavenly immortal Buddhahood (Tiānxiānfó, 天仙佛), you must complete the final nine years of cultivation by facing the wall. This is the stage of Crushing the Nothingness (Fěnsuì Xūkōng, 粉碎虛空)—Nine Years of Facing the Wall (Jiǔnián Miànbì, 九年面壁) to crush the thought of the no thought, so your spirit is able to survive forever.

In order to do so, you must again return your spirit to its center and stabilize it. the Chinese word, "Dìng" (定) is a very deep Gōngfū (功夫) which means the steadiness and firmness of the body, mind, and spirit. When this happens, the Qì will be conserved and preserved. This remains the crucial key to the spiritual baby's growth. That is why it is said: "The beginning of the exiting from the steadiness is actually the beginning of the entering steadiness." After nine years of the final stage of spiritual cultivation, Crushing the Nothingness, the spirit has matured and become completely independent. In this case, the normal human body can be given up and will not be needed any longer. This is the stage of "heavenly immortal Buddhahood." If you wish to know more about this spiritual cultivation, please refer to the book: *Qìgōng—The Secret of Youth*, published by YMAA Publication Center.

16. Songs of Embracing Singularity in Embryonic Breathing[7]

《胎息抱一歌》

The origin of a human's life is nothing else but the Original Qì (Yuánqì). If (you) know where the Original Qì resides, then (you) are not too far from the Great Dào (Dàdào). Lǎozi said: "Millions of objects, (i.e., lives) are all Embracing Singularity (Bàoyī) and live. There is no object which does not conceal the Yīn and embrace the Yáng, (i.e., contain both Yīn and Yáng)." If (you) do not know how to embrace singularity, then it will be hard to become intimate with the Dào. This is because the Dào originates from the singularity. What is the singularity? It is the Qì mother. (Two) Qìs are united (i.e., Yīn and Yáng Qì), and formed into the embryo. Once this embryo is conceived, breathing begins. Two Xuáns (i.e., key ingredients) all have their own purposes. Therefore, the classic says: "When it is in the mother's womb, there is an embryo without breathing. (This embryo) borrows the mother's breathing to grow its body. After the spirits are separated, then there is an Embryonic Breathing." Those who are learning the Dào must know the theories of the embryo and the breathing and ponder their delicate marvelousness. If one is able to reach this original root, then he can become an extraordinary (man) and verify the holiness (of the training). When a normal person holds (his) breath, the (spiritual) embryo is not firmed. (However) when a holy man retains his (spiritual) embryo, (he) does not firm (i.e., hold) his breath. When the breath is held, the chest is full and the Qì becomes chaos.

夫人受生之本，莫非元氣。若知元氣所居，方不遠於大道。老君云：‘萬物皆抱一而生，未有一物不負陰而抱陽者也。’若不知於抱一，與道難親，故道生於一也。一者，氣母。氣結成胎，胎結成息，二玄各有其旨。故經云：‘在母腹之時，有胎而無息，假母呼吸成長其身。分靈之後，胎息具焉。’學道之士，切須知胎息二理，窮其微妙。若達本原，超凡證聖。常人閉息，不固其胎，聖人存胎，不固其息。閉者，胸滿氣亂也。

Original Qì (Yuánqì, 元氣) is the inner energy converted from the Original Essence (Yuánjīng, 元精). Therefore, if you are able to know where the Original Essence is stored and how to convert it into Original Qì and keep it firmed in its residence, then you are not too far from reaching the Great Dào (Dàdào, 大道). “Lǎojūn” (老君) is the name given to Lǎozi (老子) by his Daoist followers. Lǎozi said: “When carrying and managing the vital force (Pò) by Embracing Singularity (Bàoyī, 抱一), can it be not separated?” (Chapter 10)[22] Pò (魄) is the vital force which is generated from the inner Qì and the Shén. When a person has a strong vital energy to accomplish something, it is called “Pòlì” (魄力), meaning “the strength of vigor.” Yì (一) means both the spiritual center and Qì center which are connected by the spinal cord (Chōngmài, 衝脈). The spiritual center is the Yīn center, or Mud Pill Palace, located at the center of the brain, or Upper Dāntián, where the spirit resides. The Qì center is the Yáng center where the Qì resides; it is located at the center of physical gravity (the second brain, or Real Lower Dāntián).

The spirit controls the quality of Qì manifestation, while the Qì at the Real Lower Dāntián supplies the quantity of inner Qì that supports our physical life. These two, one Yīn and one Yáng, have formalized the Singularity (Yī, 一) or the Two Poles. Though they are two physically, in function, there is actually only one singleness. When the Qì is led upward to nourish the spirit (Shén, 神), the spirit can be raised to a strong state and is called “Pò” (魄). When the Shén is energized and raised so it is able to carry and manage our lives, then it has become Yáng. That is why Shén is also called “Yángshén” (陽神). The cultivation of Shén is accomplished by cultivating the human temperament first. The cultivation of physical life is achieved by conserving and not wasting Qì, and also knowing how to build the Qì to a greater abundance. This dual practice is called “Dual Cultivation of Temperament and Physical Life” (Xìngmìng Shuāngxiū, 性命雙修). While they seem to be two things, actually they are one. This is because they are the two Poles of one life, closely related to each other and acting as one unit.

In order to reach the Dào, you must know this singularity, protect it, and cultivate it. From this singularity, the Dào of life originates. This origin is also the mother of Qì, where the Qì is converted from Original Essence. Once you are able to keep this Qì at its residence without wasting it, with the unification and harmonization of the Shén, the Spiritual Embryo can be conceived. Once the embryo is conceived, a new spirit will reside in this embryo and become independent. Therefore, the mother and the embryo each have their own spiritual center and can breathe by themselves. In order to conceive this Spiritual Embryo, you must know Embryonic Breathing. This cannot be done simply by holding the breath. The breathing should be as if it is both "there" and "not there": slender, soft, quiet, calm, and peaceful. However, in order to keep your spirit and Qì in their residences, you must know how to embrace the singularity. That means the singleness of the thought which does not have any emotional disturbance and desires.

Yānluózi said: "Swallow and then hold (the breath), then it becomes chaos by itself." Mr. Yīn said: "If you use Shén to drive the Qì, then the nose will not lose its breath." Huángtíng Classic said: "Play music three times to dance the Embryonic Immortal. Since ancient time, those holy men have practiced how to firm the Embryonic Breathing and therefore achieve the Dào. Shén (spirit) and Qì have therefore conceived the embryo, which results in the steadiness of the breathing. It is rarely heard that through holding the breathing, one has become the real (i.e., has reached the Dào)." Holy men said: "Embracing Singularity (Bàoyī) and keeping (the spirit) in its center, the embryo will naturally originate. Protect the three and return three into singleness, three are spirit, Qì, and essence." These sayings have truly revealed the deep important points of the Embryonic Breathing. Therefore, (I) write a song of Embracing Singularity (Bàoyī) which contains twenty phrases to summarize these secrets.

煙蘿子云：'咽復閉，徒自亂。'尹先生云：'但使神常御氣，鼻不失息。'黃庭經云：'琴心三疊舞胎仙，自古聖人則閉固胎息而成道。神氣胎結，其息乃定。罕聞閉息而成真也。'聖人云：'抱一守中子自沖，守三歸一神氣精是也。'斯言實露胎息之深旨，故作抱一歌二十首以訣其要。

This section of the document cites four origins which talk about Embryonic Breathing. From these four citations, we can conclude a few key points. First, you should not hold your breath if you don't understand how and why. This can only cause you mental disturbance and physical sickness. Second, the unification of the Shén and the Qì through correct breathing is the key to Embryonic Breathing. This is also the way to conceive a Spiritual Embryo. Third, in order to conceive a Spiritual Embryo, you must learn how to protect your Three Treasures (Sānbǎo, 三寶), Jīng (essence), Qì, and Shén (spirit) and keep them at the center (singularity).

When Embracing Singularity, (you) must know the origin of the "True Singularity" (Zhēnyī). The spiritual enlightenment, after all, is achieved due to (cultivation of the) Dāntián. (Through) exit and entrance (of the Qì and Shén), the deep rooted Xīn (emotional mind) can be opened (i.e., enlightened). Shén and Qì can then correspond and harmonize with each other, which results in the development of the embryonic immortal.

抱一須知真一源，神明終自有丹田。出入往來心地啟，氣神相應化胎仙。

When you practice Embracing Singularity, you must know what "the singleness" is and how to embrace it. If you don't have this knowledge, it will be like driving a car in a new city without a map. The theory is like a map which can direct you to the precise place where you want to go. Therefore, you must always keep the questions of why, what, and how in your mind.

If you wish to reach the final goal of enlightenment, you must know where the Dāntiáns are, their purposes, and the techniques. After all, without knowing these, you will not be able to keep your Shén and Qì at their residences. Consequently, you are wasting your time and effort for your cultivation. In order to locate these Dāntiáns (especially Upper and Real Lower Dāntiáns) and keep your mind there, you must first see through your emotional mind and learn to release it. Once you are able to open the gate of the emotional mind (Xīn, 心), your mind will not be attracted and bothered. This will result in the calmness and peace of your mind. Then the Shén and the Qì will naturally stay at their residences. Through the unification and harmonization of the Shén and Qì, the immortal Spiritual Embryo can be conceived.

When just learning the teaching of Embracing Singularity, it is hard to know the truth (of the practice). After diligently practicing daily for a long time, (you) will be enlightened automatically. Even though there is no mutual correspondence in the profound abyss, the clam will contain the full moon and congeal the pearl with halo (i.e., shining Holy Embryo).

抱一初傳未識真，功勤日久自通神。杳冥之內無相應，蚌含秋月暈結珍。

Even if you have thoroughly learned the theory of Embracing Singularity, you will still need time and patient, diligent practice to see the result. If you have only understood the theory and established a firm confidence in it, even though you cannot yet reach a profound level of practice, a shining Spiritual Embryo has actually already been conceived. Yǎomíng (杳冥) means "Profound Abyss" which represents the Yīn spiritual world (Yīnjiān, 陰間). The Yáng material world is called Yángjiān (陽間). A clam is able to conceive its energy inside, and therefore congeal the pearl. The full moon (Qiūyuè, 秋月) is round and shining, which implies the shining result of forming the Spiritual Embryo.

There is a marvellous door to cultivate the truth (or true Dào) by Embracing Singularity. (Through this) Mr. Xī-Yí has directly reached Kūnlún (i.e., peak of cultivation). (The practice of) marvellous breathing is not affected (whether you) recognize the Xuánpìn (or not). A single Qì must long reside at the center all the time.

抱一修真有異門，希夷直遣到崑崙。妙息不干玄牝記，時中一氣鎮長存。

Chén, Xī-Yí (陳希夷) was a well-known Daoist Qìgōng master who lived from the end of the Táng to the beginning of the Sòng Dynasty (c. 900–1000 CE) (唐末宋初). Kūnlún Mountain (崑崙山) is one of the highest mountains in the west of China. Here, Kūnlún means the head (or the brain) and implies spiritual enlightenment. Pìn (牝) represents a female animal and implies the foundation of creation, the mother of millions of objects which has the same meaning as Dào (道). Xuán (玄) means profound, mysterious, and marvellous. Therefore, Xuánpìn (玄牝) means the marvellous and mysterious Dào, the mother of creation of millions of objects. The Dào is not easy to understand, and impossible to clearly and thoroughly explain. Therefore, it does not matter how much you comprehend the Dào—to practice Embryonic Breathing, the most important thing is to keep your Qì at its residence (i.e., Embracing Singularity). Then you will conserve your inner energy and this will result in the conception of the Spiritual Embryo.

When Embracing Singularity, (you) must know how to be magnanimous within yourself automatically. (You) must not allow the breathing to be impeded at the throat. If (you) are able to comprehend the real meaning of the contents, five internal (organs) and three palaces (i.e., Three Dāntiáns) will gain peace automatically.

抱一須知自在寬，勿令氣壅在喉間。若能曉達真詮義，五內三宮自得安。

In order to embrace singularity, you must first regulate your emotional mind (Xīn, 心). You should not be attracted or disturbed by your emotional environment. The key to reaching this goal is training yourself to be magnanimous so nothing is able to bother you. Only if your mind is regulated, can your breathing be smooth and natural. Though the theory is very simple, it is not easy to really comprehend the profound meaning and make it happen. You must continue your regulating until no regulating is necessary. When this happens, your five internal Yīn organs will be harmonious and peaceful. The five internal organs include: the heart, liver, spleen, kidneys, and the lungs. According to Chinese medicine, our emotions are closely related to these five internal Yīn organs, and can influence the Qì circulation in them. Only when the mind is regulated to a peaceful and calm state, can the Qì circulating in these five internal organs also be harmonious. In addition, once you are able to regulate your emotional mind, you will be able to keep your Shén at the Upper Dāntián (Shàngdāntián, 上丹田), calm down the Fire Qì at the Middle Dāntián (Zhōngdāntián, 中丹田), and store abundant Water Qì at the Lower Dāntián (Xiàdāntián, 下丹田) or Real Lower Dāntián (Zhēn Xiàdāntián, 真下丹田).

Embracing Singularity to return (to our) origins will (allow us to) reach the primary nature of human life. (Therefore,) why (do we) give up the internal (cultivation) and focus on the external training? As long as (we are) able to firm the stalk and keep the root deep, then there is a place (i.e., opportunity) for longevity.

抱一還元達本生，何勞棄內外邊行。但能固蒂深根了，只於此處是長生。

In order to find the origin of our lives, we must cultivate our Shén and Qì internally. External physical training, though it enables us to maintain a healthy physical life, will not lead you to immortality. In order to have immortality, you must first trace back and return to the beginning of life. Only then, can you firm your root and stalk, and re-establish a foundation for your longevity and enlightenment. The "root" here means the spiritual root at the Upper Dāntián, and the Qì root at the Real Lower Dāntián. "Stalk" refers to the Thrusting Vessel (Chōngmài, 衝脈) (spinal cord) which connects the Two Poles (Dāntiáns). The Upper Dāntián, the Thrusting Vessel, and the Real Lower Dāntián constitute the central energy system of a human body. When this central energy system is strong, the immune system will function strongly, and thereby longevity can be achieved.

It is primarily extraordinary (i.e., unusual) in cultivating (our) true origins through Embracing Singularity. (You) must not allow the Shén and Qì (to be) separated from each other. Keep them together at all times whenever sitting or walking. When (the Qì and Shén are) transported to the Heaven Gate (i.e., Third Eye), the life will be extended automatically.

抱一真元本異常，勿令神氣兩分張。坐行之處長相守，運到天門生自長。

To achieve the goal of enlightenment is not an easy task. The first step is learning how to keep the Shén and Qì at their centers firmly (i.e., Embracing Singularity). Next, you must unify them, and harmonize them with each other at all times. The key to reaching this goal is to stop outside emotional attractions and disturbances to your mind. Then your mind will be calm and peaceful, and can thus pay attention to the inner feeling. This is the crucial key to the unification of the Shén and Qì.

Once you have established abundant Qì at the Real Lower Dāntián and then led it upward through the Thrusting Vessel (Chōngmài, 衝脈) (Spinal cord) to nourish the brain, the Third Eye can be reopened. The Third Eye is here called "Tiānyǎn" (天眼), meaning "Heaven Eye." The reason for this is simply that when this Heaven Eye is reopened, you will be enlightened. Your spirit will unite with the natural spirit and you will be suddenly able to feel and sense many natural occurrences which other people cannot. When you have reopened the Heaven Eye, you should also have regained the capability of telepathy which we once had a long time ago.

> *When Embracing Singularity, (you) must incorporate it (i.e., the practice) into the Five Elements (Wǔyùn). How can it be in vain if the Qì and the shape mutually correspond with each other? Since there is nothing in the empty door (i.e., Four Emptinesses), why do you still go there (i.e., long for it)? This will make (your) floating life (i.e., the life without the root) wasted and (your) practice in vain.*
>
> 抱一令歸五運中，氣形相應豈成空。空門無物何須去，虛棄浮生枉用功。

"Wǔyùn" (五運) means "the transportation of Five Elements" (Wǔxíng, 五行), and refers to the Qì exchanges among five internal organs and the four seasons. They are: Metal (Jīn, 金) (Lungs, Fall); Wood (Mù, 木) (Liver, Spring); Water (Shuǐ, 水) (Kidneys, Winter); Fire (Huǒ, 火) (Heart, Summer); and Earth (Tǔ, 土) (Spleen, Four Seasons). When you practice Embracing Singularity, you must coordinate and harmonize the five internal organs and four seasons. Only then are the Qì body and physical body able to harmonize with and balance each other. The first key to cultivation in "Embracing Singularity" is to keep the physical body strong and healthy. In order to reach this goal, you must have built up abundant Qì so the physical life can be manifested efficiently.

"Empty Door" (Kōngmén, 空門) means the door leading you to the "Four Emptinesses" (Sìdà Jiēkōng, 四大皆空). This means the illusiory world generated from the four great materials: earth, water, fire, and wind. Since they do not have meaning to the spiritual world, they are called empty. If you continue searching for these material desires and do not know how to cultivate your spiritual world, then you are wasting your life. Since a human life is short, coming and going, it is like a floating duckweed without a root (Fúshēng, 浮生).

> *To practice Embracing Singularity, (you must recognize that our lives) are just like the person in the mirror (i.e., reflection). Among the colors, it manifests the body of colors. (To avoid this false illusion, you) must start from transcending Sānjiè (i.e., Three Circles). If (you continue to) have the delusion about the dust world (i.e., emotional world or lay society), then how can (you) keep (yourself) clean from the dust?*
>
> 抱一由如鏡裡人，色中唯現色中身。從茲漸得超三界，妄塵塵更豈能塵。

When you practice "Embracing Singularity," you must first recognize that a human life is like the reflection in the mirror. All emotions and desires are only illusion. To spiritual cultivation, they mean nothing. If you are attracted by the color (i.e., material world) in the mirror, then your mind will generate the color (i.e., desires) and continue to disturb your peaceful mind. You must practice to regulate your mind gradually until you are able to jump out of "Sānjiè" (三界). "Sān" (三) means "three" and Jiè (界) means "world, boundaries, circles, and societies." According to Buddhist society, the three worlds referred to by "Sānjiè" are: 1. The world of desires (for sex and food); 2. The world of colors (material world); 3. The world of "no color" (generated from extreme calmness through meditation). The first step in regulating your mind is to get rid of the worlds of desires and colors. This will lead you to the world of "no color" which can be achieved from the calmness of the mind. Once you have reached this "no color" world, you can then focus on your spiritual cultivation of "Embracing Singularity." The final goal is to get out of these three circles and reach enlightenment. It is said in Buddhist society: "Jump out of three circles, then (you) will not be in the boundary of the 'Five Elements' (i.e., the layperson's reincarnation cycle)."[23]

"Chén" (塵) means "dust," and implies the dirty mind generated from the seven emotions and six desires. Lay society is called "Chénshì" (塵世) and means "dust world." This is the world that fills up with emotions (such as anger, hate, love, jealousy, joy, sorrow and sadness) and desires (for power, wealth, glory, dignity, and many other things).

> *When Embracing Singularity, keep the Língtái (i.e., Spiritual Station) opened every night, embryo is formalized at the embryonic (residence) (i.e., Real Lower Dāntián) in every breathing. If the Shén and Qì can be congealed and become the precious treasure, even (though) the Original Spirit (Yuánlíng) is going to be dispersed (i.e., death), they will return to (your body) eventually.*
>
> 抱一靈臺月夜開，息息之中胎在胎。神氣若凝歸作寶，元靈欲散卻還來。

"Língtái" (靈臺) means "Spiritual Platform or Station." Please do not confuse this term with Lingtai used in Chinese medicine. Though these names are exactly the same, they have different meanings in different contexts. The Língtái in Qìgōng means the "spiritual residence" located in the brain, and is also known as Língguān (靈關) (Spiritual Gate) by the Daoists, and Língshān (靈山) (Spiritual Mountain) by Buddhists. The "Lingtai" (Gv-10) in Chinese medicine is an acupuncture cavity, located on the back between the spinous processes of the 6th and 7th thoracic vertebrae (Figure 3–4).

On the basis of our scientific understanding and traditional Qìgōng practice, it is understood that when we are awake and physically active, the major Qì flow in the body stays in the Conception and Governing Vessels (Rènmài, Dūmài; 任脈・督脈).

We know from Chinese medicine that the Conception Vessel regulates the Qì circulation in the six Yīn channels, while the Governing Vessel regulates and governs Qì in the six Yáng channels. Since these twelve Qì channels distribute the Qì to the entire physical body, the Qì normally circulates strongly in these two vessels during the daytime while we are physically active.

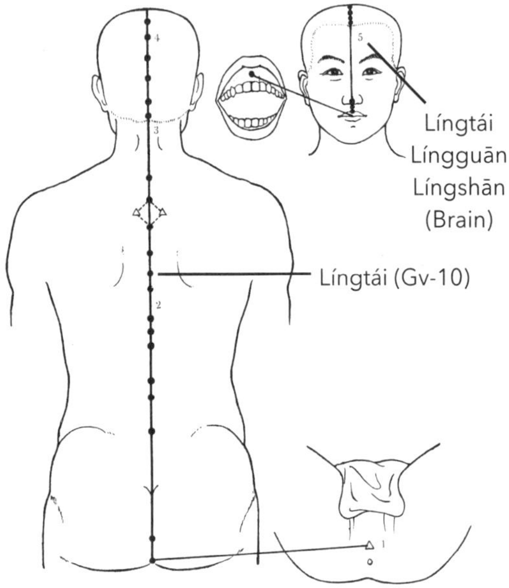

Figure 3-4. Acupuncture Língtái (Gv-10) and Qìgōng Língtái (Brain)

However, when we sleep, the major Qì flow will condense inward and circulate in the Thrusting Vessel (Chōngmài, 衝脈) (Spinal Cord). When this happens, the brain obtains Qì nourishment, and the pineal, pituitary, adrenals, and testicles or ovaries located along the Thrusting Vessel are also nourished and produce hormones. Therefore, when you train your spirit, the best time to practice is midnight, when the Qì is circulating in the Thrusting Vessel which connects the Two Poles (i.e., two brains). When you train at this time, the spirit can be nourished efficiently and raised to a high level.

When you practice, you are not only practicing the purification of your Shén but also building up the Qì at the Real Lower Dāntián through Embryonic Breathing. You should remember that these Two Poles (Upper Dāntián and Real Lower Dāntián) formalize the "singularity" of the central spiritual and physical energy. Only if you cultivate your spirit and Qì simultaneously can you reach the goal of unification and harmonization of the Shén and Qì. If you are able to condense (firm) your Shén at its residence, then you have obtained a precious result. Then, whenever your Original Spirit (Yuánlíng or Yuánshén, 元靈・元神) is attracted by the outside world, you will be able to lead it back easily and continue your cultivation.

> *The technique of Embracing Singularity must be stated correctly and clearly. (You) must not confuse the panting and relate it (to the Embryonic Breathing). The real embryo can be conceived (from interaction of the Fire Qì) at the Lí palace (i.e., heart or Middle Dāntián) which is led downward to the Lower Dāntián (to blend in with the Water Qì).*
>
> 抱一之術述正元，勿將喘息擬相干。真胎不過離宮上，直須令住下丹田。

When you practice Embryonic Breathing, your breathing must not be heavy (panting). It should be soft, natural, smooth, slender, quiet, deep, easy, and relaxed. According to the Daoist understanding, in order to conceive the Spiritual Embryo, you must lead the Fire Qì (Huǒqì, 火氣) stored at the Middle Dāntián (Zhōngdāntián, 中丹田) to interact with the Water Qì (Shuǐqì, 水氣) stored at the Real Lower Dāntián. In order to do so, you should lead the Fire Qì downward and Water Qì upward so they can meet at the Huángtíng (黃庭), where the Spiritual Embryo can be conceived. Huángtíng is a Daoist term which means the center place behind the navel area. The method of leading the Fire Qì downward and Water Qì upward is commonly called "Kǎn-Lí" (坎離) which means "water-fire" in Qìgōng practice.

> *Embracing Singularity to keep the Original (Shén and Qì) harmonious is precious and flourishing. (You) should not let the Shén and Qì apart from each other and become weird (i.e., out of place). (If you only) treat the Tǔnà (i.e., breathing) as a true essence of practice, (then it is) hard to place (your) body at the village of longevity.*
>
> 抱一元和寶易昌，莫叫神氣兩乖張。擬將吐納為真蒂，難致身於不死鄉。

"Tǔ" (吐) means "to utter" and implies "to exhale," and "Nà" (納) means "to receive" and implies "to inhale." Tǔnà (吐納) has also commonly been used as a Qìgōng practice. This is simply because the major key practice of Qìgōng is the correct way of respiration.

If you wish to have longevity, breath regulation alone will not lead you to the goal. In order to become an immortal, you must unify your Original Shén (Yuánshén, 元神) and Original Qì (Yuánqì, 元氣).

> *When Embracing Singularity, there is not even a second of pause (in practice). If the achievement can be accomplished from the six words (i.e., six healing sounds), the five internal (Yīn) organs will be clean (i.e., healthy). If (you are) able to maintain (the healthy condition) of (your) shaped body (i.e., physical body) and live long, there are always chances for (your Yīn and Yáng) interaction and for the birth (of embryo).*
>
> 抱一時中不暫停，六字功成五臟清。若留形身常住世，來來生處更交生。

To achieve enlightenment and longevity is not an easy task. It will take a long time of study and practice. Therefore, you should not be discouraged and practice discontinuously. Other than diligent practice, you also need to attend to your physical health. Only if you have good physical health can you live long, which will provide you with a longer time for your cultivation. In order to have a good physical health, first you must keep your five Yīn organs clean and healthy. These are: Heart, Lungs, Liver, Kidneys, and

Spleen. One of the key practices to keep these five organs clean, without Qì stagnation, is through making six sounds. These six sounds are: Hē (呵) (Heart), Hū (呼) (Spleen), Sì (呬) (Lungs), Xī (嘻) (Triple Burner), Xū (噓) (Liver), and Chuī (吹) (Kidneys). If you wish to know more about these six sounds, please refer to the book: *Qìgōng for Health and Martial Arts*, published by YMAA Publication Center.

> *To Embrace Singularity, (you) must always preserve the Shén (i.e., Spirit), Qì, and Jīng (i.e., Essence). From preserving these three (treasures) and returning them into one (i.e., singleness), the accomplishment will be achieved automatically. What this body's function (i.e., health and longevity) relies on is refining the Ganoderma lucidum grown in the field (i.e., Elixir Field, Dāntián) of golden room, and refining it until the crystal (i.e., Spiritual Embryo) is formalized.*
>
> 抱一惟存神氣精，守三歸一自功成。此身所為憑何住，金室芝田鍊至晶。

"Língzhī" (靈芝) is Ganoderma lucidum, a special herbal fungus. In Chinese medicine, it is believed that Língzhī has the power to extend your life. In this section, it implies the "elixir" (Dān, 丹) which can be grown at the Dāntián (丹田) (Elixir Field). Therefore, if you are able to preserve the essence, protect your Qì, and refine your Shén and unify them into a singleness, the Spiritual Embryo can be generated. Jīng (晶) is a natural crystal which usually takes a long time to formulate.

> *Embracing Singularity cannot be accomplished just living in seclusion by staying in the peaceful mountain (i.e., mind located in Kūnlún Mountain). If (you) don't have the Dào (i.e., the correct way) in (your) living, (the cultivation) is still in vain. Live long leisurely in this world with vegetarian and controlled diet to conceive the Spiritual Embryo is the way of reaching immortality.*
>
> 抱一非干守靜山，居塵無道亦徒然。長齊絕粒閑居世，結得神胎始是仙。

This section points out a few things to which you must pay attention, to reach the goal of longevity and enlightenment. The first is that unless you keep a correct lifestyle, even meditating to regulate your mind is useless. The mountain (Shan, 山) implies "Kūnlúnshān" (崑崙山) which is one of the highest mountains located in the west of China. In Daoist terminology, Kūnlún Mountain means the head, the highest place of the body.

The second thing it points out is that you must keep your life easy, without too much tension. In this way, both your mental and physical bodies will be relaxed. The third point is the importance of keeping away from eating meat. It is recognized by Chinese medical and Qìgōng societies that eating too much red meat, due to the presence of many impurities, can cause the mind's emotional disturbance and the Qì's stagnation in the body. This will result in emotional and physical illness.

Embrace Singularity so (you can) drink the sweet dew by yourself. The wind, thunder, clouds, and rains (i.e., emotional disturbances) are all over in the battle field (i.e., lay society). After cleaning and calming down the Wǔyùn (i.e., Five Internal Origins), (you) can get rid of laymen temperaments and reach the immortal village.

抱一自餐甘露漿，風雷雲雨遍疆場。五蘊肅然明靜後，齊驅凡質泛仙鄉。

The wind (Fēng, 風), thunder (Léi, 雷), clouds (Yún, 雲), and rain (Yǔ, 雨) here imply the emotional disturbances in lay society. Through these disturbances, your emotions and temperament are hard to control and cultivate. The first step in stopping these emotional disturbances is to clean the Qì circulating in the five internal organs. "Wǔyùn" (五蘊) means "five concealments," which implies the "five internal organs" (heart, lungs, liver, kidneys, and spleen). There is another interpretation. The "five concealments" of Wǔyùn are: 1. Color concealment (Sèyùn, 色蘊); 2. Perception concealment (Shòuyùn, 受蘊); 3. Thinking concealment (Xiǎngyùn, 想蘊); 4. Acting concealment (Xíngyùn, 行蘊); 5. Discriminating concealment (Shíyùn, 識蘊). All of these concealments are able to generate desire and emotional imbalance. Therefore, you must first clean away these concealments, then your temperament can be simplified and purified.

Embracing Singularity is to (apply) the real origins (i.e., Original Shén and Qì) to cultivate the true Dào. It is not necessary to put an effort in traveling clouds and water (i.e., places) to visit the immortal persons. It does not matter if the (Shén) goes or comes, always return it to its origin without any gap (i.e., break or slackening). If (you) rouse (your) cheek (i.e., agitate your emotional mind) too long, after all, will damage (your) body.

抱一真元養道真，不勞雲水訪仙君。返往元來無間得，鼓腮終久損其身。

The true Dào of cultivation is to keep, protect, and preserve the Original Shén (Yuánshén, 元神) and Original Qì (Yuánqì, 元氣) at their residences. If you know how to grasp this secret, you do not need to find a teacher. Whenever you have an emotional disturbance or a desire, the Shén will depart from its residence, and the Qì will be led away from its residence, consumed, and wasted. Therefore, the most important thing in your spiritual cultivation is avoiding any emotional disturbance to prevent yourself from generating desires.

To Embrace Singularity, (you) must always maintain the great harmony in (your body). If there is a dispute in the bird nest (i.e., emotional dispute internally), then the evil spirit will be aroused. Then the Qīpò (i.e., Seven Vital Forces) and Sānshī (i.e., Three Corpses) will bring (you) harm. If (you) keep (your) mind under the Kūnlún Mountain, then the shining moons are numerous.

抱一常令含太和，鳥窠爭敢起妖訛。七魄三尸寧有害，崑崙山下明月多。

"Qīpò" (七魄) means "Seven Vital Forces" which are related to seven emotions. The seven emotions (Qīqíng, 七情) are: happiness (Xǐ, 喜), anger (Nù, 怒), sorrow (Āi, 哀), joy (Lè, 樂), love (Ài, 愛), hate (Hèn, 恨), and lust (Yù, 慾). Sānshī (三尸), or "Three Corpses," are the three desires which could lead you to your death. They are the temptations of money, taste (i.e., food), and sex.[2]

In order to achieve longevity, you must first have harmony between the Qì body and the physical body. When this happens, all the internal organs will harmonize with each other and be healthy. To reach this harmony, you must first regulate your emotional mind and desires. If you continue to have these disputes internally, then you will bring much harm. If you are able to keep your mind at the spiritual center in the head (i.e., Kūnlún Mountain, 崑崙山), then you will be able to enlighten yourself. Under Kūnlún Mountain is the center of the valley where the spiritual Yīn center is located (i.e., Mud Pill Palace).

Embracing Singularity will allow (your) body to stay in the village of no death (i.e., longevity). Golden lotus flowers are blooming (for you) to sit on with nice and cool (feeling). There is no dregs and dirt in (your) solid abdomen (i.e., fullness of clean water Qì) and humble Xīn (i.e., mind). The jade pond (i.e., place under the tongue) is full of eight delicious juices.

抱一身居不死鄉，金蓮花發坐清涼。實腹虛心無滓穢，玉池滿注八瓊漿。

In Buddhist society, lay society, filled with emotions and desires, is considered as "emotional mud" or "dust" (Chéntǔ, 塵土). Everyone in this emotional mud has a subconscious mind of "truth" (Zhēn, 真). As long as you have this truthful subconscious mind in your deep heart, you already have a lotus seed within. If you meditate and search for spiritual cultivation, sooner or later the mask on your face will drop off, and you will step onto the first stage of spiritual cultivation, that of "self-recognition" (Zìshì, 自識). In this case, the lotus seed starts to sprout. From this self-recognition, through continuous meditation, you will step into the stages of "self-awareness" (Zìjué, 自覺), "self-awakening" (Zìwù, 自悟), and finally "freedom from spiritual bondage" (Zìtuō, 自脫). When this happens, the sprout will continue to grow out of the mud and bloom as a pure, clean lotus flower. The dirtier the mud, the bigger the flower that will bloom. This pure and clean lotus flower originates from pure thinking, with no emotional disturbance or desire, as well as a solid and abundant Qì storage at the Real Lower Dāntián. In this case, you will become a Buddha, sitting on the lotus flower with a pure mind and immortal spirit. When you have reached this stage, free from emotional and societal bondage, your body can be calm, relaxed, and cool. Consequently, the saliva, which can be used to moisten the body's dryness, will be abundantly generated in the "Jade Pond" (Yùchí, 玉池). This "Jade Pond" implies the place under the tongue which can generate an abundance of saliva during meditation.

> *There is a secret key in true interpretation of Embracing Singularity. How can those high elegant and educated gentlemen know and talk about it. Return the Shén and maintain its warmth at the embryonic origin. After (you) have obtained the marvellous key, then (you) will know the training is deep and esoteric.*
>
> 抱一真詮有秘關，高才儒士豈談宣。返神復熱胎元主，妙旨方知深又玄。

Many elegant and educated people talk about Embracing Singularity. However, they should know that the cultivation of Embracing Singularity cannot be accomplished just through talking. In order to reach the goal, you must know the secret key of maintaining your Shén (Yīn) in its residence and Qì (Yáng) at the Real Lower Dāntián. Later, when the Shén and Qì are unified and harmonized with each other, the Spiritual Embryo (Shéntāi, 神胎) will be conceived. If anyone does not know this key, then it does not matter how much he talks about it, the cultivation is still in vain.

> *To ask for longevity through Embracing Singularity is not difficult. The Qì and the shape (i.e., physical body) must correspond (i.e., harmonize) with each other mutually and (the Shén and Qì) enter Three Dāntiáns. However, how confused it can be if just talk about the matter through speaking. (To learn the truth correctly), (you) must have a personal oral instruction from a well-known (experienced) teacher.*
>
> 抱一求生不是難，氣形相應入三田。言中顯事何疑惑，親沐明師口授傳。

This last paragraph concludes that in order to achieve longevity, you must harmonize your Qì and physical body. In Qìgōng practice, the Qì body is considered the Yīn body and the physical body is considered the Yáng body. Though the Yīn body cannot be seen, it is the root of life. The Yáng body can be seen, and is the manifestation of the Yīn body. Therefore, these two bodies, seemingly two, are actually one. They are the Two Poles of the same thing: life.

You must also know how to conserve the Qì instead of wasting it. In order to preserve your Qì efficiently, you must know how to keep the Qì at the Dāntián. Only when it is necessary for physical or mental manifestation is the Qì led out for it. The more efficiently you are able to use the Qì, the longer and better your life will be. The crucial keys to reaching this goal is learning how to build up the Qì at the Real Lower Dāntián to an abundant level through Embryonic Breathing, and how to keep the Shén in its residence (i.e., Upper Dāntián) through meditation. When this happens, you will have an abundant quantity of Qì, and also a high quality of Qì manifestation.

Though talking and understanding is easy, there are many secret keys which must be taught by an experienced teacher. Knowing these secrets will shorten your training and make it more efficient and effective.

17. Secret Recording of Nourishing Life[2]

《養生秘錄》

If (one) is able to keep the "True Singularity" (Zhēnyī) (i.e., Wújí state), then the breathing will not be to and fro. It is like the fetus in the mother's womb. This is called "great steadiness."

能守真一則息不往來，如在母胞胎之中，謂之大定也。

Literally, "Zhēnyī" (真一) means "real one," "real singularity," or "real singleness." "One" or "singularity" implies the main energy pole of a human constructed by the spiritual center and the Qì center. As mentioned earlier, these two centers constitute the two energy poles of our body, and are connected via the spinal cord (Thrusting Vessel). One handles our spiritual life (Upper Dāntián) and the other supplies our physical life (Lower Dāntián). It seems there are Two Poles; however, since they are connected through the highly electrically conductive spinal cord, they function as one. That means they correspond with each other simultaneously and closely relate to each other. The Lower Dāntián belongs to Yáng, which supplies the quantity of the Qì and thus nourishes the physical life, while the Upper Dāntián belongs to Yīn, which controls the quality of the Qì manifestation. Yīn and Yáng are the two faces of the same thing, like the two inseparable poles of a magnet. It is said: "What is Zhēnyī? It means the body's Yīn (spirit) and Yáng (physical body) are unified as one."[24] The Daoist document Thesis of Retaining the Shén and Firming the Qì (存神固氣論) said: "If a human is able to place his original truth (pure mind) at the Heaven Valley (天谷) (Spiritual Valley), then it is the Dào of keeping the 'Zhēnyī.'"[25] The head is considered Heaven while the perineum is considered the "sea bottom" (Hǎidǐ, 海底). Therefore, "Heaven Valley" means the valley in the head, namely the Spiritual Valley (Shéngǔ, 神谷). When the Shén is able to stay at its residence, the Qì can then be kept at its center as well.

From this, you can see that to keep the mind at these poles means to maintain the singleness or singularity. When the mind stays at these Two Poles, the mind will not be attracted by the outside world, and the Qì can also stay at its residence without leaving and being consumed. It is said: "What is Embryonic Breathing? It is the Dào of abiding at the 'real one.' That is, Shén and the breathing are mutually relying on each other. When the Shén condenses (concentrates), the Qì will be stabilized (stay at its residence)."[26]

Therefore, it is written in the Daoist document Observing Vessels (脈望): "If one is able to abide at the 'Zhēnyī,' then the breathing (Qì) will not be to and fro." It also said: "If one is able to abide at the 'Zhēnyī,' then the real Qì will condense by itself and the Yángshén (陽神) can be gathered."[27] Though the spirit controls the manifestation of Qì, the spirit is the manifestation of the Qì, and therefore the Shén is classified as Yáng.

18. The Secrets of Spiritual Applications of All Veracious Holy Embryo (Methods of Transporting Qì)[3]

《諸真聖胎神用訣》

(御氣之法)

(If to) the top to the Níwán (i.e., Mud Pill Palace) and to the bottom to the Mìngmén (i.e., Real Lower Dāntián), two sceneries are following each other mutually, then it can save the remaining days and increase longevity. If there is no control from the Shén when exhaling, then this breathing is not complete. If there is no governing from the Shén when inhaling, again, the breathing is not complete either. If (you) are able to coordinate and harmonize the Shén and Qì mutually in every breathing, then the embryo can be conceived from concealed Qì and the Qì can be produced through Embryonic Breathing. (In this case), the embryonic Qì can be congealed internally and will never die. When it has succeeded, the male will be able to gather the Jīng (i.e., Essence) and the female is able to bear the baby. Though (the emotion) is touched by desire, it cannot compete against Shén. This is the way of returning the essence and nourishing it to the Shén. This is the breathing cultivating secret of the uppermost pure jade real (person) (i.e., those who have obtained the uppermost real Dào). If (you) are able to practice it daily, (you) will obtain its knacks (of cultivation) and gradually conform with the uppermost real Dào.

上至泥丸，下至命門，兩景相隨，可救殘老矣。若呼不得神宰，一息不全，吸不得神宰，亦一息不全。若能息息之中，使神氣相合，則胎從伏氣中結，氣從有胎中息，胎氣內結，永不死矣。功成之后，男子聚精，女子結嬰，雖動于欲，不能與神爭，是謂真返精為神也。此者乃是上清玉真修息之訣，日能行之，自得其味，漸合太上真道。

"Níwán" (泥丸) is a Daoist term, which literally means "mud pill" and implies "the brain" or "Upper Dāntián." The Spiritual Valley (Shéngǔ, 神谷) between the two hemispheres of the brain is called Níwángōng (泥丸宮) and means "Mud Pill Palace." "Palace" means the place where the Shén resides. Then, what is the physical implication of "mud pill?" I believe it refers to the pineal and pituitary glands. When these two glands are nourished with abundant Qì (bioelectricity), the hormone production can be abundant, and the body's metabolism through biochemical reaction will function smoothly. Naturally, your vital force is strong and the Shén can be high. "Mìngmén" (命門) (Life

Door) here means the Real Lower Dāntián (instead of the Mìngmén cavity in acupuncture). The Real Lower Dāntián stores the Qì, the energy for life.

This article points out that the Shén at the Upper Dāntián and the Qì at the Real Lower Dāntián are mutually coordinated and harmonized with each other. These are the two energy poles which establish the central energy system of our lives. In order to make the Shén and Qì harmonize with each other, you must know how to use Embryonic Breathing to unify them, and then the Spiritual Embryo can be conceived. In order to reach this goal, you must first keep your Shén and Qì at their residences. To reach this state, keep your mind at both the spiritual center and the Qì center. Once you can do so, the central energy will be firmed and strong.

Next, you will lead the Shén downward to unify the Qì at the Real Lower Dāntián. In this case, two Poles will be unified and become one. This is the Wújí state, the initiation of life.

19. The Secrets of Spiritual Applications of All Veracious Holy Embryo

(Secrets of Removing Hundreds of Internal Vision Barriers in Embryonic Breathing)[2,3,7]

《諸真聖胎神用訣》

（百嶂內視胎息訣）

What is Embryonic Breathing about? World people (i.e., laymen) do not know. However, many ancient virtuous persons (i.e., those who understand the Dào) have all verified its result. If (you) do not obtain this method from gaining the oral secrets, (you) will not be able to start (your) practice. (Furthermore, if) without personal instruction and (you) go ahead to do it, (you are) only the first class of fool. Even if (you) have stabilized the Xīn-monkey (i.e., emotional mind) and seized the Yì-horse (i.e., Wisdom Mind), it often wastes the Gōngfū (i.e., energy-time) and cannot achieve it greatly. If (you are one of) those who really wish to cultivate and train (Embryonic Breathing) and wish to catch the Xīn-monkey and restrain the Yì-horse, then (you) must first regulate (your) Qì and calm (your) breathing, clarify (your) Xīn, cease the worries, and forget the emotions; consequently, there is a response (i.e., result). If (you) are not doing so, then the time will pass without result and be wasted. If there is no instruction from a teacher, it is hard to know it.

且胎息者，世人不知，諸賢皆從證果。若不得此法也，把不定不得口訣，不得下手，不得親傳，把手教著尚做，不過一等愚人。便待定心猿，擒意馬，往往空費其功夫，不成大事。若真修煉之人，欲捉心猿，收意馬。先須調氣定息，然后澄心息慮忘情，乃可應也。若不如是，則空過了時光日月。不因師指，此事難知矣。

According to Chinese tradition, there are two minds in our body: the emotional mind called "Xīn" (心) (heart), and the wise, logical mind called "Yì" (意). Xīn is compared to an ape (Yuan, 猿), which, though small, makes a lot of noise and generates great disturbance. Yì is compared to a horse (Mǎ, 馬), which, though large and powerful, can nevertheless easily be restrained.

This document points out two things. First, the theory is clear, but the training methods must be obtained from an experienced master. In Chinese tradition, in order to prevent written secrets being revealed to outside people, normally there are some hidden oral secrets which allow to you connect the practice with the theory. These oral secrets are generally passed down through personal instruction between a master and a trustworthy student. Second, if you wish to reach the goal of enlightenment through Embryonic Breathing, you cannot achieve this goal by just regulating your Xīn and Yì. You must first learn how to regulate your Qì through stabilizing your breathing. Only then can your mind be clear and separated from emotional disturbance.

20. The Complete Book of Principal Contents of Human Life and Temperament

(Tàishǐ Family's Secrets of Embryonic Breathing)[2]

《性命圭旨全書》
(太始氏胎息訣)

What is the Dào? It is only a Grand Emptiness (Tàixū) (i.e., space). The heaven, the earth, the sun, and the moon are all generated from this Grand Emptiness. Therefore, the heaven and the earth are the real embryo of this Grand Emptiness and the sun and the moon are the real breathing of this Grand Emptiness. If one is able to conform with this Grand Emptiness (i.e., unification of human and nature), then the heaven and the earth constitute my embryo, and the sun and the moon are my breathing. What is contained in this Grand Emptiness is also my contents. (In this case) how can (I) be parted from the contents of the heaven, the earth, the sun and the moon, and become confused like other people?

夫道，太虛而已矣。天地日月皆從太虛中來。故天地者，太虛之真胎也。日月者，太虛之真息也。人能與太虛同體，則天地即我之胎，日月即我之息。太虛之包羅，即我之包羅。豈非超出天地日月之外，而為混虛氏其人歟。

The Dào (道) cannot be seen, and it is even impossible to describe it accurately with our limited understanding. If we force ourselves to explain it, the closest is Tàixū (太虛), meaning "Grand Emptiness." It is from this Grand Emptiness that the material world was initiated. Therefore, the heaven and the earth are actually the embryo of the Tàixū or the Dào. The natural ceaseless cycling which causes the energy change of the universe is the breathing of the universe. Similarly, a human body can be considered as heaven and earth. If we are able to unify our physical body and spiritual body with the heaven and the earth (nature), then the embryo of heaven and earth is also my embryo, and the breathing of the heaven and the earth is also my breathing. It does not matter how and what, we are part of this nature. If we are able to unite ourselves with nature, then we are able to harmonize our spirit with it.

To do this, first we must find the origin of our lives and trace back its root. This root is our Qì center and spiritual center. These Two Poles formalize a central Yīn and Yáng root which thus supplies our life both spiritually and physically. If we are able to return our spirit and Qì to these Two Poles, we will be able to reunite ourselves with nature. The spiritual center is located at the head and is considered to be the heaven, while the Qì center is situated at the lower abdominal area and is considered to be the earth.

21. The Complete Book of Principal Contents of Human Life and Temperament

(Xìngkòngzi's Secrets of Embryonic Breathing)[2]

《性命圭旨全書》
（性空子胎息訣）

My original body is round and bright originally. What is round and bright? It is my real embryo of the heaven and the earth. My original body is empty and silent originally. What is empty and silent? It is the breathing of the sun and moon in my body. Only if there is a real embryo of the heaven and the earth in my body, then the embryo of the heaven and the earth (of nature) can be blended with my embryo and therefore carry my embryo as well. Only if there is a real breathing of the sun and the moon in my body, then the breathing of the sun and the moon (of nature) is able to blend with my breathing and therefore breathe my breathing. In this case, my original body will become insubstantial emptiness. (When this happens), the insubstantial emptiness of the (natural) insubstantial emptiness will blend with my insubstantial emptiness and insubstantially empty my insubstantial emptiness.

我之本體，本自圓明。圓明者，是我身中天地之真胎也。我之本體，本自空寂。空寂者，是我身中日月之息也。唯吾身之天地有真胎矣，而后天地之胎與我之胎，相為混合，而胎我之胎。唯吾身之日月有真息矣，而后日月之息與我之息，相為混合，而息我之息。為吾身之本體即虛空矣。而后虛空之虛空與我之虛空，相為混合，而虛空我之虛空。

"Round and bright" means a mind spiritually perfect and clean, without a slight dirty thought (emotional disturbance). Then the real Spiritual Embryo can be derived in my body. My physical body was originated from emptiness and it is part of the great nature. This great nature repeats its cycle through Qì exchange (breathing). Sun and moon are the cycle of the day and month. In our body, we have the Qì cycle through breathing. In order to have a deep and profound Qì exchange and circulation, after I have entered into a deep meditative state, all material around me gradually disappears and my body becomes transparent and empty. When I have reached this stage, the natural Qì exchange and my body's Qì exchange will be unified as one.

Through Qì exchange, millions of lives are derived between the heaven and the earth. Through correct Embryonic Breathing, due to the smooth Qì exchange and circulation, a Spiritual Embryo will be generated in my body. A human body is considered as a small heaven and earth while nature is considered as great heaven and earth. When my spirit and the natural spirit have been unified, then everything is empty, since everything is originated from nothingness.

22. The Secrets of Spiritual Applications of All Veracious Holy Embryo

(Liǔzhēnrén's Secrets of Embryonic Breathing)[2,3,7]

《諸真聖胎神用訣》
（柳真人胎息訣）

Most people in this world do not know that the body we are using daily is (originated from) the creation and variation of the substances. Alas! This is (formalized by) the Qì from heaven. When the Original Essence does not weaken, then matter is formalized and becomes objects. Above, it relies on the heaven's clean Qì and therefore gathers, becoming the shape, and below, it connects with the earth's dirty Qì and condenses into a body. (In this body) is contained a "sole truth" (Yīzhēn). The world people do not recognize this and consequently leak out to outside (of the body). (This simple truth) means (the protection of) Jīng (i.e., essence), Qì, and Shén (i.e., spirit). If (you) do not know how to keep and protect these three (things), then (you) are old and near death. Those holy men (i.e., persons who have reached the Dào) will not leave (i.e., stop training) these three methods (of protecting Jīng, Qì, and Shén) even a minute in their walking, living, sitting, or lying (i.e., daily activities). After long time (of practice), the Spiritual Embryo will be conceived and (they) become immortal. It is praised as: "As a human living in this world does not know (his) root, all the time searching for the greedy mind and give up (his) original real (being) (i.e., natural temperament). If (he does) not know how to regulate the real breathing and Qì so as to nourish (his) original Yáng, till today (i.e., consequently), the heaven will be angry and sickness will still tackle (his) body."

夫人往往在世間，不知自身日用，物所造化也。噫！乃上天之氣也。元精不衰，物結成器，上依天之清氣，聚而成形，下接地之濁氣，凝而成體，內包一真。世人不識，故泄于外，乃精、氣、神也。若不守此三者，老死近矣。聖人常不離此三法，行住坐臥，久結成胎神仙矣。頌曰：‘為人在世不知根，一向貪心棄本真。不管元陽真息氣，至今天怒病纏身。’

All living objects are the products of the heaven and the earth Qì (natural Qì). In all of them, there is an essence concealed within. Through absorbing the natural Qì, they are able to grow and formalize the shape (physical body). This is also true for a human. After the embryo is conceived, through absorbing the natural Qì, it grows into a baby. After being born, through conservation and training of this essence, and continuously absorbing the natural Qì, and cultivation of our spirit, we are able to extend our lives and reach the goal of spiritual enlightenment. Therefore, these Three Treasures (Sānbǎo, 三寶) or Three Origins (Sānyuán, 三元), Jīng (精) (essence), Qì (氣), and Shén (神) (spirit) are the true values of our lives. They seem to be three items, but are, in fact, only one. They are all related to each other and cannot be separated.

Generally, a human's mind is greedy and the thoughts have been contaminated by emotional desires such as glory, dignity, power, jealousy, etc. When our emotional mind continues to disturb us, we will continue to lose our Original Essence, affect our smooth Qì circulation, and dirty our originally pure human spiritual being. In this case, it does not matter how much you regulate your breathing and Qì, you will eventually become sick and lose your life.

The key to Embryonic Breathing is learning how to protect Original Essence, maintain smooth Qì circulation, and raise the spiritual vitality. In order to keep your mind steady and calm at the Upper and Real Lower Dāntiáns, the most important thing is learning to regulate your emotional mind. In summary, this paragraph offers you a crucial key to Embryonic Breathing: regulating your emotional mind and continuing to search for the truth in protecting your Original Essence, Qì, and Shén.

23. The Righteous Rules of Heavenly Immortality

(The Straight Discussion of Embryonic Breathing)[2]

《天仙正理・胎息直論》

When a human being is just beginning to formalize, it is only a combination of two Qìs (i.e., Yīn and Yáng Qìs) and it is as empty as the air. Therefore, there is no embryo and also no breathing. It is because of mother's respiration, the embryo is formalized. When the embryo is formalized, it begins the Embryonic Breathing. It is marvellous that the embryo's respiration follows the mother's respiration and therefore, breathing all day without feeling stagnation (of the oxygen). This is achieved not from the (embryo's) mouth or nose respiration. Since there is only a connection through navel and thus as if there is no breathing at all. This is the scene of the real Embryonic Breathing.

夫人身初時，只二氣合一為虛空中之氣而矣，無胎也，亦無息也。因母呼吸而長為胎，因胎而長為息，及至胎全妙在隨母呼吸而為呼吸，所以終日呼吸而不逼悶，此緣不由口鼻呼吸，只臍相通，故能似無氣息一般，此真正胎息景也。

It is believed that a new life is originated from the combination of Yīn and Yáng Qìs. Yīnqì implies the Qì coming from the mother, while Yángqì implies the Qì coming from the father. Since Qì is an energy which does not have material form, it is empty. If there is no materialized form, there is no life yet and thus no breathing. Later, as the embryo is conceived and grows, it breathes following the mother and obtains oxygen and nutrition from her. This is how Embryonic Breathing occurs.

In this article, it is implied that the Qì originated from the Original Essence (Yuánjīng, 元精) is Yīnqì (i.e., water Qì) while the Qì generated from the Post-Heaven Essence is Yángqì (Post-Heaven Qì, 後天氣) (i.e., Fire Qì). When these two Qìs are unified at the Huángtíng (黃庭), the spiritual embryo can be conceived and formed. In order for this embryo to grow, you must continue the Yīn Qì nourishment. This Yīnqì is considered as the mother's Qì, which is able to nourish the Spiritual Embryo and allow it to grow. However, in order to generate abundant Yīnqì (Original Qì), you must learn how to protect and conserve your Original Essence (Yuánjīng, 元精). To reach this goal, you must keep your mind at the center without being attracted by the outside world. Through the correct slender and soft breathing, the embryo can be grown in the Huángtíng cavity.

24. The Secrets of Spiritual Applications of All Veracious Holy Embryo

(Hǎichán Zhēnrén's Secrets of Embryonic Breathing)[2,3]

《諸真聖胎神用訣》

（海蟾真人胎息訣）

What is the Original Qì (Yuánqì)? It is the mother of the heaven and the earth, the root of the Great Dào (Dàdào), and the (original natural) quality of Yīn and Yáng. In objects, it is named "the Qì of purity and benefit." In human, it is named "Original Qì." This means the human physical life and temperament. Each day and night, there are thirteen thousand and five hundred respirations and often the Real Qì (i.e., Original Qì) leaks through nose and mouth during these respirations. Those holy men (i.e., persons who have reached the Dào) who practice Embryonic Breathing always take in (the Qì) and (store it in Real) Dāntián, therefore, the air is out and in slenderly, the mind is steady and body is peaceful, consequently, gain longevity. What is longevity? It is the (result of) mutual harmonization of the Xīn, Shén, and Qì. It belongs to the truth of the Dào.

夫元氣者，天地之母，大道之根，陰陽之質。在物名淳利之氣，在人名元氣者也，乃性命也。凡一晝一夜，一萬三千五百息，常常口鼻泄了真氣。聖人久煉胎息者，常納于丹田，故微微出入，定自身安而得長生。長生者乃心與神氣相合，與道同真也。

Original Qì (Yuánqì, 元氣) is the root of all lives in this Great Nature (Dàdào, 大道). When it is manifested, it determines the Yīn and Yáng qualities of all objects.

Naturally, we humans also have this Original Qì, which is converted from Original Essence (Yuánjīng, 元精) in our bodies. If you are able to protect and preserve the Original Essence, the Original Qì converted from it will be abundant and pure. This implies that you will have a long and healthy life.

The key to Embryonic Breathing is through soft and slender breathing. Normally, we have 13,500 respirations each day. Since there are 86,400 seconds each day, that means it takes about 6.4 seconds for each respiration. This document explains that our Original Qì continuously leaks to the outside world through respiration. In order to protect and preserve our Original Qì, we must slow down our breathing and extend our respiration. Original Qì is also called "Zhēnqì" (真氣) which means "Real Qì." When the breathing is slow, the Xīn can be calm and the physical body will be relaxed and peaceful. Then the mind can be unified and harmonized with Shén and Qì. This is the key to conceiving a Spiritual Embryo.

In summary, the keys to reaching longevity through Embryonic Breathing are: 1. Slow, soft, and slender breathing; 2. Keep the mind in its extreme calm state (i.e., Wújí state at the Real Lower Dāntián); 3. Harmonize your mind with Shén and Qì.

25. The Secrets of Spiritual Applications of All Veracious Holy Embryo (Lǎngránzi's Secrets of Embryonic Breathing)[2,3]

《諸真聖胎神用訣》

(朗然子胎息訣)

Whoever wishes to cultivate his human nature (i.e., temperament), (should) burn incense and enter into an (isolated) room, sit quietly with profound Xīn (i.e., emotional mind), bite the teeth and gather the Shén. Calm the Yì horse and tame the Xīn monkey and place them together at (the Real) Dāntián. Nourish them with warm (Qì). Do not allow the internal vision out. It is just like a commander marches his soldiers. The Shén is the commander and the Qì is the army. Where the Qì arrives, the Shén also arrives. Two things mutually chase each other, not allow to separate. (Thus,) ten thousand sicknesses will not be related, and thousands disasters all exterminated. If those who wish to study the Dào have already gained this method, (they) should practice diligently.

凡修性之人，焚香入室，靜坐冥心，叩齒集神。定意馬，伏心猿，都收在一處，放在丹田，令溫養之，內視勿出。如元帥行軍，神是主，氣是軍，氣到處神到，二物相逐，不得相離，萬病不干，千災皆滅。學道之人，若得此法，勤而行之。

This document emphasizes that the important key to practicing Embryonic Breathing is to place your Yì and Xīn at the Real Lower Dāntián and gradually build up the Qì there, to nourish the mind with Qì. The key to reaching this goal is to keep the vision inward (internal vision). That means paying attention to internal feeling and cutting off all feeling and vision connecting with the outside world. This kind of internal feeling practice is called "Nèishì Gōngfū" (內視功夫) and means "The Gōngfū of internal vision." It is called "Gōngfū" (功夫) because it will take a lot of time, effort, and practice to reach a profound level of this inner feeling.

The place you meditate must be quiet and not have any disturbance. When you sit, keep your mind in the Yīn side. This is called "Míngxīn" (冥心). Míng (冥) represents the Yīn Space (Yīnjiān, 陰間) (spiritual world), which is opposite to the Yáng Space (Yángjiān, 陽間) of the material world. Xīn (心) is the emotional mind that links you together with the emotional and material world. If you are able to keep your mind at the Real Lower Dāntián, you will be able to cut off your mental connection with the outside world, conserve your Qì and store it there. If you can do so, you will be healthy and the Shén will be high. This is the key to health and longevity. If your mind is away from this center, it will lead your Qì away, and naturally, consume the Qì.

26. The Secrets of Spiritual Applications of All Veracious Holy Embryo

(Líshān Lǎomǔ's Secrets of Embryonic Breathing-Continuum)[2,3,7]

《諸真聖胎神用訣》

（續驪山老母胎息訣）

Classic said: "The heaven and the earth are the thieves of the million objects, million objects are the thieves of humans, and humans are the thieves of the million objects." These three ways are mutually adverse with each other, which results in the loss of the real Qì, essence, and Shén, consequently the Embryonic Breathing cannot be formalized. Therefore, those who cultivate human nature (i.e., temperament) do not love million objects, and thus their human temperament will not be stolen naturally. Therefore, it is said: "'Běnfèn' (i.e., Keeping Honest)." What those Daoists do is, I don't want what is yours, you don't want what is mine, and I just simply keep what I have already (acquired) honestly (Shǒufèn). Then, what is Shǒufèn (i.e., keep what I already have)? It is without exit and without entrance, always keep myself (i.e., my human nature being) at its root and origin, not moving and not still, not going and not coming, as if it is there and as if it is not there. (I am just like) a dead living human, then immorality is near.

經云：'天地，萬物之盜；萬物，人之盜；人萬物之盜。' 故三道相反，走失了真氣精神也，不成胎息。故修性之人，不愛萬物，自不盜你本性也。故云：'本分。' 道人我不要你底，你不要我底，只守分。守分者何也？乃是不出不入，常守本源，不動不靜，不來不去，似有似無，是箇死的活人，仙道近矣。

When millions of objects die, they lose their essence and Qì to the heaven and earth, therefore, the heaven and the earth are the thieves of millions of objects. Humans consume the essence and the Qì of millions of objects (i.e., air, food, substance) and therefore, humans are the thieves of millions of objects. When humans die, the essence and Qì return to nature and are consumed by the millions of objects (i.e., animals and plants) and therefore, millions of objects are also thieves of humans. These are the natural cycles.

In order to practice Embryonic Breathing and achieve longevity, we must first restrain emotional desires, conserve the essence, and keep the mind at the Real Lower Dāntián. In this case, your mind will not be attracted by the outside world, and consequently, your essence and Qì can be kept in their residences. "Běnfèn" (本分) means: keep "what you deserve" or "fulfill what you should fulfill." "Shǒufèn" (守分) means "to keep what you should keep" and do not go beyond it. Therefore, it implies to protect, to keep, and to preserve your Original Essence and be precious in keeping your Qì at its residence, the Real Lower Dāntián. When you treat yourself like a dead person, your emotions will not be touched and attracted by the outside environment. In this case, you have regulated your mind and are able to keep it at the Real Lower Dāntián.

In conclusion, the keys of longevity are: 1. Keep the mind at the Real Lower Dāntián, not on outside attractions and events; 2. Protect and preserve your Original Essence and Qì.

27. The Secrets of Spiritual Applications of All Veracious Holy Embryo (Xiāoyáozi's Secrets of Embryonic Breathing)[3]

《諸真聖胎神用訣》
（逍遙子胎息訣）

To cultivate means to establish a strong will and to nourish. Nourish means to take care, to tame, and to reach the truth sincerely. Those who wish to cultivate the breathing must first cultivate their essence; if they wish to cultivate the essence, they must first cultivate their Shén; if they wish to cultivate their Shén, they must first cultivate their temperaments; if they wish to cultivate their temperaments, they must first cultivate their physical lives. What the temperament and life mean, it means the Shén and Qì, the soul (Hún) and vigorous energy (Pò), Yīn and Yáng, Kǎn and Lí. After practicing for a long time, the Holy Embryo (Shèngtāi) can be formed. This is the real Embryonic Breathing.

夫修者，志也，養也。養也，頤也，伏也，真也。凡欲養息，先須養精；凡欲養精，先須養神；凡欲養神，先須養性；凡欲養性，先須養命。性命者，乃是神氣也，魂魄也，陰陽也，離坎也。久而行之，結成聖胎，乃真胎息也。

In order to cultivate anything, you need a strong will to accomplish it. Without this, you will fail. Therefore, the first step of practicing Embryonic Breathing is establishing your confidence and a strong commitment to yourself. Next, you must understand that the cultivating process is long and time-consuming. The formation of a Spiritual Embryo is achieved through continuous Qì nourishment, which is done through correct breathing. Once this Spiritual Embryo is conceived, it is truthful, pure, simple, and restrained as a baby. Therefore the goal of nourishment is the truth, the purity, and the simplicity of this Spiritual Embryo.

To cultivate Embryonic Breathing correctly, first you must learn how to firm your essence, to conserve it and refrain from wasting it. In order to do this, first firm your spiritual center. For this, first regulate your temperament, retrain your desires, and control your emotions. This is the inner side (Yīn side) of a human being. However, you must also have a strong physical body (Yáng side) to support your life. Without it, you will be sick, and your mind will be scattered, emotional, and confused. Therefore, the temperament (Yīn) and the physical health (Yáng) are the two most important things for your training. The way to reach this goal is through cultivation of Shén and Qì. When the Shén and Qì are cultivated, the soul (Hún, 魂) (Yīn) and vigorous energy (Pò, 魄) (Yáng) can be strong. This is the way of Yīn and Yáng balance.

To summarize, this article emphasizes the importance of dual cultivation of both mental and physical bodies. It also points out that the entire success of Embryonic Breathing practice depends on how much you are able to cultivate your internal mentality first.

28. The Secrets of Spiritual Applications of All Veracious Holy Embryo (Yānmèngzi's Secrets of Embryonic Breathing)[3]

《諸真聖胎神用訣》（煙夢子胎息訣）

Those who are moving are originally moving, and those who are still are originally still. There was no such moving or stillness in ancient time originally. However, the origin of the movement and stillness is initiated through the unsteady thinking of all lives. Ancient wise men taught us how to stabilize (i.e., calm down) the breathing. (When this happens,) the Shén will follow (the Qì) and Qì is stabilized. Consequently, the Qì stays (at its residence) and the Shén is stable. If the Qì is agitated, the Xīn (i.e., emotional mind) will be excited. When the Xīn is excited, then the Shén will be fatigued (easily). Those who wish to cultivate the Dào, if they do not practice Embryonic Breathing, then there is an origin of the movement and stillness. In this case, how can they enter the door of "Wúwéi" (i.e., doing nothing). Therefore, they are lost.

夫動者本動，靜者本靜，古者本無動靜，且動靜一源，蓋為一切眾生妄想不定，聖人留教，教人定息。神隨氣定，氣住神定。若氣動心動，心動神疲。凡修道之人，不行胎息，則有動靜之源，怎入無為之門戶也，走失了也。

The movement (or excitement) and stillness (or calmness) here means the mind's behavior. Movements are considered Yáng, while stillness is considered Yīn. At the beginning of human history, humans were the same as all other animals, behaving naturally and following the Dào of nature. There was no desire or emotional bondage. Therefore, there was no distinction of movements or stillness of the mind. Everything was done in a natural way.

However, later humans created seven emotions and six desires, and the mind became active. Since then we have learned how to lie, to play tricks, to love, to hate, to be jealous, to be angry, etc. Consequently, we have been trapped in human emotional bondage. The seven emotions or compassions (Qīqíng, 七情) are: happiness (Xǐ, 喜), anger (Nù, 怒), sorrow (Āi, 哀), joy (Lè, 樂), love (Ài, 愛), hate (Hèn, 恨), and lust (Yù, 慾). The six desires (Liùyù, 六慾) are the temptations generated from the six roots: the eyes, ears, nose, tongue, body, and mind. Once we have generated these emotions and desires, the mind actively leads the Qì away from its residence and consumes it. In order to preserve the Qì and allow it to stay at its residence (i.e., the Real Lower Dāntián), you must know how to keep your mind away from those human emotions and desires so you are able to calm down your mind. Only when your mind has been calmed, can your Shén be condensed, focused, and cultivated.

In order to reach this goal, the first step is to stabilize your breathing and make it peaceful and calm. Then the physical body will be relaxed, and the oxygen and Qì consumption will be reduced to its minimum. The mind will also be centered and calm. Only then can the Shén be focused and raised to a high level. Once you are able to do so, you will have returned to the beginning stage of life and behave like a baby. This is the stage of no movement (action), of stillness of the mind. It is the stage of Wúwéi (無為) (doing nothing) and Wújí (無極) (no discrimination of Yīn and Yáng).

29. The Secrets of Spiritual Applications of All Veracious Holy Embryo

(Zhāng, Guǒ-Lǎo's Secrets of Embryonic Breathing)[3]

《諸真聖胎神用訣》

（玉云張果老胎息訣）

What is the embryo? It is (the fetus grown) in the palace (i.e., womb) (the place) where the life is originated. Through breathing, the Qì is received at the Yuánhǎi (i.e., Original Ocean) which is located one cùn and three fēn under the mother's navel and named "Dāntián" (i.e., Elixir Field). After accepting the real essence (i.e., sperm), the shape (i.e., embryo) is formalized and begins to receive the Qì of the heaven and the earth. After one month, it is (the size) as a (tiny) pearl, two months as a dewdrop, three months as a peach or plum, this results from the pure and simple harmonious Qì. The embryo is in mother's womb; when mother exhales, he exhales, and when mother inhales, he inhales. When ten months period is up, the Qì is abundant, the six emotions are generated and (the mind is) toward outside, does not return his vision (i.e., feeling) and pay attention to his origin, without pro-

tecting the inner breathing (i.e., Qì), consequently, there is life and death. Therefore those holy men said: "I should not indulge my Sānshī (i.e., three origins of temptations), the (activity of) six emotions ceases and (the mind is) always kept at the Dāntián through breathing, keep there without slightly retreating (i.e., slackness). Those who cultivate the Dào, must first cultivate the entrance (i.e., way) of keeping the Xīn (i.e., emotional mind) calm." Also said: "To end (i.e., terminate) the Xīn so as to cultivate the Dào, then effort can be saved and (immortality) can be reached easily; for those who do not end the Xīn first and cultivate the Dào, then in vain and useless. First, (you) must end the origin of the Xīn, then (your mind) can be steady by itself. Consequently, the dragon and tiger (i.e., Yīn and Yáng) can be tamed and controlled, the success of immorality can be reached."

夫胎者，受生之宮也。息氣納于元海，在母臍下一寸三分，名曰丹田。受真精成形，納天地之氣，一月如珠，二月如露，三月如桃李，此名淳和之氣朴也。子在母胞胎之中，母呼則呼，母吸則吸，至于十月氣足，而生六情轉于外，豈于返視元初，不守內息，故有生死。故聖人云：'我不縱三尸，六情常息于丹田，守而無退。凡修道之人，先修心靜之門。'又云：'了心修道，則省力而易成；不了心修道，修道者返費功而無益。先了心源，然後自定，自然龍虎伏覲，仙道必成矣。'

"Yuánhǎi" (元海) means "Original Ocean." This is the Lower Dāntián (Xiàdāntián, 下丹田) (Lower Elixir Field) or Qìhǎi (Co-6) (氣海) (Qì Ocean) which is able to produce the Original Qì (Yuánqì, 元氣) without limit, like an ocean. One cùn (寸) of Chinese length equals one-third of a decimeter and one fēn (分) equals one-third of a centimeter. Sānshī (三尸) means "three corpses" and are the three desires which could lead you to your death. They are the temptations of money, taste (food) and sex. Liùqíng (六情) is a special Buddhist term that means "six compassions" derived or generated from the eyes, ears, nose, tongue, body, and mind.

This paragraph explains that in order to formalize a Spiritual Embryo, you must learn how to lead the Qì to the Real Lower Dāntián. In order to do so, you must first know how to regulate your emotional mind (Xīn, 心). If your mind is tempted and excited, the Qì will be led away from its residence. In this case, the Spiritual Embryo cannot be conceived. Therefore, the first step in cultivation is to end the activities of the emotional mind (Xīn, 心).

The location of (the Lower) Dāntián is one cùn and three fēn under the navel and is the palace site (i.e., main location) which controls three hundred and sixty key positions (of the body). The essence, brightness (i.e., righteousness of the mind), and the Shén protect the Original Qì (Yuánqì). There is a Spiritual Turtle (Shénguī) inside who utters and receives the Original Qì, keeps the breathings to and fro. There are thirteen thousand and five hundred respirations each day and night. The Original Qì has been leaked from the mouth and the nose, consequently the evil Qì has entered and invaded (the body), thus sicknesses are initiated. (Lower) Dāntián is the origin of the Qì's production. Named as "Dāntián" (i.e., Elixir Field), second named as "Jīnglù" (i.e., Essence Path), third named as "Qìhǎi" (i.e., Qì Ocean), fourth named as "Shǒugōng" (i.e., Abide in the Palace), fifth named as "Dàyuán" (i.e., Great Origin), sixth named as "Shénshì" (i.e., Spiritual Residence), seventh named as "Yuáncàng" (i.e., Original Treasure), eighth named as "Cǎibǎo" (i.e., Picking the Treasure), ninth named as "Wùjǐ" (i.e., Earth), and tenth named as "Běngēn" (i.e., Original Root). All these names mean the residence of the grand harmonious Original Qì. If (you) know how to preserve the Essence and Qì at the (Lower) Dāntián, then (you) will gain the Dào of longevity. Those who wish to cultivate the Dào, it does not matter if they are walking, stopping, sitting, or lying down, they should always absorb and contain the Real Breathing (i.e., Embryonic Breathing) at the Dāntián, then the Original Qì can be preserved firmly. After practicing for a long time, immortality can be reached. This is the Embryonic Breathing of the Truthful Persons (i.e., those who have reached the truth of the Dào).

夫丹田者，在臍下一寸三分，是元氣之宮位，管三百六十坐，精光神守護元氣，內有神龜一坐，吐納元氣，往來呼吸，一晝一夜，一萬三千五百息，皆元氣于口鼻中泄出，故引入邪氣，所侵而生病也。丹田者，生氣之源。一名丹田，二名精路，三名氣海，四名守宮，五名大源，六名神室，七名元藏，八名採寶，九名戊己，十名本根。皆是太和元氣，居止之處。若存精氣于丹田，則得長生久視之道。凡修行之人，行住坐臥，常含納真息于丹田，則得元氣成實，久煉而成仙矣。斯乃真人之胎息也。

"Shénguī" (神龜) means "Spiritual Turtle." Turtles can live for a long time. It is believed this is because they know how to keep their physical body calm, still, and their Shén centered. Therefore, "Spiritual Turtle" often implies the immortality of the Spiritual Embryo which resides at the Real Lower Dāntián. The key to forming this Spiritual Turtle is through profound Embryonic Breathing. When the Original Qì is able to stay at its residence, the Spiritual Embryo can be conceived.

After so many thousands of years of Qìgōng study in countless schools, there are many names for the Qì's residence (i.e., Qì Origin or Dāntián). This article points out only ten of many.

3.3 About the Dāntián (Guānyú Dāntián, 關於丹田)

1. Dialogue of Golden Elixir
《金丹問答》

Brain is Upper (Elixir) Field (Shàngdāntián), the Xīn (i.e., heart) is the Middle (Elixir) Field (Zhōngdāntián), and Qìhǎi is Lower (Elixir) Field (Xiàdāntián). If (one) is able to turn around the situation through catching the pivotal function of the dipper's handle, then the circulation between the top (i.e., Upper Dāntián) and the bottom (i.e., Lower Dāntián) will be just like the circulation of the heavenly river.

腦為上田，心為中田，氣海為下田。若得斗柄之機斡旋，則上下循環如天河之流轉也。

In Chinese Qìgōng society, the exact positions of the three Dāntiáns are often confusing and controversial. Due to more than two thousand years of independent study by different groups such as the medical, scholar, Buddhist, Daoist, and martial arts families, different names or locations are also somewhat different. Therefore, you should not be confused and simply believe just from one of the ancient documents. As long as you calm down and use the logical mind to analyze them, you will have no doubt about where the three Dāntiáns are.

As explained in Chapter 2, "Dān" (丹) means "Elixir" and "Tián" (田) means "Field." Therefore, Dāntián means the place in the body where the elixir can be grown or stored. Elixir implies the Qì which is able to offer you health and longevity. Generally speaking, there are three recognized Dāntiáns: Upper Dāntián (Shàngdāntián, 上丹田), Middle Dāntián (Zhōngdāntián, 中丹田), and Lower Dāntián (Xiàdāntián, 下丹田). The Lower Dāntián can again be subdivided into False Lower Dāntián (Jiǎ Xiàdāntián, 假下丹田) and Real Lower Dāntián (Zhēn Xiàdāntián, 真下丹田).

The authors of most of the documents believe that the Upper Dāntián is located at the central point between the two eyebrows and about three inches directly inward. In the document Embracing Simplicity (Bàopǔzi, 抱朴子) it is said: "The space between the two eyebrows, one inch inward is Míngtáng (明堂), two inches inward is Dòngfáng (洞房), and three inches inward is Shàngdāntián (上丹田) (Upper Dāntián)."[28] This is the center of the brain at the bottom of the Spiritual Valley (Shéngǔ, 神谷). It is where the pineal and pituitary glands are located. These two glands are called "Níwán" (泥丸) (Mud Pills) and this central area of the brain is called "Níwángōng" (泥丸宮) which means "Mud Pill Palace" in Daoist society. From this center, unlimited Qì can be produced. As known today, due to hormone production in the pineal and pituitary glands, the body's biochemical reaction and metabolism can be smoothly carried out and the Qì in the body can be abundant, with the Spirit of Vitality (Jīngshén, 精神) raised to a higher level.

Some others believe the entire brain is the Upper Dāntián. Eastern Medical Advices of Maintaining Health (Dōngyī Bǎojiàn, 東醫保鑒) said: "Brain is Upper Dāntián... is the residence of the concealed Shén."[29] The valley-like space between the two lobes of the brain is called "Shéngǔ" (神谷) (Spiritual Valley) or "Tiāngǔ" (天谷) (Heaven Valley) where the "Gǔshén" (谷神) (Valley Spirit) resides. This valley acts as an energy chamber that allows your thinking to vibrate and resonate with the surrounding energy and communicate with other natural spirits. The front end of the valley is the "Heaven Eye"

(Tiānyǎn, 天眼) or "Heaven Gate" (Tiānmén, 天門) and is what the Western world calls the "Third Eye." It is believed that we humans had this third eye, just as other animals do, and it was open for us to communicate with other spirits through telepathy a long time ago. Later, when we learned how to lie, cheat, and play tricks on each other, in order to hide our secrets behind the mask, we closed the third eye and stopped the brain from communicating directly through telepathy.

According to Buddhist and Daoist societies, when this third eye is reopened, we will be enlightened and will suddenly comprehend the meaning of life and nature. Naturally, we will regain our capability of telepathy and resume reading other peoples mind's. When this happens, you must retire to the mountains and keep away from the masked human society. In order to reach this spiritual enlightenment, you must learn how to build up abundant Qì in the Real Lower Dāntián and lead it upward through the Thrusting Vessel (Chōngmài, 衝脈) (spinal cord) to nourish the brain. When the brain has been energized to a higher level, the Third Eye will be reopened.

The Upper Dāntián has also been called "Shàngdǎo" (上島), "Shàng Tǔfǔ" (上土釜), or "Shàng Tiānguān" (上天關), among other names. To avoid complexity, we will not explain all of these alternative names here.

Generally, the Middle Dāntián (Zhōngdāntián, 中丹田) is believed to be located on the Shānzhōng (膻中) area which is the center between the nipples. In the Daoist document Embracing Simplicity, Inner Chapter, Dìzhēn Roll (Bàopǔzi Nèipiān. Dìzhēnjuǎn, 抱朴子內篇・地真卷), it is said: "Under the heart is Jiànggōng (絳宮) (Crimson Palace), Jīnquè (金闕) (Golden Palace), and Middle Dāntián."[30] Therefore, Middle Dāntián is also called Jiànggōng or Jin Jue. This has also been mentioned in the document Eastern Medical Advice for Maintaining Health (Dōngyī Bǎojiàn, 東醫保鑒): "The heart is Jiànggōng, Middle Dāntián... is the residence of storing Qì."[31] In Chinese Qìgōng, it is known that the Middle Dāntián is the residence of the "Fire Qì" (Huǒqì, 火氣), while the Lower Dāntián is the residence of the "Water Qì" (Shuǐqì, 水氣). The Fire Qì is produced from the air and food essence taken into our bodies after the birth and therefore called "Post-Heaven Qì" (Hòutiānqì, 後天氣). The Water Qì is converted from the Original Essence (hormones) from the kidneys (adrenals and testicles) and therefore called "Pre-Heaven Qì" (Xiāntiānqì, 先天氣).

In actuality, behind the Middle Dāntián area is the diaphragm. Through the diaphragm's up-and-down movement, we are able to take in oxygen and get rid of carbon dioxide. Due to this heavy exercise occurring in every second of our lives, the diaphragm is thought to be made of highly electrically conductive tissue. On the top and the bottom of the diaphragm are the fasciae, which are poor electric conductors.[32] When a good conductor is sandwiched between two poor conductors, the charges can be stored as in a battery. I believe that this is how this area is able to accumulate Qì (bioelectricity).

The Middle Dāntián has also been called "Huángtáng" (黃堂), "Tǔfǔ" (土府), and "Huángtíng" (黃庭), etc. Again, we will offer no further interpretation for these names.

There are many names for the Lower Dāntián such as "Qìhǎi" (氣海) (Qì Ocean), "Guānyuán" (關元) (Key Origin), "Mìngmén" (命門) (Life Door), "Shénlú" (神爐) (Spiritual Furnace), "Tiāngēn" (天根) (Heaven's Root), "Línggǔ" (靈谷) (Divine Valley), etc. It is named so because the Lower Dāntián is the root and the origin of our physical and spiritual lives. You should remember that it (Yáng pole) is one of the Two Poles which constitute our body's central energy system. The other pole, the Yīn pole, is the Upper Dāntián. These Two Poles are connected by the Thrusting Vessel (Chōngmài, 衝脈) (Spinal Cord), a very highly electrically conductive material. Therefore, though physically there are Two Poles, in function, they are actually one, because they correspond and synchronize with each other.

According to Daoist Qìgōng practice, there are actually two Lower Dāntiáns, one is called "False Lower Dāntián" (Jiǎ Xiàdāntián, 假下丹田) and the other is called "Real Lower Dāntián" (Zhēn Xiàdāntián, 真下丹田). The location of the False Dāntián is located about three inches below the navel. In the document Eastern Medical Advices of Maintaining Health (Dōngyī Bǎojiàn, 東醫保鑒), it is said that: "The place three inches under the navel is Lower Dāntián... it is the residence of storing the essence."[33] This place is also commonly called Qìhǎi (氣海) (Qì Ocean) by Chinese medical society. This place is also often called "Elixir Furnace" (Dānlú, 丹爐) since it is able to produce elixir (Qì). This False Dāntián is located on the Conception Vessel (Rènmài, 任脈) which is connected with the Governing Vessel (Dūmài, 督脈) at the Huìyīn (會陰), thus connecting the path of Small Cyclic Heaven Circulation (Xiǎozhōutiān, 小周天) (Figure 3–5). Through this circulation, the Qì can be distributed to the twelve primary Qì channels to support the physical body's life and activities. Therefore, whenever the Qì is built up to a higher level at the False Dāntián, the Qì will be distributed immediately, and cannot be stored to an abundant level. The Daoists called it the False Dāntián, because if it were a Real Lower Dāntián, it should be able to store the Qì to an abundant level.

Then where is the Real Lower Dāntián? In the document *Seventh Bamboo Slips of the Bamboo Bookcase* (*Yúnjí Qīqiān*, 云笈七籤), it is said: "What is Dāntián? It is the root of a human('s life), the hidden place of the essence and Shén, the origin of five Qìs (i.e., five internal Yīn organs), and the residence of the embryo. Males use it to conceal the essence and females use it to preserve the liquid. It is the place for production of the baby and the door of unification and harmonization of Yīn and Yáng. It is located three inches underneath the navel (in the body) attached to the spine, and the root of two (internal) kidneys."[34] From this document, we can see the place of the Real Lower Dāntián is recognized as the place underneath the navel and in front of the kidneys.

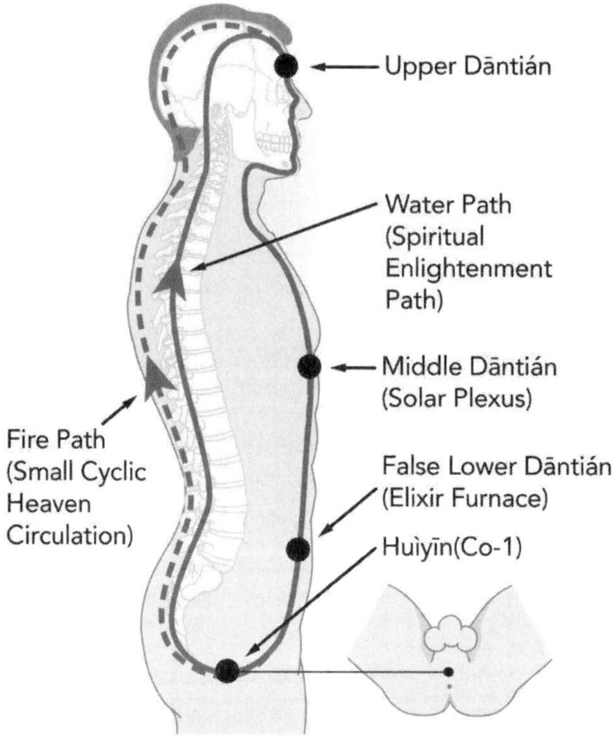

Figure 3-5. The Water and Fire Paths of Qì Circulation

2. Observing Vessels[2]
《脈望》

Dāntián, is the root of life. This is the reason why those Daoists who ponder (i.e., meditate) for their spiritual (cultivation) and Buddhists who meditate for (their Buddhahood), all gather the real Qì (i.e., Original Qì) under the navel. There is a Spiritual Turtle (Shénguī) in the Dāntián who inhales and exhales this Real Qì (Zhēnqì). This respiration is not the breathing through the mouth and nose. The mouth and the nose are only the doors for respiration. Dāntián is the origin of the Qì and is the place for those holy men to begin their cultivation. This is the place where they keep and store the "Real Singularity" (Zhēnyī), therefore, it is called "Embryonic Breathing."

丹田，性命之本。道士思神，比丘坐禪，皆聚真氣于臍下，良由此也。丹田內有神龜，呼吸真氣，非口鼻之呼吸也。口鼻只是呼吸之門戶，丹田為氣之本源，聖人下手之處，收藏真一所居，故曰胎息。

Meditation is called "Dǎzuò" (打坐) or "Zuòchán" (坐禪). It does not matter whether those who meditate are Daoists or Buddhists, when they meditate they all learn how to keep the mind inside the body and the body relaxed. In this way, they are able to store the Qì to a higher level at the Lower Dāntián, which is located under the navel.

"Zhēnyī" (真一) means "Real One" or "True Singularity." This real one means the central Qì system that is constituted by the Two Poles: the Yáng pole at the Real Lower Dāntián, that provides the quantity of the Qì and the Yīn pole at the Upper Dāntián, which controls the quality of the Qì's manifestation (life). Physically, there are Two Poles. In function, however, they are one, and are only Two Poles—the Yīn and Yáng—of the same thing (Real One). If you are able to keep your mind in this "Real One" or "True Singularity," you will be able to raise up your Spirit of Vitality (Jīngshén, 精神) and also establish an abundant storage of Qì.

As explained in Section 2–2, the air (Kōngqì, 空氣) we inhale through the nose is called "Shàngcéngqì" (上層氣) which means "Upper Level Qì" or "Wàiqì" (外氣) which means "External Qì." The bioelectricity stored at the Real Lower Dāntián is called "Xiàcéngqì" (下層氣) which means "Lower Level Qì" or "Nèiqì" (內氣) (Inner Qì.) Please review Section 2–2 for more detail.

3. Classic of Difficulties; 66th Difficulty
《難經・六十六難》

> *The site between (the place) under the navel, and between the kidneys, where the Qì is initiated, is the life of a human and the origin of Qì in the Twelve Primary Qì Channels. Yáng, Xuán-Cāo explained: "The site between (the place) under the navel, and between the kidneys is Dāntián. Dāntián is the root and foundation of a human."*
>
> 臍下腎間動氣者，人之性命也，十二經之根本也。楊玄操注：'臍下腎間動氣者，丹田也。丹田者，人之根本也。

From this document, it is believed that the Dāntián is below the navel, and that means the abdominal area. However, it is also between the kidneys. Here, you should know that the Chinese define kidneys as internal kidneys (Nèishèn, 內腎) and also external kidneys (Wàishèn, 外腎). Internal kidneys are the same kidneys as defined by Western medicine. However, "external kidneys" means testicles or ovaries. All of these places are capable of producing "Original Essence" (Yuánjīng, 元精) (hormones).

This document talks about the Real Lower Dāntián, which is considered to be the "second brain" located in the intestines. This place is able to store Qì or bioelectricity to an abundant level, and can be considered the bio-battery of the human body. This place is the root of human physical and spiritual life.

4. Muscle/Tendon Changing Classic; Appendix
《易筋經・附錄》

Huángtíng: The place which the immortals use to form the elixir. Huángtíng Classic said: "Underneath the heart, above (i.e., in front of) the kidneys, spleen on the left, and the liver on the right. The life door (Shēngmén) is in the front, the closed door (Mìhù) is in the rear, they are connected like a ring, it is white like cotton with an inch diameter. It encloses the Essence and the refinement of the entire body... This place is opposite the navel and is the root of a human life."

黃庭：神仙結丹處。曰：〝心下腎上，脾左肝右，生門在前，密戶居后，其連如環，其白如綿，方圓徑寸，包裹一身之精粹。・・・其處與臍相對。人之命脈根蒂也。〞

"Huángtíng" (黃庭) (Yellow Yard) is also called "Yùhuánxué" (玉環穴) (Jade Ring Cavity). The name "Jade Ring" is first used in the book *Illustration of the Brass Man Acupuncture and Moxibustion* (*Tóngrén Yúxuè Zhēnjiǔtú*, 銅人俞穴針灸圖) by Dr. Wáng, Wéi-Yī (王唯一). The Daoist book *Wánglù Shíyú* (王錄識餘) said: "In the Illustration of the Brass Man Acupuncture and Moxibustion it was recorded (that) within the body's cavities of viscera and bowels, there is a Jade Ring (Yùhuán, 玉環), (but) I do not know what the Jade Ring is." Later, the Daoist Zhāng, Zǐ-Yáng (張紫陽) explained the place which the immortals use to form the elixir: "The Heart is on the top, the kidneys are underneath, spleen is on the left, and the liver is on the right. The life door (Shēngmén, 生門) is in the front, the concealed door (Mìhù, 密戶) is in the rear—they are connected like a ring, it is white like cotton with an inch diameter. It encloses the essence and the refinement of the entire body. This is the Jade Ring."[35]

"Shēngmén" (生門) means "Life Door", namely the navel which allows a fetus to absorb the supplies for its life. "Mìhù" (密戶) means "Concealed Door" which implies the Mìngmén (Gv-4) (命門) cavity located between L2 and L3 vertebrae (Figure 3–6). It is said in *Classic of Huángtíng's External Scene* (*Huángtíng Wàijǐngjīng*, 黃庭外景經): "Above Mìngmén, there are two esoteric marvellous apertures, left is Xuán (玄) and right is Pìn (牝) (two internal kidneys).

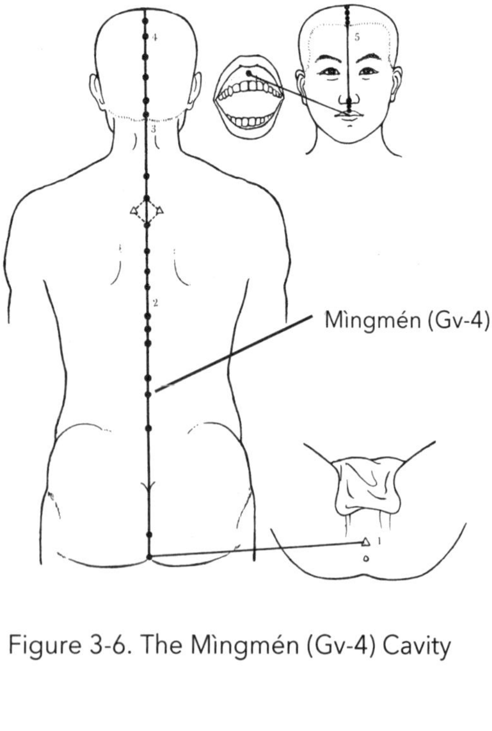

Figure 3-6. The Mìngmén (Gv-4) Cavity

There is an empty place between named 'Huángtíng.'"[36] From this, we can see that Huángtíng actually is the second brain where the guts are. This place is also called "Real Lower Dāntián" (Zhēn Xiàdāntián, 真下丹田) or the bio-battery of a human body. This place is able to store the Qì or bioelectricity to an abundant level.

5. The Complete Book of Principal Contents of Human Life and Temperament

(About Large and Small Tripod and Furnace)

《性命圭旨全書》
（大小鼎爐說）

Huángtíng is the tripod, Qìxuè (Qì cavity) is the furnace. Huángtíng is just on the top of the Qìxuè, mutually connected with numerous Luo (i.e., secondary Qì channels), and is the meeting place of hundreds of Qì vessels (and channels) in a human body. Original Qì (Yuánqì) is dense between these two cavities (i.e., between Huángtíng and Qìxuè) and is called "Small Tripod Furnace." If "the position of Qián is the tripod and the position of the Kūn is furnace," then it means the Níwán (i.e., Upper Dāntián or brain) is the tripod and the Lower (Real) Dāntián is the furnace. This is called "Big Tripod Furnace."

〝黃庭為鼎，氣穴為爐。黃庭正在氣穴上，縷絡相連，乃人身百脈交會之處。〞元氣氤氳二穴之間，謂之〝小鼎爐。〞〝乾位為鼎，坤位為爐。〞即泥丸宮為鼎，下丹田為爐，謂之〝大鼎爐。〞

Chinese Daoists liked to think of the training of longevity cultivation as the method of purifying elixir in the tripod above the furnace. Elixir implies the Qì circulating in the body. When it is cultivated and manifested correctly, you can obtain health, longevity, and even spiritual enlightenment.

Through thousands of years, Daoists continued their search for the tripod and furnace, to be able to accumulate the herb inside the tripod and then purify it through cultivation. They identified the two most important places and called them "Small Tripod Furnace" (Xiǎodǐnglú, 小鼎爐) and "Big Tripod Furnace" (Dàdǐnglú, 大鼎爐).

In "Small Tripod Furnace," the Real Lower Dāntián is considered the furnace since it provides the energy for cooking, while the Huángtíng (黃庭) is the tripod, believed to be the place for producing the Spiritual Embryo. Since the "Real Lower Dāntián" is able to store the Qì to an abundant level and distribute it to the entire body, it is the center which connects with all Qì channels and vessels.

In "Big Tripod Furnace," the head or Upper Dāntián which is located at the Qián (乾) position of the human Trigram (Bāguà, 八卦) is the tripod, while the Lower Dāntián area (including the Real Lower Dāntián) located at the Kūn (坤) position of the human Trigram is the furnace. The Lower Dāntián provides the quantity of the Qì while the Upper Dāntián, through meditative cultivation (refining the elixir), enables the Qì manifestation to reach a higher level of efficiency. Consequently, the quality of physical and spiritual life can be improved. Please refer to Section 1–10 for a description of tripod and furnace.

6. Testimonial Thesis of Golden Immortality 《金仙証論》

Those who wish to pick up the herb (i.e., Qì) and transport it (i.e., circulate it) in the Cyclic Heaven (i.e., Small and Grand Circulations), should start the fire from Qì cavity Kūn furnace (i.e., Lower Dāntián). Ascend it to the Qián head as the tripod and descend it to the abdomen as the furnace. This is what the ancient people said about using Qián and Kūn as the tripod tool. When there is a rise and fall of the Shén and Qì, then the Qì is existing in tripod. Note: "Qián is at the top and is the tripod while Kūn is at the bottom and is the furnace. Whenever there is a Shén and Qì, then there is a furnace and tripod. If there is no Shén and Qì, then there is no furnace or tripod."

采藥運周天者，當從氣穴坤爐而起火，升乾首以為鼎，降坤腹以為爐。即古人所謂乾坤為鼎器者是也。見神氣之起伏，而鼎氣在是矣。注：〝乾在上為鼎，坤在下為爐。有神氣即有爐鼎，無神氣即無爐鼎。〞

In Daoist Qìgōng society, Qì is commonly thought of as herb (Yào, 藥) (elixir). Traditionally, Daoists were searching for the way of longevity through the purification and refinement of herbs and called it Dān (丹) (elixir). Later, they realized that the elixir was actually concealed in the body and was the Qì circulating in the body.

From the previous document, it is understood that the Lower Dāntián (including the Real Lower Dāntián) is the large furnace that produces the Qì (fire) while the Upper Dāntián is the tripod where the Shén resides and receives the Qì so it can be raised up to a higher spiritual state.

In order to reach this goal, you must understand that the Lower Dāntián provides the quantity of the Qì while the Upper Dāntián, through Shén, controls the quality of the Qì manifestation (physical and spiritual life). Therefore, in order to reach a high level of achievement of immortality cultivation, Shén and Qì must be unified and harmonized with each other. This training is called "the unification and harmonization of Shén and Qì" (Shénqì Xiànghé, 神氣相合) in Qìgōng practice.

Theoretically, in order to reach the goal of longevity and enlightenment, you must have a strong, healthy physical life and a high level of spirit. The way to achieve healthy physical life is through Small Cyclic Heaven (Xiǎozhōutiān, 小周天) (Muscle/Tendon Changing Qìgōng) meditation practice. The method of reaching spiritual enlightenment is from spiritual Grand Cyclic Heaven meditation (Dàzhōutiān, 大周天) (Marrow/

Brain Washing Qìgōng). If you are interested in these two subjects, please refer to the book: *Qìgōng—The Secret of Youth*, published by YMAA Publication Center.

3.4 Regulating the Breathing (Tiáoxí, 調息)

1. Dào Dé Jīng
(Chapter 5)[1]
《道德經・五章》

Heaven and Earth (i.e., Nature) does not have benevolence, therefore, all millions of objects (i.e., lives) are treated just like Chúgǒu. Those holy men do not have benevolence, therefore, the populace are treated as Chúgǒu. Between the Heaven and the Earth, is it just like the Tuóyuè? Empty but cannot be bent (i.e., resources cannot be exhausted), the more it moves, the more it produces. If (we) talk too much about it, then it will be often limited (i.e., parted from the Dào). Therefore, it is better if (we) keep (ourselves) at the center (i.e., neutral thinking).

天地不仁，以萬物為芻狗；聖人不仁，以百姓為芻狗。天地之間，其猶橐籥乎？虛而不屈，動而愈出。多言數窮，不如守中。

Nature does not have emotions such as love, hate, glory, happiness or sadness. Even though millions of objects living in this nature are full of emotions and limited life, to nature, they are just like the sacrificial offering, Chúgǒu (芻狗). Chúgǒu were sacrificial dogs that were made from straw and used for ceremonies of worship in ancient China. The holy men cultivated their emotional minds to the neutral state, and were therefore not touched by any emotional disturbances from lay society. All events are only part of natural occurrences.

The space between the heaven and the earth is just like Tuóyuè (橐籥). Tuóyuè is the bellows that was used to assist the air circulation in ancient times. This implies that through the natural Qì circulation, millions of lives are living within and relying on it to survive. Though it is empty, the flow of air can never be exhausted. The more you act, the more the flow of the air will be generated.

All of these principles are the natural rules and the Dào of nature. The more we talk about it, the farther it is separated from nature. Therefore, you should think about it and comprehend it with your natural instinct. In this case, you will be able to feel it and understand it from your heart.

From the Qìgōng point of view, the head is considered as heaven (Qián, 乾) while the abdominal area is considered as earth (Kūn, 坤). The space between is where the lungs are located which is just the space of the natural heaven and earth. In this space, the Qì (Kōngqì, 空氣) (air) circulates and keeps millions of cells alive. The mind (or the Shén) is the motive force which makes the internal Qì (bioelectricity) move or stop. The more the mind acts, the more the Qì circulation is excited and out of control. Therefore, in order to calm down the body and keep the Qì at its residence, you must keep your mind centered at the neutral state. When this happens, there is no emotional disturbance no matter what happens around you. Your mind is not moved away from this center.

2. The Question from A Buddhist Guest about Listening to the Heart
《聽心齋客問》

Expanding the bellows means to regulate the real breathing. When exhaling, then the air exits and when inhaling, the air enters. When exiting, then it is like the earth Qì's ascending, and when entering it is like the heaven Qì's descending. This is the same as the heaven and the earth. Therefore, isn't the space between the heaven and the earth just like the wind bellows?

鼓橐籥，曰調真息。呼則氣出，吸則氣入，出則如地氣上升，入則如天氣下降，與天地同。故天地間，其猶橐籥乎？

As mentioned, "Tuóyuè" (橐籥) means "the bellows" that was used to assist the air circulation in ancient times. Breathing is considered as a strategy in Qìgōng practice, which is able to make the Qì circulate smoothly in the body. The lungs are considered as the air bellows while the Lower Dāntián is considered the Qì bellows. When the air is taken in by the lungs, the Qì is sunken to the Lower Dāntián like the Qì descending in nature. When the air is expelled by the lungs, the Qì in the Lower Dāntián is rising up and being distributed to the body like the Qì ascending in nature. The human body is a small microcosm of heaven and earth. The tricky key to taking in the air and expelling it is the nose, while the "piston" of the Qì bellows in the Lower Dāntián is at the Huìyīn (Co-1, 會陰) (Perineum). Once you know how to regulate your breathing to a natural way (regulating without regulating), it is called "Real Breathing" (Zhēnxí, 真息).

3. An Essay about Regulating the Breathing
(The Complete Book of Zhūzi, Song Dynasty)
《調息箴》
(朱子全書・宋・朱熹撰)

The tip of the nose has white, I observe it (i.e., pay attention to it) all the time and all the places. Allow it soft, gentle, and pliant. When calmness has reached its extremity, it hisses like a spring fish in the pond. When action has reached its extremity, it is harmonized like hundred insects' torpidity. Open and close harmoniously and its marvelousness is unlimited. What else is able to preside? It is achieved from not presiding. The clouds lying in the sky and the heaven (i.e., nature) cycling as it is. Who dares to question it? Keeping in one place harmoniously. (Then, able to live) one thousand and two hundred years.

鼻端有白，我其觀之，隨時隨處，容與猗猗。靜極而嘘，如春沼魚，動極而翕，如百蟲蟄。氤氳開闔，其妙無窮，誰其尸之？不宰之功。雲臥天行，非予敢議，守一處和，千二百歲。

The white at the tip of the nose means the air. I should always pay attention to how I breathe, to be able to regulate it until it is soft, gentle, and pliant. When I am extremely calm (inhale to a profound level), then I exhale like a fish in the spring time. When I am extremely active (exhale to an efficient level), then I retain it calmly and harmoniously like insects' torpidity or dormancy. If I am able to breathe this way harmoniously, what else can I improve? All of the success depends on regulating without regulating. Once I have reached this state, it is like the clouds in the sky, and nature repeating its cycles. Who else dares to say I am wrong? When I am in this state, I am able to keep my mind at the "Real Lower Dāntián' (Zhēn Xiàdāntián, 真下丹田) harmoniously. In this case, there is nothing strange in being able to live one thousand and two hundred years.

This clearly implies that in order to obtain longevity, you must learn two important things. First, regulate your breathing until no regulating is necessary. Second, keep your mind at the "Real Lower Dāntián" so the Qì can be kept at its residence. This means "Embryonic Breathing" (Tāixí, 胎息).

4. Regulating the Breathing[2]

(Original Truth of Using No Herbs, Qīng Dynasty)

《調息》

(勿藥元詮・清・汪昂輯)

The method of regulating the breathing has been thoroughly studied by three educational groups (i.e., Buddhism, Daoism, and Confucianism). (When reaching) the great achievement, (it) is able to enter the Dào and (when reaching) the small achievement, (it) is able to preserve health. Therefore, Sanskrit documents (i.e., Buddhist records from India) teach us to use the eyes to look at the nose tip, count the breaths in and out internally. This is the beginning practice of Stopping Vision (Zhǐguān) (attraction by sight). Zhuāngzi in his book Nánhuájīng *said: "A sage will breathe through the soles." Great Yì (i.e., Yìjīng, The Book of Changes) explains in its trigram which stated: "When getting dark, gentlemen enter Yànxí (i.e., meditation or profound breathing)." Wáng, Lóng-Xī said: "The ancient sages had deep breathing without sleeping. Therefore, it is said when getting dark, (they) enter the Yànxí." The method of Yànxí is when it is getting dark, the ears do not hear, the eyes do not see, the four limbs are not moving, and the heart (i.e., emotional mind) does not have thinking or worry. It is just like a seed fire. The Pre-Heaven's Original Shén and Original Qì gather to nourish each other mutually. The real Yì is soft as cotton, open and close naturally. (The self-being) exists in the same body (i.e., space or dimension) as insubstantial emptiness. Therefore, it is able to live as long as insubstantial emptiness. Those world people (i.e., laymen) are bothered with daily management, the spirit is bound and tired. It depends on the single night sleep to be able to be used during the day. A point of spiritual light (i.e., self-subconscious spiritual being) all covered by the Post-Heaven's dirty Qì. This is, the Yáng falls into the Yīn.*

調息一法，貫徹三教，大之可以入道，小用可以養生。故迦文垂教，以視鼻端，自數出入息，為止觀初門。莊子《南華經》曰：〝聖人之息以踵。〞大易隨卦曰：〝君子以向晦入晏息。〞王龍溪曰：〝古之聖人，有息無睡，故日向晦入晏息。〞晏息之法，當向晦時，耳無聞，目無見，四體無動，心無思慮，如種火相似，先天元神元氣，停育相抱，真意綿綿，開闔自然，與虛空同體，故能與虛空同壽也。世人終日營擾，精神困憊，夜間靠此一睡，始夠一日之用。一點靈光，盡為后天濁氣所淹，是謂陽陷于陰也。

The techniques of regulating the breathing in Qìgōng practice have been popularly studied and practiced in three major philosophic schools, namely Buddhism, Daoism, and Confucianism. Breathing is considered to be the strategy of Qìgōng practice. If you practice correctly, you may gain good health and longevity. In Buddhist and Daoist societies, through correct breathing practice, the Qì can be stored and led upward to the brain to nourish the Shén for enlightenment. Entering the Dào (Rùdào, 入道) means to enter the path of searching for the truth. The Daoists who have comprehended the truth of nature are called "Truthful Persons" (Zhēnrén, 真人).

Regulating the breathing in Buddhist society is considered a crucial key to regulating the mind. In order to stop the mind from continuous attraction and wandering in meditation, first place your attention at your breathing (use the eyes to look at the nose tip) (Yǎnguānbí, 眼觀鼻) and then count the breathing. From this you make the breathing deeper and calmer. Slowly, the thoughts connecting with the surroundings, the past, present and future will be stopped. In Buddhist meditation, this method is called "stopping the vision" (Zhǐguān, 止觀). Remember, when it is said: "to use the eyes to look at the nose tip," it does not mean physically you are using the eyes to look at the nose. It simply means to bring in your attention from outside attraction, to concentrate on your breathing (i.e., nose).

The Daoist scholar Zhuāngzi (莊子) said: "A sage breathes through the soles." This means the Two Gates' breathing through the Yǒngquán (K-1, 湧泉) cavity. Later, it was developed into Four Gates breathing (two Yǒngquán and two Láogōng at the palms), and finally reached the practice of "Five Gates" breathing (Wǔxīn Hūxī, 五心呼吸). Not only that, *Yìjīng* said: "When getting dark, gentlemen enter the Yànxí (晏息) (Meditation or profound breathing)." This reveals that one of the best times for regulating the breathing is during or after sunset. At this time, nature and the body are turning from Yáng to Yīn state. If you practice regulating the breathing at this time, you can easily calm down your physical and mental body and reach a profound level of meditation. This is also mentioned by Daoist Wáng, Lóng-Xī (王龍溪). He implies that ancient sages (who have reached the Dào), through practicing regulating the breathing, did not have to sleep or needed just a little sleep, because they were able to obtain a deep level of rest from meditation.

The way of "Yànxí" (晏息) is, during or after sunset, to stop the ears from attractions by the noises around you. Close your eyes to stop the vision which can therefore allow you to enhance your feeling instead of looking. Keep the body extremely calm and relaxed. The mind should not worry or think. It is just like a tiny fire (little Yáng within Yīn) in the darkness. When this happens, the subconscious mind (Yīn mind) will be awakened while the conscious mind (Yáng mind) will be calm. In this case, the Original Spirit (Yuánshén, 元神) will be raised and harmonized with the Original Qì (Yuánqì, 元氣). When you are in this deep profound meditative level, your Shén will unify with the natural Shén. This is different from normal people who must rely on the night's sleep to overcome their tiredness. Even during sleeping, their minds are still confused by the dreams generated from human emotion and desires. In this case, the healthy mind and body will degenerate quickly, that is, the Yáng falls into the Yīn.

5. The Method of Regulating the Breathing[2]

(Original Truth of Using No Herbs, Qīng Dynasty)

《調息法》

(勿藥元詮・清・汪昂輯)

The method of regulating the breathing is: do not be restricted by the timing, sit (anywhere and anytime) you wish. The body is balanced and upright, and allow it to be comfortable and natural. Do not lean and curve (forward) (i.e., bowing forward). Take off the clothes and ease the belt to make sure (the body) is regulated properly. Circle the tongue in the mouth several times. Gently and slowly release the dirty air (from the lungs) and then gently and slowly take in (the air) from the nose. Repeat three to five times or one to two times. When there is saliva generated, swallow it. After biting the teeth a few times, the tongue touches the palate of the mouth. The lip and the teeth are closed, two eyes are closed like the new moon. Then gradually begin regulating the breathing. Do not pant and do not be coarse. Either count the exhalation or inhalation, from one to ten, from ten to hundred. Restrain (your) mind in counting and do not be disordered. If the mind and the breathing have harmonized with each other mutually and the random thoughts are generated no more, then stop counting and allow it be natural. The longer (you are) able to sit, the more marvellous it will be. If wish to raise up the body, (you) must slowly and comfortably extend your arms and legs. (You) should not raise up suddenly. If (you) are able to practice this intelligently, the various sceneries appearing in the calmness are peculiar. This is able to direct (you to the path of) enlightening (your) mind and comprehending the Dào. It is not just for preserving health and extending life.

調息之法，不拘時候，隨便而坐，平直其身，縱任其體，不倚不曲，解衣緩帶，務令調適。口中舌攪數遍，微微呵出濁氣，鼻中微微納之，或三、五遍，或一、二遍，有津咽下；叩齒數通，舌抵上齶，唇齒相著，兩目垂簾，令朧朧然；漸次調息，不喘不粗，或數息出，或數息入，從一至十，從十至百，攝心在數，勿令散亂，如心息相依，雜念不生，則止勿數，任其自然，坐久愈妙。若欲起身，須徐徐舒放手足，勿得遽起。能勤行之，靜中光景，種種奇特，直可明心悟道，不但養身全生而已也。

From the same source as the last one, this is another paragraph describing the method of regulating the breathing. From here, you can see that there are many methods of regulating the breathing, though the principles and the theory remain the same. These principles and theory are: keeping the body relaxed (regulating the body), keeping your mind calm and profound (regulating the mind), and breathing softly, deeply, and naturally (regulating the breathing). In order to regulate your breathing to a profound level, you must also regulate your body and mind. They must harmonize and coordinate with each other. The key to regulating the breathing is not to hold it, but to regulate it until it can be natural, smooth, and slender.

6. Four Demeanors of Regulating the Breathing[2]

(Original Interpretation of Using No Herbs, Qīng Dynasty)

《調息四相》

(勿藥元詮・清・汪昂輯)

There are four demeanors in regulating the breathing. Those when they breathe, there is a sound, it is classified as the wind breathing. If the wind persists, then (the Qì and the mind are) dispersed. Those when they breathe, there is no sound but when obstructed in the nose, it is classified as panting breathing. If the panting persists, then (the Qì and the mind are) stagnant. Those when they breathe, there is no sound and no stagnation but to and fro has the shape, it is classified as the Qì breathing. If (the mind) keeps in the Qì, then fatigued. (Those when they breathe) do not have sound and stagnation, (the air) exits and enters softly, as if it is existing and as if not existing. The Shén and the breathing are mutually relying on (i.e., harmonized with) each other. This is the demeanor of (real regulating) the breathing. When the breathing is truly regulated, then the mind is steady, the real Qì can be to and fro (naturally). This will allow (you) to capture the variations of the heaven and the earth (i.e., nature). Every breath returns to its origin. This is the stalk (root) of life.

調息有四相：呼吸有聲者風也，守風則散；雖無聲而鼻中澀滯者喘也，守喘則結；不聲不滯而往來有形者氣也，守氣則勞；不聲不滯，出入綿綿，若存若亡，神氣相依，是息相也。息調則心定，真氣往來，自能奪天地之造化，息息歸根，命之蒂也。

This paragraph explains how, from the demeanors of a meditator, we can tell how correct and how deep his breathing is. Those who breathe heavily will make noise. When this happens, the Qì is dispersed and not gathered. Those who breathe without smoothness and uniformity, the Qì circulation will be stagnant. Those who pay too much attention to their breathing will be fatigued. Only those whose breathing is soft, slender, uniform, deep, natural and smooth, the Shén will be peacefully harmonized with the Qì circulation. When this happens, the Original Spirit (subconscious mind) will be awakened, which allows you to trace back the origin of our lives. Dì (蒂) means "stalk" of a fruit or flower. Here it means the key passage connecting to the life.

7. Lízhēnrén's Sixteen Marvellous Longevity Secret Words

(Eight Notes of Life Abidance, Míng Dynasty)

《李真人長生一十六字妙訣》

(遵生八箋 ·明·高濂撰)

Once inhaling, immediately lift up (the perineum) to return the Qì to the navel (i.e., Lower Dāntián); once lifting, immediately swallow (the saliva to allow) the water and fire to meet each other.

一吸便提，氣氣歸臍；一提便咽，水火相見。

Kǎn (坎) (water) means the water Qì produced from the Original Essence (Yuánjīng, 元精), while Lí (離) (fire) means the Fire Qì generated from the Post-Birth Essence (food and air). When these two sources meet each other, the Shén can be raised up to a higher level.

These sixteen words in Chinese reveal the secret of how to make the Fire Qì and water Qì meet and interact with each other. This secret is at the Huìyīn (Co-1, 會陰) cavity (perineum). When you inhale, gently lift up your perineum and lead the Qì to the Lower Dāntián. Immediately right after the inhalation, swallow your saliva and lead the Qì down to the Lower Dāntián. From this sentence, we can see that Reverse Abdominal Breathing should be used for this practice.

8. Recording of Marvellous Relations of Temperament, Heaven, Wind, and Moon[2]

(Teaching the Dào Between Teacher and Students)

《性天風月通玄記》

（師徒傳道）

There is a movement within the calmness and the fire is burning. This is the best time to train Dàfǎn (i.e., Great Returning). When (you) pick up this correct timing, it is called "herb" (i.e., elixir). In (the refinement of) the herb, there is a fire. If asked what is "martial fire?" Then, it is the great action of the strong wind. If asked what is the "scholar fire?" Then, it is the soft, continuous, and slender Embryonic Breathing.

靜中一動火正燃，此時正好煉大返。采時謂之藥，藥中有火焉。若問武火，大舉巽風；若問文火，胎息綿綿。

There are four steps in spiritual cultivation in Daoist society: A. Refining the Essence (Semen) and Converting it into Qì (Liànjīng Huàqì, 煉精化氣); B. Purifying Qì and Converting it into Shén (Liànqì Huàshén, 煉氣化神); C. Refining Shén and Returning it to Nothingness (Liànshén Fǎnxū, 煉神返虛); D. Crushing the Nothingness (Fěnsuì Xūkōng, 粉碎虛空). This training process is called "Dàfǎn" (大返) (Great Returning), meaning to "return the human temperament to the natural state." This term also means the re-unification of the human spirit with the spirit of nature (Tiānrén Héyī, 天人合一).

When your physical body has reached its extremely calm state, you will bring your Shén downward to the Real Lower Dāntián to unify with the Qì. When this happens, through Embryonic Breathing, the Qì (fire) can be established. Once this fire is built to an abundant stage, the Qì is led upward to Huángtíng (黃庭) (tripod) to conceive the Spiritual Embryo. There are two ways of building up the fire to an abundant level. One is called "Martial Fire" (Wǔhuǒ, 武火) and the other is called "Scholar Fire" (Wénhuǒ, 文火). In Martial Fire practice, you use heavy and faster breathing with the coordination of the abdominal up and down movements. This kind of breathing is called "Xùnfēng" (巽風) and means "Great Wind." When this happens, the fire can be built up to an abundant state in a short time. This kind of breathing is commonly used in external martial arts. Here, you should understand that, since in the martial fire practice your physical body is more tensed and the breathing more shallow, the fire built up will be consumed immediately into physical manifestation. Therefore, through martial fire practice, it is harder to keep the fire built up internally for "Internal Elixir" (Nèidān, 內丹) Qìgōng practice.

To build up the fire (Qì) to an abundant level and use it for the cultivation of internal elixir, you must use scholar fire. In scholar fire practice, your breathing is deep, slender, soft, and long. It is said in Anthology of Daoist Village (Dàoxiāngjí, 道鄉集): "What is scholar fire? It is as if it stays, as if it exists. There is no decease (perish) and there is no assistance." It is the state of "extremely slender when uttering (exhaling) and extremely soft when receiving (inhaling)."[37]

9. The Complete Book of Principal Contents of Human Life and Temperament[2]

(Xǔ, Qī-Yán's Secrets of Embryonic Breathing)

《性命圭旨全書》

（許棲岩胎息法）

Those who cultivate the Dào should always observe self internally, send away Sānshī (i.e., Three Corpses), and get rid of Liùzéi (i.e., Six Thieves), receive the Qì in Dāntián, stabilize the Xīn (i.e., emotional mind) in Awakened Ocean (Juéhǎi). When the Xīn is steady, then the Shén is peaceful. When the Shén is peaceful, the Qì stays (at its residence). When Qì stays, then the embryo will grow. The growth of the embryo is due to the residence (i.e., the existence) of the breathing. If there is no breathing, there is no embryo and if there is no embryo, there is also no breathing. When the breathing stays (i.e., exists), the embryo will grow and (this is) the holy mother and spiritual baby. Therefore, it is said that when the Embryonic Breathing is steady, the metal and the wood will interact and when the Xīn and Yì are peaceful, the dragon and the tiger will meet together.

凡修道者，常行內觀，遣去三尸，驅除六賊，納氣于丹田，定心于覺海。心定則神寧，神寧則氣住，氣住則胎長矣。胎之長者，由于息之住也。無息不胎，無胎不息。住息長胎，聖母神孩。故曰胎息定而金木交，心意寧而龍虎會也。

"Nèiguān" (內觀) means "Internal Observation." Ancient documents often speak of "Gōngfū of internal vision" (Nèishì Gōngfū, 內視功夫). It is called Gōngfū simply because it will take you a long time and great effort of practice to reach a profound level of internal observation (internal feeling). Only if you look internally, will you be able to understand yourself both physically and mentally. Therefore, if you wish to reach a profound level in your Qìgōng practice, you must first learn to feel internally. Remember, feeling is a language that allows communication between your mind and body. The more sensitive and clear your feeling is, the more you will be able to cultivate your being.

"Sānshī" (三尸) (Three Corpses) are also commonly called "Sānchóng" (三蟲) (Three Worms). These are: the worm of desire which likes treasures and precious things; the worm which likes the tastes, easily loses its temper, and despises those who are good and kind; and the worm that likes sex and makes one confused. If you know how to avoid these three worms, then you are able to stabilize your mind and keep it calm. "Liùzéi" (六賊) means: eyes, ears, nose, tongue, body, and emotional mind (Xīn, 心), which could disturb your feeling and increase your six desires (Liùyù, 六慾).

If you wish to cultivate your Embryonic Breathing, you must first learn how to calm down your mind and keep it clean and pure. When this happens, you will be able to reach the awakening stage of your cultivation. When you awaken, you will see through millions of human emotional affairs and occurrences. Since these affairs and events are so abundant and confused, there is no limit to your awakening. That is why this state of awakening is called "Juéhǎi" (覺海) which means "Awaken Ocean."

Once your mind is regulated, your Shén will be able to stay at its residence (Upper Dāntián). The trick of regulating your mind is through the correct way of breathing. When this happens, the metal (Jīn, 金) and wood (Mù, 木) will harmonize with each other smoothly. Metal implies the lungs or the breathing, while the wood implies the liver which relates to the Shén. Through correct breathing, the Shén can be condensed and brought to a high level of concentration. With the calm mind, dragon and tiger (i.e., Yīn and Yáng) will meet and interact with each other. When this happens, the holy Spiritual Embryo (Shèngtāi, 聖胎) can be conceived at the Huángtíng (黄庭).

10. Miscellaneous Secrets of Embryonic Breathing[3]

(Mr. Yánlíng's Collections in New and Old Qìgōng Classics)

(Tang Dynasty)

《胎息雜訣》

（延陵先生集新舊服氣經・唐・延陵先生集）

One of the classics said: "Just leading the (air) Qì in and out (i.e., breathing) slowly, consequently, the Original Qì (Yuánqì) will not exit as well. In this case, the internal Qì and external Qì (i.e., air Qì) will not be mixed together, this is what is named as 'Embryonic Breathing.'" However, those beginners who just start this Gōng (i.e., Gōngfū), though the internal Qì has already been steadily firmed, the nose should still allow the (air) Qì in and out slenderly. Do not let (the air) reach to the throat (only) and return (to the nose). This will make the Qì adverse and full and this will result in the Qì's rising upward. Therefore, it (i.e., the breathing) should not be suppressed and restrained (this way). If it happens, then allow (the air) out slenderly, smoothly, and comfortably. After the breathing has been regulated, then again seal (i.e., control the breathing). (You) must allow it (i.e., air) to exit and enter through the nose slenderly and slowly. (You) must not let it reach the throat and suppress it with great effort. (You) just need to practice for a while, then (you) will suddenly feel comfortable and natural. In this case, the internal and external are harmonious. If (you) have reached this stage, then even (if you) have completed the Thousand Breathings, (you) will not be tired.

一經云：但徐徐引氣出納，則元氣亦不出也，自然內外之氣不雜，此名胎息。然初用功之人，閉固內氣訖，亦鼻中微微通氣往來，使令不至咽喉而返，氣即逆滿上沖，不可抑塞。如此，則徐徐放令通暢，候氣調，即復閉之。切在徐徐鼻中出入，勿令至喉，極力抑忍，為之須臾，忽然自得調暢，內外泰矣。到此，即千息亦不倦矣。

"Yuánqì" (元氣) means "Original Qì" which is produced from "Original Essence" (Yuánjīng, 元精). In Chinese medical and Qìgōng societies, it is believed that the "Original Essence" is the essence of your physical life and spiritual life which you inherited from your parents. If you are able to conserve this essence and also know how to convert it into Qì efficiently, then your life span can be extended significantly.

As explained in section 2-2, Chinese Qìgōng and medical societies distinguish between two Qìs. One is called "Wàiqì" (外氣) and means "External Qì." This Qì is the Qì (energy) of the air. The air is called "Kōngqì" (空氣) and means "Qì of Space." When this air enters the body, it can be converted into "Nèiqì" (內氣) that means "Internal Qì" (bioelectricity) circulating in the body. The chamber that takes in and repels the external Qì in the body is the lungs, the diaphragm is the pump (or piston) and the nose and the mouth are the door for the air to enter and exit. This Qì is also commonly called "Shàngcéngqì" (上層氣) and means "Upper Layer Qì." Please refer to Section 2-2 for details.

When the "External Qì" is absorbed into the blood system, through the biochemical reaction processes, the food (glucose) can be converted into "internal energy" or "Internal Qì." We should understand that the more oxygen we have, the more efficiently this biochemical reaction can be accomplished. That is why whenever we need to manifest more power (for example, pushing a car or lifting a heavy weight), we must first inhale deeply so we can take in more oxygen. The more oxygen is provided, the more power can be manifested. Once the "Internal Qì" is produced, then it can be stored in the Real Lower Dāntián. Therefore, the Real Lower Dāntián is the storage or bio-battery of the "internal energy or Qì." The abdominal area and the Huìyīn (Co-1) (會陰) cavity are the pump (or piston) of the Qì's in and out. This Qì is also commonly called "Xiàcéngqì" (下層氣) and means "Lower Layer Qì."

From the above, you can see that the "External Qì" and "Internal Qì" are not the same but are closely related to each other. When the external Qì is absorbed appropriately, the production and usage of the internal Qì can be significantly more efficient. In order to increase the efficiency of converting the external into internal Qì, at the end of the inhalation, you normally hold the breath for a few moments. For example, when you push a car or lift a heavy weight, you first inhale deeply and then exhale while manifesting your power. When you reach the end of the manifestation, you normally hold your breathing in order to increase the power to its maximum. In the same way, if you wish to store the Qì in the body, once you inhale all the way, you hold your breath for a while.

However, you should not hold it too long and choke yourself or even feel uncomfortable. If you experience any unease and discomfort, your body will be tensed up, increasing the consumption of oxygen and Qì. Naturally, in this case, you are not storing the Qì but consuming it. This is not desired in Embryonic Breathing.

In order to lead the Qì to the Real Lower Dāntián and keep it there, you must be in an extremely relaxed and mentally calm state. The first task is to neutralize your emotional mind. When this happens, your Shén will not be wandering around, and can be condensed at its residence. With this highly focused Shén (quality of life) at the Upper Dāntián and the abundant storage of Qì (quantity of life) at the Real Lower Dāntián, you are able to reach the goal of longevity and enlightenment.

> *In addition, (classic) said: "The marvelousness of Embryonic Breathing is that there is no thinking and no worries. The bodies (i.e., spiritual and physical bodies) are in harmony with nature. The Xīn (i.e., emotional mind) is like dead ash and the shape (i.e., physical body) is like dried wood. In this case, (the Qì circulating in) hundreds of meridians and vessels will be flowing without obstruction, the joints will be opened wide. However, if there are hundred initiations of worries and concerns, initiated and exterminated constantly, then if (you) wish to reach the final Dào, (you are) wasting (your) time and effort. This will not lead (you) to success at the end." This Dào is immensely delicate and extremely marvellous, it can be successfully achieved only by those who have separated from laymen society. If (you) have not parted from fame and wealth, then all the effort will be in vain. Another classic said: "After completing the practice of swallowing Qì, then seal (i.e., control your) Qì and keep (your) mind there (Dāntián). Yì is like flowing water. When the front wave is gone the coming wave has arrived." Whenever (you) have finished (your) Gōng in Embryonic Breathing, all the joints are opened wide, (the Qì circulating in) hair is smooth and comfortable. When this happens, then inhale (the air) slenderly from the nose and image it exits through hundreds of pores, gone without returning (i.e., skin breathing). The air arrives continuous and simply lead it inward without letting it out. But remember, it must be slow and gradual. Though it is said that to lead the air in and not out, what (you) are leading will not be obstructed at the throat. (Simply) let it be dispersed slowly. In this case, the internal Qì will not be dispersed and lost.*
>
> 又：〝胎息之妙，切在無思無慮，體合自然，心如死灰，形如枯木，即百脈暢，關節通矣。若憂慮百端，起滅相繼，欲求至道，徒費艱勤。終無成功。〞此道至微至妙，出塵之士，方可為之，未離名利之間，徒勞介意。一經云：〝咽氣滿訖，便閉氣存想，意如流水，前波已去，后浪續起。〝凡胎息用功后，關節開通，毛髮疏暢，即依此，但鼻中微微引氣，想從四肢百毛孔出，往而不返也，后氣續到，但引之而不吐也。切在于徐徐。雖云引而不吐，所引亦不入于喉中，微微而散。如此，內氣亦不流散矣。

As explained in the last paragraph, in order to reach the goal of Embryonic Breathing, you must first regulate your mind to the neutral state. It is believed in Chinese medicine that your emotions closely influence the Qì circulation in your body. In order to conserve the Qì and prevent it from leaving its residence and being wasted, the first task is to avoid emotional disturbance, so that the Qì can circulate smoothly in all channels. Not only that, when your mind is in a neutral and free state, your breathing will be smooth, natural, calm, deep, and slender. This will allow the oxygen and carbon dioxide to be exchanged more efficiently, and also allow the internal Qì to be converted to stay in the Real Lower Dāntián. However, if your breathing is shallow, then the body's metabolism will not be efficient, and naturally the Qì converted will not be abundant. In addition, if your mind is disturbed, the consumption of the Qì will be increased and this will result in its exhaustion.

Pay attention to your inhalation and allow the air to be taken in slowly and profoundly. Then simply allow the air to exit slowly by itself. When this happens, the internal Qì can be built up and kept internally.

3.5 Regulating the Mind (Tiáoxīn, 調心)

1. The Complete Book of Principal Contents of Human Life and Temperament; Development of Heaven and Human's Unification, Picking up the Herb and Returning it to the Pot 《性命圭旨全書・天人合發，采藥歸壺》

Nothing in the heart (i.e., mind) is Xū (i.e., emptiness), no initiation of the thought is Jìng (i.e., calmness). Approaching Xū to its extremity and maintaining Jìng to its final sincerity. Yīn and Yáng will interact with each other naturally. When Yīn and Yáng are interacting, then the Yáng essence is produced.

心中無物為虛，念頭不起為靜，致虛而至于極，守靜而至于篤。陰陽自然交媾，陰陽一交而陽精產矣。

This document explains two main concepts of the Wújí state which were originally written of by Lǎozi. *Dào Dé Jīng* (道德經), Chapter 16, states: "Approaching the nihility (i.e., nothingness or emptiness) to its extremity and maintaining the calmness with sincerity."[38] This is the state of returning your spiritual being to the beginning of life which is originally complete emptiness and calmness. "Xū" (虛) means "emptiness" (nihility) and "Jìng" (靜) means "calmness." Therefore, Xū here means to empty the mind so there is nothing there to be bothered by. Jìng means to keep the mind calm so new thoughts will not be initiated.

When you have reached this Wújí state, your mind is in its neutralized state. This allows the interaction of Yīn and Yáng. When the Yīn and Yáng interact, the new life will be initiated. The Yīn here means the Shén while the Yáng is the Qì. When these two interact with each other, the Yáng Essence (Yángjīng, 陽精) of the life will be generated. This is the state of "crushing the nothingness" (Fěnsuì Xūkōng, 粉碎虛空) in Daoist cultivation.

2. The Righteous Rules of Heavenly Immortality; Straight Discussion of Pre-Heaven and Post-Heaven Two Qìs 《天仙正理・先天后天二氣直論》

Those who apply this Qì, how do they know it (i.e., the practice) is the truth of pre-heaven (i.e., true pre-heaven practice)? When calmness (Jìng) and emptiness (Xū) have reached to their extremities, there is no single slight thought involved in the consciousness. This is the real state of truthful pre-heaven (practice).

夫用此氣者，由何以知先天之真也。當靜虛至極時。亦未涉一念覺知，此正真先天之真境界也。

Pre-Heaven truth (Xiāntiān Zhī Zhēn, 先天之真) means the truthful state before birth. In this stage, the mind is simple and pure, extremely calm and sincere. However, how do you know that you have reached this state of extreme calmness and nihility in your practice? The way to know this is if there is not even a tiny thought existing or initiating in your conscious mind. Then your subconscious mind (Pre-Heaven truthful mind) will be awakened and active.

In Chinese Qìgōng society, the conscious mind is classified as Yáng and is believed to be generated by the brain since birth. However, the subconscious mind is classified as Yīn and is born with you. The conscious mind and memory are generated from education (or brainwashing) by the environment, and are not truthful. Often, there are thick masks on our faces to cover the untruthful fact of this conscious mind. However, the subconscious mind is truthful, and is connected with your spiritual memory which can be sensed and felt only when your physical body is calm and activity of your conscious mind has ceased.

In order to return to the stage of Pre-Birth, you must first cease activity, both physically and mentally. Then the subconscious mind will be acting, and direct you to the true path of spiritual cultivation.

3. The Complete Book of Principal Contents of Human Life and Temperament; Hēng Anthology 《性命圭旨全書・亨集》

When the physical body does not move, the Xīn (i.e., emotional mind) will be peaceful automatically. When the Xīn does not move, the Shén will abide automatically.

身不動而心自安，心不動而神自守。

The first step in keeping your Shén at its residence (the Upper Dāntián) is to keep your physical body calm and relaxed. Whenever the body is acting or tensed, the Qì is excited and manifested into external forms. This will also cause the mind to be disturbed and moved away from its center. Once the emotional mind can be calm and centered, then your mental body can also be centered, steady, and peaceful. Then you have provided favorable conditions for the Shén to stay at its residence.

4. Concealed Treasure of Dao; Thesis of Sitting Forgetfulness 《道藏・坐忘論》

The Xīn (i.e., mind) is the master of the entire body, the commander of hundred spirits. When it is calm, wisdom is generated and when it is moving, then confusion is initiated. Bewildered or not is decided within the moving (i.e., excitement) or the calmness (of the mind).

夫心者一身之主，百神之帥，靜則生慧，動則生昏，欣迷動靜之中。

Xīn (心) is the emotional mind while Yì (意) is the logical Wisdom Mind. Xīn is classified as Yáng (陽) since it excites and energizes the mental and physical bodies. Yì is classified as Yīn (陰) since it allows you to keep the emotional mind under control and direct your thinking and behavior to the correct path. Therefore, Xīn is the initiation of the thought which decides the entire body's action. It is like the commander who controls the entire army. The Yì is like a minister who offers advice and directs the commander's decision to the correct path. When the commander is calm, he will be willing to accept the advice and consider it, thus, acting wisely. However, if a commander is excited and aggressive, then his mind will be confused and bewildered. Therefore, the first step in meditation is using the Yì to calm down the Xīn. When the Xīn is calmed down, then the action or cultivation can be correct and effective.

5. Thousands of Golden Important Prescriptions for Emergency; Scroll #27, Temperament Cultivation 2 《備急千金要方・卷二十七・養性》

Too much of longing, then the Shén will be precarious. Too much of obsession, then the will can be dispersed. Too much of desires, the aspiration will be bewildered. Too much of laboring, then the shape (i.e., physical body) will be weary. Too much of talking, then the Qì is exhausted. Too much of laughing, then the internal organ (i.e., heart) can be damaged. Too much of worry, then the Xīn (i.e., emotional mind) is fearful. Too much of joy, then the Yì (i.e., Wisdom Mind) will overreact. Too much of delight, then make mistakes and confused. Too much of anger, then (the Qì circulation in) hundreds of meridians are not steady. Too much of indulgence, then (the mind is) strongly fascinated and ignore (others). Too much of wickedness, then emaciated without joy. If these twelve too much (i.e., things) cannot be removed, then Guardian and Managing (Qìs) will lose their control, the blood and Qì will circulate disorderly. This is the basic cause of losing the life.

多思則神殆，多念則志散，多欲則志昏，多事則形勞，多語則氣乏，多笑則臟傷，多愁則心懾，多樂則意溢，多喜則忘錯昏亂，多怒則百脈不定，多好則專迷不理，多惡則憔悴無歡。此十二多不除，則榮衛失度，血氣妄行，喪生之本也。

From Chinese medical and also scholar Qìgōng, it is known that the Qì circulation in the internal organs is closely related to the emotions. For example, too much excitement and happiness can make the heart too Yáng and thus trigger a heart attack. Too much sadness can make the lungs too Yīn, and too much anger can disrupt the smooth circulation of liver Qì. (Table 3–1) Therefore you must first understand the relationship between your emotional mind and the Qì status in the body. This document lists twelve emotional disturbances for your reference.

Guardian Qì (Wèiqì, 衛氣) is the Qì spread on the surface of the entire body's skin. When this Qì is strong and abundant, the immune system will be effective and powerful, so you will not get sick easily. Managing Qì (Yíngqì, 營氣) is the Qì required for the internal organs' normal functioning. Whenever this smooth circulation is disrupted, then illness of the internal organs will be initiated. Therefore, the first step in regulating your Qì is regulating your emotional mind (Xīn, 心).

	WOOD 木	FIRE 火	EARTH 土	METAL 金	WATER 水
Direction	East	South	Center	West	North
Season	Spring	Summer	Long Summer	Autumn	Winter
Climactic Condition	Wind	Summer Heat	Dampness	Dryness	Cold
Process	Birth	Growth	Transformation	Harvest	Storage
Color	Green	Red	Yellow	White	Black
Taste	Sour	Bitter	Sweet	Pungent	Salty
Smell	Goatish	Burning	Fragrant	Rank	Rotten
Yīn Organ	Liver	Heart	Spleen	Lungs	Kidneys
Yáng Organ	Gall Bladder	Small Intestine	Stomach	Large Intestine	Bladder
Opening	Eyes	Tongue	Mouth	Nose	Ears
Tissue	Sinews	Blood Vessels	Flesh	Skin/Hair	Bones
Emotion	Anger	Happiness	Pensiveness	Sadness	Fear
Human Sound	Shout	Laughter	Song	Weeping	Groan

Figure 3-5. The Water and Fire Paths of Qì Circulation

6. The Complete Book of Principal Contents of Human Life and Temperament; Concealed in Qì Cavity, All Marvelousness Returns to its Roots [2]

《性命圭旨全書・蟄藏氣穴，眾妙歸根》

(If you are) capable of reaching the deep and profound breathing like a Truthful Person (Zhēnrén) (i.e., Daoist who has reached the Dào), then the Xīn and breathing will be interdependent, which will thus result in a regulated breathing and a calmed Xīn.

合真人深深之息，則心息相依，息調心靜。

"Zhēnrén" (真人) means "truthful person." Daoists often call themselves "Zhēnrén" since they are aiming for "the truth of the Dào." One of the major trainings to reach the goal of enlightenment is through regulating the breathing. When the breathing has reached a profound level of Embryonic Breathing, it is called "Zhēnxí" (真息) and means "Real Breathing" or "True Breathing." In this stage, your emotional mind is extremely calm and harmonized with the breathing. This is simply because when the mind is emotionally disturbed, the breathing will be fast, and when the mind is peaceful and stays at the Real Lower Dāntián (Zhēn Xiàdāntián, 真下丹田), the breathing will be calm, slender, and peaceful. Not only that, when the breathing is faster and excited, the emotional mind will also be disturbed. Therefore, the emotional mind (Xīn, 心) and breathing (Xí, 息) must be interdependent and harmonized with each other (Xīnxí Xiāngyī, 心息相依).

7. The Question from A Buddhist Guest about Listening to the Heart[2]

《聽心齋客問》

(Our) Xīn (i.e., emotional mind) has been attached with (laymen) affairs for a long time, once it is attached to the (laymen) environment, it cannot be independent (easily). Therefore, (we) must use the Gōngfū of regulating the breathing (Tiáoxí) to restrain this Xīn and allow the Xīn and breathing to mutually depend on each other. The word of regulating (Tiáo) does not mean using the Yì (i.e., Wisdom Mind). It is only using one exhalation and one inhalation (i.e., respiration) to keep the thought there. Once the Xīn is able to separate from the (laymen) environment, then there is no body, and neither it nor I exist. Then there is no breathing needing to be regulated. It is so soft as if it is existing (and as if it is not). After a long time (of practice), it will become proficient naturally.

心依著事物已久，一旦離境，不能自立。所以用調息功夫，拴系此心，便心息相依。調字亦不是用意，只是一呼一吸系念耳。至心離境，則無人無我，更無息可調，只綿綿若存，久之，自然純熟。

"Xīn" (心) means "emotional mind" (Yáng mind), which is commonly analogized as "monkey" while "Yì" (意) means "Wisdom Mind" (Yīn mind), which is often analogized as "horse" (Xīnyuán Yìmǎ, 心猿意馬). Though the monkey is small and weak, it is able to generate a great disturbance, whereas, although the horse is large and powerful, it can be calm and easily restrained. In order to regulate the monkey mind, you will need a banana to lead the monkey into a cage and lock it there. This banana in Qìgōng practice is the breathing. When you regulate the emotional monkey mind, you cannot just use your Yì to restrain it. The more you intend to restrain it, the worse it will be. It is just like when you cannot fall asleep, the more you intend to sleep, the more awake you will be. The way to reach the goal of regulating the emotional monkey mind is simply to pay attention to the breathing. The more you are able to regulate your breathing to a profound, slender, calm, and soft stage, the more easily the emotional mind can be controlled. Once your emotional mind has been restrained, then regulation of the breathing is no longer important since it has become natural. This is the stage of "Embryonic Breathing."

8. Collection of Neutral Harmony
《中和集》

(If we) carefully look at the writings by those holy men in Three Teachings (Sānjiào) (i.e., Three Schools), the word of Xí (i.e., ceasing) is the simplest and most straightforward. If (you are) able to put (your) Gōngfū in ceasing, then (you) will not need too much effort to reach Buddhahood and immortality. To cease the feeling of affinity (Yuán) so (you) can reach the pivotal function of original Chán. To cease the Xīn (i.e., actions of emotional mind) so (you) can comprehend and understand the theory of Confucianism profoundly. To cease the breathing so (you) can reach the marvellous Dào of condensing the Shén. These three ceases are mutually required from each other without any conquest.

諦觀三教聖人書，息之一字最簡直。若于息上做功夫，為佛為仙不勞力。息緣達本禪之機，息心明理儒之極，息氣凝神道之玄，三息相須無不克。

"Sānjiào" (三教) means "Three Teachings" or "Three Schools." These three schools are Buddhism, Confucianism, and Daoism. All of these three schools talk about the methods of "ceasing" (Xí, 息). Literally "Xí" means "to stop" or "to cease" any action or initiation of something. Here, it means the stage of "regulating without regulating" (Bùtiáo Értiáo, 不調而調). This implies that when regulating is no longer necessary, all of the regulating processes will naturally cease.

The key practice of Buddhists is to cease the "affinity" (Yuán, 緣) with the affairs of lay society. When this affinity ceases, then the emotional mind will be calm and peaceful. Then the Shén, which is related to the subconscious mind, will be awakened, and

Buddhahood can be achieved. This kind of cultivation in Buddhism is called "Chán" (禪). The Buddhist document, The Transliteration of Wisdom Garden (Huìyuàn Yīnyì, 慧苑音義) said: "Chán, it means to calm down the Xīn to ponder."[39] It is the method of stabilizing the Xīn's activity (i.e., meditation).

The cultivation of "ceasing" in the Confucian school is to cease the Xīn's activity so the scholar philosophies can be comprehended. These philosophies include the relationship between humans, as well as between nature and humans. When these philosophies are understood, the mind can be peaceful and calm.

However, to the Daoists, the "ceasing" means to cease the regulating process of the breathing. In order to reach this goal, you must learn the method of "Embryonic Breathing" with the condensed mind. This is the necessary path to reach the goal of enlightenment.

9. Four Books; Great Study
《四書・大學》

Confucius said: "Only knowing (how to) cease, can you then have steadiness. When there is steadiness, then (your mind) can be calm. When (your mind is) calm, then (you) can be peaceful. When (you are) at peace, then (you) are able to ponder. When (you) ponder, then (you) will gain."

孔子曰：〝知止而后有定，定而后能靜，靜而后能安，安而后能慮，慮而後能得。〞

To the Confucian scholar, the final goal of meditation is to gain understanding of the meaning of life and the rules of nature. In order to comprehend this deep philosophy, you must go through a few necessary procedures. The first step is to stop or to cease (Zhǐ, 止) the initiation of a thought. Only then will your mind be steady and under control, both calm and peaceful. Once you have reached this state of peace, then your mind is clear for you to ponder. Through deep pondering, you will comprehend the reason for all events around us.

10. Anthology of Daoist Village [2]
《道鄉集》

"Once (you) can be calm, then pay attention to the Lower Dāntián. Where (your) eyes (i.e., focus) are, that is where (your) Xīn (i.e., emotional mind) should follow. When Xīn and eyes have reached the place and ceased, then the Xīn and the breathing should accord to each other and gradually enter the Great Steadiness (Dàdìng)." Also, "The Shén can be stabilized through coordination with the breathing. The breathing can be peaceful through coordination with the Shén. Both accord with each other, then the Great Steadiness can be reached."

〝能靜時觀照下田，目之所在，心亦隨之，心目得其所止，而后心與息依，漸入大定。〞又〝神依息而定，息依神而安，互相依附，始歸大定。〞

"Eyes" implies to focus and pay attention, and means the Yì (意). It is often said in ancient documents that: "The eyes observe (Guan) the nose (i.e., breathing), and the nose observes the Xīn (i.e., emotional mind).[40] Guān (觀) here means "to observe," or "to pay attention." Therefore, the first part of this sentence means to restrain your eyes or pay attention to your breathing. The second part implies that through the breathing, the emotional mind can be watched and regulated.

In Chinese Qìgōng society, it is often said: "Xīn-ape and Yì-horse" (Xīnyuán Yìmǎ, 心猿意馬). According to Chinese tradition, there are two minds that can be classified as Yáng and Yīn; the emotional mind called "Xīn" (心) is Yáng while the Wisdom Mind called "Yì" (意) is Yīn. Xīn literally means "heart", because the heart is related to our emotional disturbance. For example, if your mind has too much emotional disturbance it prevents you from falling asleep. If you are instead able to pay attention to your breathing and keep your mind at the Lower Dāntián, you will be able to regulate the "emotional monkey" and fall asleep.

When your emotional mind is under control, then can you stabilize your Shén and keep it at its residence. In this case, the Shén and the breathing will be mutually harmonized and accord with each other. This is called "Great Steadiness" (Dàdìng, 大定) in Qìgōng meditation practice. In Buddhist society it is said: "When the Xīn (i.e., emotional mind) for Buddhism is clear and bright, it is called 'Dàdìng.'"[41] This implies the calm and peaceful state of mind, where the body is extremely relaxed. The Shén and the physical body harmonize and coordinated with each other, leading to steadiness and calmness of both mental and physical bodies.

11. Theory of Evaluating Wisdom
《智度論》

Justify (i.e., Regulate) the Xīn (i.e., emotional mind) to where it should be. Cease the worry (i.e., mind of affinity) and condense (i.e., stabilize) the Xīn. When the Xīn is steady at one place without moving (i.e., being disturbed), thus, it is called "steadiness." Justify (the Xīn) so it can accept the solution through observation (i.e., self-investigation), thus it is called "acceptance" (Shòu). To regulate the violence (i.e., aggressive actions) of the Xīn, and to straighten the curve (i.e., intricacy) of the Xīn, and stabilize its dispersion (i.e., distraction), thus it is called "regulating, straightening, and stabilizing." To justify the actions of Xīn and allow it to accord to the rule as it should be, thus it is called "justify the Xīn to the proper place." Cease the mind's affinity and worry so as to condense and focus the thought of Xīn, thus it is called "cease the worry and condense the Xīn."

正心行處，息慮凝心，心定于一處而不動，故曰定；正受所觀之法，故曰受；調心之暴，直心之曲，定心之散，故曰調直定；正心之行動，使合于法之依處，故曰正心行處；息止緣慮，凝結心念，故曰息慮凝心。

In Buddhist society, "Dìng" (定) (steadiness of the emotional mind and the physical body) is always emphasized in meditation. The process of entering this steadiness is called "Rùdìng" (入定) (Entering the Steadiness). In order to do so, you must first cut off any emotional disturbance and keep your mind at the Upper and the Real Lower Dāntián. The Upper Dāntián (brain) is the residence of the Shén and the Real Lower Dāntián (second brain) is the residence of the Qì. When the Qì can be kept at its residence, the physical body can be calmed without stimulation or excitement. When the Shén can be condensed at its residence, the mind will be calm and clear.

In order to reach the above goals, you must learn how to face your emotional mind, analyze it, understand it, and then learn how to remove the mask from your face. Only when these affinities of Xīn can be removed, can your mind then be steady and kept at one place. This is the method of reaching "Steadiness" (Dìng, 定).

12. Great Conveyance in Hundred Methods of Comprehension; Discussing Sincere Advice[2]
《大乘百法明門·論忠疏》

When observing the environment (i.e., situation), if one is able to concentrate (his mind) without dispersion (i.e., distraction), it is the "Xìng" (i.e., natural temperament), (thus) the wisdom can be built upon. Therefore, if (one only) observes the gain or loss, (he) will not enter the situation (i.e., the root). (It must be) from stability of the Xīn and not allow it to be from dispersion. If (one) follows this, there (he) will make decision from wisdom.

于所觀境令人專注不散為性，智依為業。謂觀得失，俱非境中，由定令心不散，依斯便有決擇智生。

"Dàchéng" (大乘) in the title of this document means "Great Conveyance." "Chéng" (乘) means the Buddhist teaching, a conveyance to bring the truth to men and help them. Comprehending the meaning of life and the truth of nature is called "Wù" (悟) (enlightenment).

To comprehend the human temperament (Xìng, 性) is not easy. You must first inspect, analyze and understand all of the events or affairs occurring around you carefully and accurately. Once you have established this capability, you will be able to concentrate and ponder. From this, wisdom can be generated, and you will be able to comprehend the human temperament.

If you only pay attention to the consequence of what has happened without knowing how to trace its cause or origin, then you will never understand the origin of the problem. In this case, you will not be able to comprehend the meaning of life and reach spiritual enlightenment. The first crucial key to reaching this concentration of the mind and wisdom is to have a stabilized Xīn. When the Xīn is calm and stable, you will be wise and your judgment will be accurate. This is the way to reach the Dào of wisdom.

13. Theory of Evaluating Wisdom[2]
《智度論》

What does it mean "stabilizing the Xin?" It means there is only one Xīn without disorder. When disordered, then the Xīn cannot see through the fact and truth. It is just like the wave on the water which makes (you) unable to see the face (in the reflection). It is just like lighting a lamp in the wind, cannot be lighted.

定心者，定名一心不亂。亂，心中不能得見事實，如水波蕩，不得見面；如風中燈，不能得點。

In order to reach spiritual enlightenment, you must first comprehend the meaning of life. The first task here is to stabilize your Xīn (心) (emotional mind). Only when the emotional mind can be kept calm and steady can your Wisdom Mind (Yì, 意) be clear in its judgment. Otherwise, if the emotional mind is in disarray and out of control, you will not be able to see yourself clearly. It is like being unable to see the reflection of your face clearly, when the emotional mind has generated ripples on the surface of the water. This emotional mind is also like the wind which keeps you from lighting your lantern of enlightenment.

14. The Inner Mental Method of Reaching the Heavenly Immortality Through Golden Elixir[2]
《天仙金丹心法》

Establish a determination, straighten out the morals, repent the errors, shift toward goodness, build up the foundation, train self, install the furnace, pick up the herb, start the fire, cease the fire, conceive the embryo, nurse the baby, accumulate good deeds, train the Gōng, face the wall, and spiritual ascending.

立志，端品，悔過，遷善，築基，煉己，安爐，採藥，起火，熄火，結胎，養嬰，積行，行功，面壁，飛升。

According to Daoist society, these are the sixteen steps of training to reach the final goal of spiritual enlightenment. First establish a strong will aiming for your goal. Next, re-evaluate your morality by removing the mask on your face and facing your true self. According to Buddhism, in order to reach this goal, you must learn Self-Internal Vision

(Zìguān, 自觀) that allows you to see yourself clearly, the step of Self-Recognition (Zìshì, 自識). To enter the Self-Internal-Vision (Rùguān, 入觀) is to analyze and understand yourself. You must first understand your Xīn so you can see your human temperament (Míngxīn Jiànxìng, 明心見性) (Liǎowù, 了悟), and only then can you face the truth.

Having recognized and understood the real you, then you learn how to change your morality towards goodness and truth. Only then can you establish a firm foundation for your spiritual cultivation. If your subconscious mind remains at the stage of laymen morals, with an untruthful mask on your face, then you will not be able to face the truth. You must learn to remove the mask on your face, first by facing the Self Inner-Comprehension (Zìwù, 自悟) or Self-Awareness (Zìjué, 自覺). Only then, can you find the way to awaken your Shén, the stage of Self-Awakening (Zìxǐng, 自醒).

Once you are able to wake up your Shén (related to the subconscious mind), then you will find the way to set your Shén free from spiritual bondage. This is the stage of Self-Spiritual-Freedom (Zìtuō, 自脫). To reach this enlightened stage, you must convert the Original Essence into Qì (Liànjīng Huàqì, 煉精化氣), convert (nourish) the Qì to the Shén (Liànqì Huàshén, 煉氣化神), and then refine your Shén and lead it into emptiness (Liànshén Fǎnxū, 煉神返虛). Finally, you must crush the emptiness (Fěnsuì Xūkōng, 粉碎虛空) so as to establish an independent Shén that is able to survive even if the physical body is dead. To Buddhist society, this is the stage of Buddhahood. When you have reached this stage, your spirit will gain eternal life and will not be reincarnated into a human form again.

Train the self (Liànjǐ, 煉己), install the furnace (Ānlú, 安爐), pick up the herb (Cǎiyào, 採藥), start the fire (Qǐhuǒ, 起火), and cease the fire (Xíhuǒ, 熄火); these are the trainings of converting the essence into Qì. Conceive the embryo (Jiétāi, 結胎), nurse the baby (Yǎngyīng, 養嬰), and accumulate good deeds (Jīxíng, 積行); these are the trainings of converting the Qì into Shén. In order to establish an independent Shén, you must train the Gōng (Xínggōng, 行功). Face the wall (Miànbì, 面壁) is for crushing the emptiness, and finally spiritual ascending (Fēishēng, 飛升) means the separation of the spiritual body and the physical body.

15. Anthology of Daoist Village
《道鄉集》

Those talks (in Dào Dé Jīng) such as: "when there is a Xīn (i.e., intention), it is used to observe the ways (i.e., constant changes) of nature; when there is no Xīn (i.e., no intention), it is used to observe the marvelousness of nature," are actually the applications of the Dào. In addition, (the sentence) of "when having (the Xīn), it is to observe the ways (of nature)" is again the application of (the sentence): "when without having (the Xīn), it is to observe the marvelousness (of nature)." Furthermore, (the sentence of) "without having (the Xīn), it is to observe the marvelousness (of nature)" is again the main core (of the sentence): "when having (the Xīn), it is to observe the ways (of nature)." (You) must understand that (the sentence of) "when having (the Xīn), it is to observe the ways (of nature)" means there is an action and is the time of returning the Qì to nourish the Shén. "Without having (the Xīn) so as to observe the marvelousness (of nature)" is doing nothing. There is no body around and no self, no mountain, rivers, grass, or wood. It is the timing of no consciousness and no feeling. This means the extreme calm and peaceful conscious state of "approaching the nihility (i.e., nothingness or emptiness) to its extremity and maintaining the calmness with sincerity." Follow this extreme calmness, then a Yáng (state) can be generated and therefore the marvellous lives can be conceived.

有心觀竅，無心觀妙等語。乃道之功用也。有欲以觀竅，又為無心觀妙之用。無心以觀妙，又為有心觀竅之體。要知有欲觀竅有為也，神返氣自回之時也。無欲觀妙無為也，無人無我，無山川草木，混混然不知不覺之時代也。指〝致虛極，守靜篤。〞之意識活動的寧靜，靜而后一陽生，萌發奇妙生機。

The first sentence originated from Lǎozi's *Dào Dé Jīng* (道德經), Chapter 1. It is said: "Always keep nothingness, so as to observe the marvelousness (of nature). Always having, so observe the returning (recycling or ending) of million objects."[42] The word Qiào (竅) is actually the word Jiǎo (徼) which means returning to its root. Therefore, "Qiào" (竅) implies "the changes or variations of the nature." When you have a heart (Yǒuxīn, 有心) (intention) to observe the changes of nature, then your mind is paying attention to it and pondering on it. However, when your mind is not paying attention to (Wúxīn, 無心) (no intention) the changes of nature, you are experiencing the marvellous manifestation and interplay of natural power and forces. All of these are the applications of the Dào. This is simply because the Dào itself cannot be interpreted and talked about. Once you talk about it, you are using the limited human knowledge to judge the great nature. In this case, the Dào will not be accurate. All we try to observe and understand is not the Dào itself, but its applications.

However, when you have an intention to observe the natural changes and variations, it is due to the experience you have gained from nature in which you do not pay attention. Thus, the intention of observing the applications (consequences) of experiencing, originated without intention. Naturally, the experience without intention is the cause and the root of observation with intention.

To approach the goal of Embryonic Breathing, you must begin with an intention which allows you to observe the changes and variations of your Qì and Shén. However, the final goal of Embryonic Breathing is the doing of no-doing, the intention having disappeared. You are able to approach the Dào and experience nature. When this happens, you are able to trace back to the root of life.

The first step is to observe the Xīn (心) (emotional mind) and understand its behavior. From this you learn to understand yourself. This is the process of regulating, and your intention is present. However, after you have regulated your mind into a neutral state, you regulate it without regulating. Then, your intention is not there any more, and you have approached the Dào of nature and will find the original human nature. That is why all of the Buddhist or Daoist societies have focused on the regulating of the Xīn (心). It is said in the document, Important Script of Similar Contents (Tóngzhǐ Yàochāo, 同指要鈔), that: "The religious doors (i.e., styles), in generations, all considered 'observing the Xīn' (Guānxīn, 觀心) is the most important (in cultivation)."[43]

Only after you are able to cease the activity of Xīn, can you then calm down and keep peace within. Then your mind is clear and Shén will stay at its residence, and you will be able to see through the cycling of nature (creations and variations). Lǎozi (老子) (Dào Dé Jīng, Chapter 16) said: "Approaching the nihility (nothingness or emptiness) to its extremity and maintaining the calmness with sincerity. Millions of objects (lives) are in actions which allow me to observe their cyclic repetitions. Though there are so many objects, each individual must repeatedly return to its root (origin). When it returns to the root, it means 'calmness.' When it is calmed, then it means 'repetition of a life.'"[44]

16. The Complete Book of Principal Contents of Human Life and Temperament; Nourishing the Origin, Precious Key of Saving and Protecting the Life 《性命圭旨全書・涵養本源・救護命寶》

It is marvellous that the (key) method of Observing the Xīn (Guānxīn) is on the sole key gate, Língguān (i.e., Spiritual Gate). When a human begins to conceive (his) life through feeling (i.e., receiving) the Qì, endowed with a tiny Original Yáng (Yuányáng) from heaven and the earth (i.e., nature) and derived into this key gate so as to conceal the Original Shén. It is completely empty within, but extremely insubstantial and utmost bright. It is the master of our lives. Truthfully, when (we) have it, (we are) alive and without it, (we are) dead. Alive, dead, flourishing, and withering, all depend on this (Spiritual Gate). Scholars called it Lingtai (i.e., Spiritual Platform), Daoists called it Língguān (i.e., Spiritual Gate), and Buddhists called Língshān (i.e., Spiritual Mountain).

觀心之法，妙在靈關一竅。人自受生感氣之初，稟天地一點元陽，化生此竅，以藏元神。其中空空洞洞，至虛至明，乃吾人生生主宰。真所謂有之則生，無之則死。生死盛衰，皆由這個。儒曰靈臺，道曰靈關，釋曰靈山。

To observe the Xīn (Guānxīn, 觀心), you must remove the mask from your face and encounter the real you, and understand your thinking and actions. In order to do so, you must first build a strong Yì (意) (Wisdom Mind) that allows you to analyze your

Xīn and then restrain it. The key to reaching this goal is to keep your Yì at the Língguān (靈關) (Upper Dāntián). "Língguān" (靈關) (Spiritual Gate) implies "Spiritual Valley" (Shéngǔ, 神谷) between the two lobes of the brain, the residence of the spirit. This place is called "Língtái" (靈臺) (Spiritual Platform) by scholars, "Língshān" (靈山) (Spiritual Mountain) by Buddhists. Although this place is empty, the power manifested there can be mighty and marvellous.

17. Zhìyóuzǐ; Collection of Important Papers[2]
《至游子・集要篇》

Do not be afraid of the initiation of a thought but be afraid of the delaying of its perception (i.e., awareness).

不畏念起，惟畏覺遲。

The thoughts generated related to the past, the present, and the future can be emotionally disturbing, preventing you from keeping your mind in a calm state. Therefore, the first step in regulating the mind is to stop the thoughts which are lingering in your mind. You must also stop the initiation of a new thought.

However, it is not easy to stop the initiation of a new thought. You must have an awareness so you are able to stop this new thought from getting deeper and wider. This awareness is the first step in eliminating its initiation.

18. The Complete Book of Principal Contents of Human Life and Temperament; The Rules of Training the Shape by Jade Liquid
《性命圭旨全書・玉液煉形法則》

If (you) wish to cease the initiation and termination of Xīn (i.e., emotional mind), (you) must begin from the thought of no thought.

欲除生滅心，必自無念始。

To stop the initiation of a new thought or the disturbances of old thoughts lingering in your mind, the best way is learning how to keep the mind empty and think nothing. However, in reality, it is not possible since when you think of nothing, you are thinking of something. Therefore, the common way of regulating the mind is paying attention to the breathing. Slowly and gradually allow the breathing to become softer and more slender until it is as though it were there and yet as though it were not there. When this happens, you are in the state of deep meditation of no thought.

19. Anthology of Daoist Village[2]
《道鄉集》

Today, I would like to teach you the method of ceasing the thought. For example, when my Xīn is looking at the water, my thought will be on the water; when my Xīn is looking at the moon, my thought will be on the moon; assuming if my eyes (i.e., attention) are focused in looking at the Qì cavity (Qìxuè, Dāntián), my Xīn will be on the Qì cavity.

余今傳汝止念之法。譬如我心看水，此念即在水上；我心看月，此念即在月上；設想此眼光專看氣穴，我心即在氣穴矣。

This article talks about the key trick of stopping the thought is paying attention to the Qìxuè (氣穴). "Qìxuè" means "Upper Dāntián" or "Real Lower Dāntián." Naturally, the way of doing so is through the breathing. Once you pay attention to the breathing and keep your mind at the Dāntián, the thought will disappear gradually.

20. Zhuāngzi, Laymen World[2]
《莊子・人間世》

With a sole will, do not listen with ears but listen with Xīn (i.e., sincere mind); do not listen with Xīn but listen with Qì. Listening ceases at the ears and Xīn is stopped in accordance (Fú). What is Qì? It is insubstantial and attached to (i.e., existing in) all objects. Only (following) the Dào can you gather this insubstantial (Qì). What is this insubstantial? It is (obtained from) the purification of Xīn (Xīnzhāi).

若一志，無聽之以耳而聽之以心；無聽之以心而聽之以氣。聽止于耳，心止于符。氣也者，虛而待物者也。唯道集虛，虛者心齋也。

In order to regulate your emotional mind (Xīn, 心), you must stop your listening contact with the outside world and pay attention to your emotional mind. Once you can bring your thoughts from outside to inside of your body, then you should pay attention to your Qì through breathing. "Fú" (符) means "to accord," "to match," "to harmonize," "to coordinate," or "to cooperate." This means the way of stopping the activities of Xīn is through the coordination of breathing.

In order to gather the Qì at the Dāntián, you must first have a calm and non-disturbed Xīn. "Xīnzhāi" (心齋) means "purified Xīn" and implies a simply calm and sincere mind. Only then, the Qì can be preserved at its residence. This is the way of Dào (道).

21. The Complete Book of Principal Contents of Human Life and Temperament; Hen Anthology[2]

《性命圭旨全書・亨集》

If there is an initiation of a thought, then everywhere is fire. The quiet place where the millions of affinities (of the thoughts are ceased), then the spring can blossom.

一念動時皆是火，萬緣寂處即生春。

This sentence emphasizes two important things in regulating the mind. The first is to stop the initiation of a thought. When the thought is initiated, then the mind is excited and becomes Yáng (fire). The second is to cut off all of the thoughts which are lingering in your mind.

22. Wéimó Classic[2]

《維摩經》

"To restrain the Xīn (i.e., emotional mind) from its emotional affinity is called stop. To see deep and reach far clearly is called observation." It is also said: "Every thought returns to one (i.e., the origin) is called stop, and everything can be discriminated clearly is called observation."

〝系心于緣謂之止，分別深達謂之觀。〞〝念念歸一為止，了了分明為觀。〞

These two sentences explain the meaning of "Zhǐguān" (止觀), which literally means "to stop the observation" and implies that the observation of the Xīn's activities is stopped. In order to do so, you must have regulated your emotional mind to a stage where the regulating is no longer necessary.

The first phrase explains that, in order to reach this goal, you must first stop the emotional affinity with the outside world. This is the meaning of "stop" (Zhǐ, 止). Once you have reached the stage where your mind is so clear and profound that it allows you to analyze the situation through observation and thus you are able to stop the old thought and the new thought's initiation, then it is called "observation" (Guān, 觀) (see through thoroughly).

The second phrase explains that when you bring all of the disturbing thoughts into a place and pay attention to it, this is called "stop" (Zhǐ, 止). Naturally, this place is the Dāntián (Embracing Singularity). That implies that if you are able to pay attention to the Dāntián (either Upper Dāntián for Shén or Real Lower Dāntián for Qì) and coordinate with your deep breathing, all of the disturbing thoughts will be replaced with one thought—thus, the disturbing thoughts can be stopped. To see through thoroughly so your mind is clear and calm is called "observation" (Guān, 觀).

23. Anthology of Daoist Village
《道鄉集》

"The real meaning of Buddhahood which has been handed down (to us) is: observation is stopped." "What is observation? It means to place my vision warmly on the ultimate goodness." "What is stop? It means to place and stop (i.e., focus) my real intention at the ultimate goodness."

〝佛之真傳，在于觀止。〞〝觀者何？將我目光，溫煦于至善地之義也。〞〝止者何？將我真意止于至善地之義也。〞

According to Buddhist society, there are three observations (Sānguān, 三觀): 1. Observing Emptiness. It is to observe the emptiness of all natural laws and events. 2. Observing Falseness. It is to observe the falseness of all natural laws. 3. Observing Between. It is to observe non-emptiness and non-falseness of the natural laws. This means to keep the neutral viewpoint. It also means double observation.[45] "Zhǐguān" (止觀) (Stop Observation) is the way of reaching "Guānzhǐ" (觀止) (Observation is Stopped). In order to reach this, you must first have observed and analyzed all of the events and natural occurrences. Once you have seen through all of the events in your mind, then nothing will bother you. Then you have reached the stage of "Guānzhǐ."

This document explains that the best way of reaching "Guānzhǐ" is simply paying attention to cultivating your self-mind until the stage of ultimate goodness. When you pay attention to all of the goodness, then nothing bothers you. You are kind, righteous, and gentle. Then you have no inner conflict in your emotional mind. That means you are free from the affinity of emotions and desires.

24. Thesis of Buddha Ground
《佛地論》

All laws (i.e., natural rules) and all different appearances (i.e., manifestations of nature) are able to bloom and be awakened by themselves. If (we are) also able to bloom and awaken from all emotional bondages, just like being awakened from sleep and like the blooming of lotus flower. Therefore, it is called 'Buddha'.

于一切法，一切種相，能自開覺，亦開覺一切有情，如睡夢覺醒，如蓮花開，故名佛。

This is talking about the definition or the feeling of Buddhism. It is like how a lotus flower emerges from the emotional mud and blooms. It is like having just woken up and suddenly realized that every occurrence or emotional bondage is unreal, as if it were happening in a dream.

Buddha means to achieve awareness and wisdom. For example, to awaken through understanding, to awaken through observation, to awaken through knowing about the reasons (causes) for all laws and natural rules, and being able to discriminate them clearly. It is like just being awakened from sleep, and is called awakening through realization. Comprehend the vexations through observation so they are not harmful. It is like observing and sensing thieves in laymen society. Therefore, it is called the awakening through observation.[46] "Thieves" refers to the emotions and desires which can steal away the purity of your heart and spirit.

According to Buddhist society, we are born and grow in the human emotional mud or dust (Chéntǔ, 塵土) (human matrix). We have created dignity, glory, pride, happiness, sadness, jealousy, and all kinds of desires. We learn how to lie and place a mask on our face. However, we all experience significant spiritual pain living in this human matrix. We have been blinded by the mud and our hearing has been blocked by it. Nothing is clear in our minds. The conscious mind is active while the subconscious mind which is connected to the Shén is in its sleeping state. When this happens, we are dreaming in the human matrix and are not awakening.

Nevertheless, each of us has a lotus seed. Through meditation, this lotus seed will bud and start to grow from deep in the mud. Gradually, our subconscious minds will grow through meditation. After meditating a long time, this lotus flower will push you out of the human mud and you will see everything clearly. To waken your Shén, you must learn to bring all thoughts to your Shén center and to keep the Shén there. This spiritual center (Upper Dāntián) is called "Spiritual Mountain" (Língshān, 靈山). In this mountain, there is a Spiritual Valley (Shéngǔ, 神谷) where the Valley Spirit (Gǔshén, 谷神) resides.

There is a song in Buddhist society which says: "Do not search far for Buddha since he is in the Spiritual Mountain. Where is the Spiritual Mountain? It is actually in your mind. Everyone should have a pagoda at Spiritual Mountain so (he) is able to cultivate (his) being under the pagoda at this Spiritual Mountain."[47] Pagoda (Tǎ, 塔) implies good deeds you have done, and the comprehension of nature which you have accumulated in your spiritual cultivation.

In *The Complete Book of Principal Contents of Human Life and Temperament* (*Xìngmìng Guīzhǐ Quánshū*, 性命圭旨全書), it is said: "When learning the Dào, (you) must first learn to comprehend your own Xīn (emotional mind). The deep hidden place of your own Xīn is the hardest place to find. Once you have found it and no more other places can be found, then you will have comprehended that the layman's Xīn can be just like that of a Buddha."[48] This entire paragraph implies that the Xīn of awakening is in a place deeply hidden within yourself. Once you have found it, then this Xīn is nothing special and is just like a layman's Xīn. This means every layman's Xīn, once awakened, can be just like a Buddha's.

25. Dào Scriptures; Fifteenth Religious Thesis of Chóngyáng[2]
《道藏・重陽立教十五論》

The world with desires, the world with colors, and the world with no color are the three worlds. When the Xīn (emotional mind) has forgotten (been isolated from) the worries and the thoughts that are hanging around, then (you) have passed the territory of desiring world. When the Xīn has forgotten the surrounding environment (laymen world), then (you) have passed the color world (material world). When (the Xīn) is not attached to anything (illusion) but emptiness, then (you) have passed the world of no color.

欲界、色界、無色界，此乃三界也。心忘慮念，即超欲界；心忘諸境，即超色界；不著空見，即超無色界。

This paragraph explains the three worlds (Sānjiè, 三界) defined in Buddhist society. These three worlds are: the world of emotional bondage and desires; the world of layman activities and material existence (color world), and the world of imagination and fantasy. When your Xīn can be separated from these three worlds, then you have reached the stage of regulating your mind.

26. The Secrets of Spiritual Applications of All Veracious Holy Embryo
(Yúzhēnrén's Secrets of Embryonic Breathing)[2,3,4]
《諸真聖胎神用訣》
（于真人胎息法）

Those who wish to cultivate their temperaments must first stabilize their Xīn and Qì. When Xīn and Qì are stabilized, the Shén can be condensed (i.e., focused). When Shén is condensed, then the Xīn is peaceful. When Xīn is peaceful, then the Qì can ascend upward (to nourish the brain). When Qì has ascended upward, then the surrounding environment will be empty. When the surrounding environment is empty, then it (i.e., the entire being) is pure and quiet (i.e., calm). When it is pure and quiet, then there are no objects (i.e., emptiness) around. If there is no object (in the mind), then (the cultivation) of life can be completed. When the life is completed, the Dào can be derived. Once the Dào is derived, then all appearances (i.e., illusion generated from desires and emotions) can be cut off. If the appearances can be cut off, then the consciousness can be bright (i.e., clear). When the consciousness is clear, then the Shén can be communicative (i.e., enlightened). The classic said: "When the Xīn is communicative, then millions of methods are also communicative. When the Xīn is calm, then millions of occurrences are all eliminated. This is the door to achieving real stability of Rúlái (i.e., Buddha)." (Therefore), those who cultivate the Dào must first cultivate the methods of stabilizing the Xīn. Once the methods of stabilizing the Xīn can be obtained, then it is not difficult to return the elixir, the golden liquid (Jīnyè) (saliva) will not be far, and immortality can be achieved.

凡所修行，先定心氣，心氣定則神凝，神凝則心安，心安則氣昇，氣昇則境空，境空則清靜，清靜則無物，無物則命全，命全則道生，道生則絕相，絕相則覺明，覺明則神通。經云：‘心通萬法皆通，心靜萬法皆滅，此一門如來真定者也。’凡修道者，先修心定之法，既得定法，還丹不遠，金液非遙，仙道得矣。(亦見于性命圭旨全書；王方平胎息訣)

This document talks about the sequential consequences of cultivation. From stabilization of Xīn and Qì to the Shén's condensing. From the Shén's condensing results the peace of Xīn. From peaceful Xīn, the Qì can ascend upward to nourish the brain. When this happens, the surrounding environment will disappear, and you will be set free from emotional bondage and the desires of the material world. If there is no object in the mind, then the cultivation of human temperament can be completed. This will result in the unification of human Shén and the Dào. Finally, it will lead you to spiritual enlightenment. "Jīnyè" (金液) means "golden liquid" which implies the generation of precious saliva during Enlightenment Grand Cyclic Heaven meditation. This implies the Qì has been successfully led upward to nourish the brain.

27. The Secrets of Spiritual Applications of All Veracious Holy Embryo

(Yuánxiàn Zhēnrén's Secrets of Embryonic Breathing) [2,3,4]

《諸真聖胎神用訣》

（元憲真人胎息訣）

Those who wish to study Embryonic Breathing through Wúwéi (i.e., doing nothing) can only be reached through (cultivation of) a pure and calm Xīn. It is also named "Zhēnrú" (i.e., Real Buddhahood). (In this state,) there are no objects (i.e., emptiness) at all originally. It is just like the Grand Nihility (Tàixū): no to or fro, no up or down, no moving or still, very quiet and simple. It shares the same body as the real emptiness (i.e., coexistence) and has the same origin as Great Dào (Dàdào), and is able to meet the original face (of life). If (you) wish to cultivate the Great Dào, (you) must cultivate Wúwéi. The mind is clear and insubstantial, quiet but not quiet, calm but not calm, the Xīn is clean and isolated from the surrounding environment. When the Xīn and environment are both forgotten, then (you) have entered the real Dào of Wúwéi. Those who cultivate this method, the (refinement of) elixir can be achieved. (In this case,) the Qì can be stabilized naturally and the Embryonic Breathing can be achieved.

夫學無為胎息者，只是本清靜心也。亦名真如，本無物也。有若太虛相似，無去無來，無上無下，非動非靜，寂寂廖寥，與真空同體，與大道同源，與本面目相逢者也。若修大道，當修無為，其心清虛，寂而無寂，靜而無靜，心澄境謝，心境雙忘，則入無為真道也。學道之人，若修如是法門，則其丹自成，自然氣定而得胎息矣。

"Wúwéi" (無為) means "doing nothing," and implies "regulating without regulating." Therefore, every thing has become natural. It happens without any intention or desires. In order to reach the goal of Embryonic Breathing where no regulating is necessary, you must have a clear and calm mind. "Zhēnrú" (真如) means "Real Buddhahood." Once you have reached the stage of regulating without regulating your mind, you will then regulate your breathing until it has reached the stage of as if it is there and as if it is not there. When this happens, your spirit and the natural spirit will be united. This is the way of "Great Dao" (Dàdào, 大道). Dào is great, so it is often called "Great Dào."

28. The Secrets of Spiritual Applications of All Veracious Holy Embryo (Kàngcāngzi's Secrets of Embryonic Breathing)[2,3,4]

《諸真聖胎神用訣》(亢倉子胎息訣)

When (you) cultivate (your Shén) to enter the Dào, (you should) cease (your) Xīn (i.e., emotional mind) and not let it be disordered; the Spirit of Vitality (Jīngshén) should not be scattered (or dispersed); cease the Shén and do not let it be vigilant (i.e., active); cease snoring (i.e., heavy breathing) and do not let (the air) out (too fast); cease the words and not talk; cease the blood's circulation (from being too exciting) and not allow it be stagnant; cease the spittle and do not spit it far; cease tears and do not let it be discarded; cease anger and do not let events bother (you); cease the Shén and do not let it worry; cease resentment and do not keep it (in your mind); cease the ego and do not dispute (with others); and cease the misfortune and do not keep it in (your) mind. If a person can do so constantly whenever he is walking, residing, sitting, or lying (i.e., daily life), his Xīn (i.e., emotional mind) will be happy by itself and the accomplishment can be achieved naturally. If (you) do not cultivate these rules (of regulating), the efforts will be in vain and end up with no result. If (you) do the above rules, the elixir will be completed. (In addition,) if (you) are able to forget both movement and stillness (i.e., forget the activity of the mind and body), then the Dào can automatically be gained without asking for it.

凡修煉入道，息心勿亂，精神勿泄，息神勿惕，息鼾勿出，息言勿語，息血勿滯，息唾勿遠，息涕勿棄，息嗔勿惱，息神勿憂，息怨勿念，息我勿爭，息害勿記。若人行住坐臥，常持如是，其心自樂，自然成就。不修此理，枉費其功，終無成法。但日日如是，其丹必就，若動靜雙忘，道不求自得矣。

This document points out that in order to regulate your mind and enter the Dào of cultivation, you must first regulate the thinking and behaviors of your daily life. Only if you are able to do so, can you then have a peaceful Xīn. This is a crucial key to cultivation.

29. The Secrets of Spiritual Applications of All Veracious Holy Embryo

(Xuánhú Zhēnrén's Secrets of Embryonic Breathing)[2,3]

《諸真聖胎神用訣》

（玄葫真人胎息訣）

(To cultivate) the Great Dào (Dàdào), (you) must use the emptiness (Kong) as the origin (of cultivation). It is marvellous (if you are able) to cut off (the mind of) the appearances (i.e., material world), approach the original root, calm and stabilize the Tàisù (i.e., Grand Simplicity), absorb the Qì and store it at the (Real Lower) Dāntián, refine the Shén in the Jīnshì (i.e., Golden Residence, Upper Dāntián), and stabilize the Xīn (i.e., emotional mind) deeply at the sea of consciousness (Juéhǎi). When the Xīn is stable, the Shén will be tranquil. When the Shén is tranquil, then the Qì will stay (at its residence). When Qì stays, then the Xīn will be naturally delighted. (You) should keep (your mind) at the Zhēnxí (i.e., Real Breathing, Embryonic Breathing) at all times. It is also said: "When Shén and breathing are stabilized, the Jīn (i.e., metal) and Mù (i.e., wood) will intercourse. When Xīn and Yì are tranquil, the Lóng (i.e., dragon) and Hǔ (i.e., tiger) will meet together. This is the real (cultivation) of Internal Elixir (Nèidān) and the applications of Embryonic Breathing. Those who cultivate the Dào, if (they) wish to live long without dying, (they) must first refine (their) Xīn." Zhēnrén (i.e., Truthful Person who has achieved the Dào) said: "What is Xīn? It is one inch and three centimeters under the lungs and is called 'Jade Kettle' (Yùhú). There is a sole Qì of white nihility within." Classic said: 'To generate the whiteness in the nihility, one name is "Jade Kettle," second name is "spiritual residence (Shénshì)," third name is "Jade Hall" (Yùguǎn), fourth name is "crimson palace" (Jiànggōng). Within it, there is a Buddha who could save those who suffer, there is an immortal who does not die, there is an efficacious precious Buddha, there is an incarnation of life, there is a grand sole Zhēnrén (i.e., Truthful Person or Buddha), and there is a Zhēnrén who saves those who suffer. (You should) always keep (your) Original Qì (Yuánqì) and don't let it be dispersed. When the elixir is congealed, it is as big as a grain, the color is like gold. It is named as "Bǎolín" (Precious Jade). If one is able to know it, discriminate it, recognize it, and seal his Liùmén (i.e., Six Doors), always keep (his) original truth, Embryonic Breathing will be achieved automatically and live long without dying.

夫大道以空為本，絕相為妙，達本元，靜定太素，納氣于丹田，煉神于金室，定心于覺海。心定神寧，神寧則氣住，氣住則自然心樂。常于百刻之中，舍守于真息。又云：'神息定而金木交，心意寧而龍虎會，此內丹之真，胎息之用也。凡修道之人，若要長生不死，先須煉心。' 真人曰：'心者，在肺之下一寸三分曰玉壺，內有虛白一氣。' 經云：'虛中生白，一名玉壺，二名神室，三名玉館，四名絳宮，中有救苦天尊，中有不死之神，中有靈寶天尊，中有元始符命，中有太一真人，中有救苦真人。常持元氣，勿令失散，丹砂結就，大如黍米，色如黃金，一名寶琳。若人識得、辨得、認得，塞其六門，常守天真，胎息自成，延年久而不死矣。

In order to find the real Dào, you must first empty your mind. This is simply because the Dào itself is empty and there are no material or emotional desires. If you wish to understand and reach the Dào, the first step is to stop the mind which is attached to the material world and emotional disturbance. In order to establish a firm root of life, you must keep your mind in the state of Grand Simplicity (Tàisù, 太素) (emptiness), accumulate the Qì at the Real Lower Dāntián to an abundant level, refine your Shén until it is focused, and stays at the Upper Dāntián. "Jīnshì" (金室) means "Golden Residence" and implies "the brain" or "Upper Dāntián."

To reach this goal, you must first stabilize your Xīn through the awakening of life. When the Xīn is stabilized, the Shén can be peaceful. Then the Shén and Qì will stay at their residence, and you will be able to unify the Shén and Qì at the Real Lower Dāntián to reach the state of "Wújí" (無極). This will allow you to return yourself to the origin or the root of life. "Jīn" (金) means "metal" and implies "lungs" since lungs belongs to metal in the Five Elements (Wǔxíng, 五行). "Mù" (木) means "wood" and implies "liver" since liver belongs to wood in the Five Elements. According to Chinese medical science, the lungs associate with your breathing and the liver associates with your Shén. Therefore, when your mind is calm and peaceful, the Shén can be condensed and the breathing can be slender, soft, and uniform. This is the key to Embryonic Breathing.

"Yùhú" (玉壺) means "Jade Kettle," "Shénshì" (神室) means "Spiritual Residence," "Yùguǎn" (玉館) means "Jade Hall," and "Jiànggōng" (絳宮) means "Crimson Palace." All these alternative names imply "heart" (Xīn, 心). "Liùmén" (六門) means "Six Doors" and implies two eyes, two ears, nose, and mouth, the six organs of sense.

30. The Secrets of Spiritual Applications of All Veracious Holy Embryo

(Hóuzhēnrén's Secrets of Embryonic Breathing) [2,3,4]

《諸真聖胎神用訣》

（侯真人胎息訣）

What is the real sole rule (of cultivation)? It is not to separate from its Běnyuán (i.e., Original Root). What is Běnyuán? Then, it means a sole Xīn (i.e., simplicity of emotional mind). (If the Xīn) does not move and does not transport away (i.e., apart), then the Xīn is (at) the origin. (If the Xīn) does not stop (its activities) and does not stay (at the origin) (i.e., unsteady), then the origin (of problems) will be (initiated from) Xīn. When the Xīn is tranquil and calm, then the Great Herb (Dàyào) (i.e., elixir) can be completed; when the Xīn is bewildered and disordered, then it will result in the production of great thief (Dàzéi) which is able to take away (your) essence (Jīng), to steal (your) Shén, to damage (your) furnace (i.e., Lower Dāntián), to make (you) lose the herb (i.e., elixir), and bring disaster to (your) body, and finally end (your) life. Those who are cultivating the Dào must first cultivate the methods of keeping the Xīn calm. When the Xīn is calm, then it can be stabilized. When the Xīn is stabilized, then the Shén will be peaceful, lead (Qiān) and mercury (Gǒng) will be mutually delighted with each other, and the dragon (Lóng) and tiger (Hǔ) will marry. After practicing cyclic heaven for plenty of number (i.e., time), the essence will be increased, the Qì will be enhanced, and the Shén will be nourished. If these three things are completed, then millions of spirits (i.e., all existing spirits) can gather and meet at the Dāntián, Qì and blood can circulate around the entire body smoothly, and the Dào of longevity can be achieved freely and unfettered. It is also said: "how to keep (your mind) clear and tranquil, (you) must first clean (your) Shén, stop worries, forget self, extinguish the surrounding environment, and embrace the real (i.e., truth). This is what the marvellous tranquil Dào should be."

夫真一法界者，不離于本源。本源者，則是一心也。不動不行，心則是源；不停不住，源則是心。其心清靜，則成大藥；其心惑亂，則成大賊。奪其精，盜其神，敗其爐，失其藥，患其身，喪其命也。凡在道之人，必先修心靜之法。但于心靜，必得定心。心定則神安，鉛汞相投，龍虎親也。周天數足，添精、益氣、養神。此三法若全，則萬神感會于丹田，氣血周流于遍體，逍遙于長生之道。又云：如何清靜，當澄其神，絕其慮，忘其我，滅其境，抱其真，此謂妙靜之道。

This article emphasizes that the most important thing in spiritual cultivation is to keep the emotional mind (Xīn) in its extreme simplicity (emptiness). When the Xīn can be calm and peaceful, then the Qì (elixir) can be accumulated to an abundant level. However, if the Xīn is confused and emotionally disturbed, then you will lose your essence, Qì, and Shén. Therefore, you must first learn how to stabilize your Xīn. Only then can the Shén be peaceful and stay at its residence, and the Shén and the Qì (Yīn and Yáng) interact with each other at the Real Lower Dāntián. Lead (Qiān, 鉛) and mercury (Gǒng, 汞), dragon (Lóng, 龍) and tiger (Hǔ, 虎) imply Yīn and Yáng.

31. The Secrets of Spiritual Applications of All Veracious Holy Embryo

(Central Lǎojūn's Secrets of Embryonic Breathing)[3,4]

《諸真聖胎神用訣》
（中央老君胎息訣）

What is the original root that establishes the heaven and the earth (i.e., nature)? It is generated from Yīn and Yáng. The clean Qì is the heaven and the dirty Qì is the earth. The clean Qì is Xīn while dirty Qì is kidneys. (Humans) are distracted by laymen affairs, which gives rise to the Xīn's actions, thus the cleanliness and the dirtiness are not able to be distinguished. How do we know this theory? Whenever there is an action and movement, the eyes see and the ears hear, thus the five thieves (Wǔzéi) have caused the loss of Zhēnyuán (i.e., Real Origin). The Xīn is lost due to the eyes (i.e., seeing), thus, the Xīn is touched and the Shén is fatigued. In addition, the Xīn is also lost due to the ears (i.e., hearing). This Xīn then sends sounds into the kidneys, the Shén is labored and Xīn is annoyed, and thus damaged. If the mind is touched, then the Original Qì is leaking, consequently, the practice of Embryonic Breathing cannot be achieved. Then, how can (we) reach the goal? If a person sits quietly, the mind does not act, all thoughts cease and (the disturbances generated from) emotions are all forgotten, the Qì and the Shén are thus regulated uniformly and smoothly. After a long time (of practice), immortality can be reached automatically.

夫本立天地，生于陰陽，清氣為天，濁氣為地，清氣為心，濁氣為腎。被世牽惹，引動人心，故清濁不分也。怎曉此理哉！每動作處，經行處，眼見耳聞，五賊送了真元。眼送于心，心動神疲，又被耳送于心，心送音聲入腎，神勞心煩壞了也。若動念，則泄真氣，故胎息不成矣。如何得成？若人靜坐，念心不動，息念忘情，氣神調勻，久而自成仙矣。

Xīn (心) is the origin of our actions. This Xīn was originally clean and pure at the beginning of our lives. However, when we grow up, through our organs of sense, this Xīn gradually becomes contaminated by the five thieves (Wǔzéi, 五賊), and our thinking and internal organs become dirty. "Five thieves" are "five emotions" that are related to the five internal organs: anger-wood (liver), happiness-fire (heart), pensiveness-earth (spleen), sadness-metal (lungs), and fear-water (kidneys). "Zhēnyuán" (真元) means "Real Origins" and implies the "Original Essence, Qì, and Shén" (Yuánjīng, Yuánqì, and Yuánshén, 元精、元氣、元神).

In order to conserve our Qì and extend our lives, we must first regulate our Xīn. Then the breathing can be slender, soft, natural, and smooth, which is the necessary requirement for Embryonic Breathing.

32. The Secrets of Spiritual Applications of All Veracious Holy Embryo

(Chén, Xī-Yí's Secrets of Embryonic Breathing)[3]

《諸真聖胎神用訣》

（陳希夷胎息訣）

From Dào, the youths (i.e., new lives) are derived, youths are (then) derived into elders, elders are (then) derived into sickness, from sickness, deaths then result, (and finally), from deaths spiritual (energy) is derived. From this spiritual (energy), millions (of living) objects are derived; from (the existing) Qì, living spiritual beings can be created; from (parents') essence, the shape (i.e., physical body) can be formalized. When these, essence, Qì, and Shén are derived (correctly), (a human) can be refined into a real immortal. Therefore, it is said: "To conserve the essence, to nourish the Shén, and to refine the Qì, these three items are the three virtual spirits of nature. (One) must know it." Zǐ (i.e., 11 p.m.–1 a.m.), Wǔ (11 a.m.–1 p.m.), Mǎo (5–7 a.m.) and Yǒu (5–7 p.m.), four timings, are the four doors for the Yīn and Yáng's entrance and exit. Stabilize the Xīn and do not be touched, it is called "Chán." The

Shén is transportable and changeable in millions of ways, it is called "Líng." The wisdom is able to comprehend millions of affairs, it is called "Huì." The Dào has returned to its root and harmonized with Qì, it is called "Xiū." When the Real Qì (Zhēnqì) has returned to its origin, it is called "Liàn." When the dragon and tiger have intercourse, it is called "Dān." When three Dāns (i.e., three Dāntiáns) cooperate with each other, it is called "Liǎo." If those who cultivate their temperament are able to understand these roots, the path of entering the Dào will be near.

夫道化少，少化老，老化病，病化死，死化神。神化萬物，氣化生靈，精化成形，神、氣、精三化，煉成真仙。故云：'存精、養神、煉氣，此乃三德之神，不可不知。'子午卯酉四時，乃是陰陽出入之門戶也。定心不動，謂之曰禪；神通萬變，謂之曰靈；智通萬事，謂之曰慧；道元合氣，謂之曰修；真氣歸元，謂之曰煉；龍虎相交，謂之曰丹；三丹同契，謂之曰了。若修行之人，知此根源，乃可入道近矣。

It is the Dào that conceives our lives; born as a child, we grow up becoming an adult, getting old, becoming sick, and finally we die becoming Shén. This is the repetition of the natural cycle. It is the Shén that allows the Dào to again derive millions of living objects. It is due to the existence of Qì that all of these living objects can exist. It is also due to the essence, that the material forms are sustained. Therefore, if you wish to become an immortal, you must refine and train your three treasures (Sānbǎo, 三寶): essence (Jīng, 精), Qì (氣), and spirit (Shén, 神).

Many practitioners believe that when you meditate to train your three treasures, the best times are: Zǐ (子) (11 p.m.–1 a.m.), Wǔ (午) (11 a.m.–1 p.m.), Mǎo (卯) (5–7 a.m.), and Yǒu (酉) (5–7 p.m.). This is because the natural Qì changes at these times. Zǐ (子) (11 p.m.–1 a.m.), the natural Yīn is changing into Yáng; Wǔ (午) (11 a.m.–1 p.m.), the natural Yáng is changing into Yīn; Mǎo (卯) (5–7 a.m.), dawn; and Yǒu (酉) (5–7 p.m.), dusk. *In The Complete Book of Principal Contents of Human Life and Temperament* (*Xìngmìng Guīzhǐ Quánshū*, 性命圭旨全書), it is said: "Zǐ, Wǔ, Mǎo, and Yǒu are the four doors for Yīn and Yáng's exit and entrance."[49]

However, many others believe that you should not be restricted to these four times. Once you have reached a profound level of meditation, you may use any time for your cultivation. The key is learning how to create "Alive Zi Timing" (Huózǐshí, 活子時). That means the Zi timing is alive and can occur at any time and any place. Then how do we define this "Alive Zi Timing?" It is said: "When you practice Qìgōng, the shape (physical body) and the Shén are peaceful and calm, the Shén is condensed and stays at the Qì cavity (Upper Dāntián) and at the same time, (you) feel the Qì's action (aliveness) in the (Real Lower) Dāntián. This is the time of the interaction of Yīn and Yáng."[50] It is also said in the document, Observing Vessels (Màiwàng, 脈望), that: "When (you) begin to establish the elixir foundation (to produce the elixir), (you) should not be restricted to the Zǐ and Wǔ. When this is a (Qì) movement (generated in the Real Lower Dāntián) within the calmness, then it is the time to produce Guǐ (i.e., kidneys), this is the time called "Alive Zǐ Timing."[51] "Guǐ" (癸) implies "kidneys," and means the production of the Original Essence (i.e., hormone).

"Chán" (禪) is a Buddhist term and means meditation in which the mind is free from any emotional bondage. "Líng" (靈) is a super-psychic capability that allows you to communicate with nature of other spiritual beings. "Huì" (慧) means the wisdom generated from accumulation of experiences and knowledge. "Xiū" (修) means to accomplish the cultivation which allows you to return to the root (i.e., origin) of the Dào. "Liàn" (煉) means to refine the Shén and Qì so the Original Qì (Yuánqì, 元氣) can be returned to its origin. Only then will the Yīn and Yáng interact to produce the elixir (Dān, 丹). Once you are able to lead the Qì upward to the Upper Dāntián and keep the Shén there, all three Dāntiáns are unified, coordinated and in harmony with each other, then it is the end of human emotions. That is the training of "Liǎo" (了). In order to reach this stage, you must first calm down your Xīn located at the Middle Dāntián, so the Qì can be preserved and stored at the Real Lower Dāntián, and the Shén can be condensed at the Upper Dāntián.

3.6 Regulating the Spirit (Tiáoshén, 調神)

1. Dào Dé Jīng

(Chapter 6)[1]
《道德經・六章》

The Valley Spirit (Gǔshén) does not die, then it is called "Xuánpìn." The door (i.e., key) to reaching this "Xuánpìn" is the root of heaven and earth (i.e., nature). It is very soft and continuous as if it were existing. When it is used, it will not be exhausted.

谷神不死，是謂玄牝。玄牝之門，是謂天地根，綿綿若存，用之不勤。

The spirit (Shén, 神) resides at the space between the two hemispheres of the brain. This space acts as a valley between mountains, which is able to trap energy and generate resonant vibrations in the valley, that correspond with the energy outside the valley. Thus, the Shén residing in this valley is called "Valley Spirit" (Gǔshén, 谷神) and the valley in which the Shén resides is called "Spiritual Valley" (Shéngǔ, 神谷). It is understood that the Shén residing in this valley governs the energy vibration of the entire body and thus controls the Qì status and its manifestation. When this Shén is strong, the Qì manifestation in your life will be strong, and consequently you will have a long and healthy life (i.e., immortality).

"Xuán" (玄) means "Original" (Yuán, 元), and "Pìn" (牝) refers to female animals and means "mothers." Therefore, "Yuánpìn" means the "Origin or Root of Lives."

When the Valley Spirit is centered (i.e., condensed) and functions actively, the life force is strong. Actually, "Xuánpìn" (玄牝) is what is called "Tàijí" (太極) (Grand Ultimate) in *Yìjīng* (*Book of Changes*). This Tàijí is the Dào (道) of lives in the great nature. Therefore, we can conclude that "Xuánpìn" is: "the root of creation, variation, bearing, and raising of millions of lives, and is the mother of millions of objects of heaven and earth. It is another name for 'Dào'."[52]

The door to reaching this "Xuánpìn" is the key to reaching natural Shén (i.e., heaven and earth). The Shén is very soft and continuous as though existing, and yet without existing. The Shén cannot be seen but felt through cultivation. When it is used, it will not be exhausted.

According to Daoist and Buddhist society, in order to reach the natural Shén, you must re-open your third eye. The Third Eye is called "Tiānmù" (天目) (Heaven Eye), or "Yùmén" (玉門) (Jade Gate) by religious societies, and Yìntáng (M-HN-3, 印堂) (Seal Hall) by Chinese medical society. The document, Wǔdāng's Illustration of Cultivating Truth (Wǔdāng Xiūzhēntú, 武當修真圖): "(the place) under the Míngtáng (明堂) (Ézhōng, M-HN-2, 額中) (central area of forehead), above the midpoint of the line connecting the two eyebrows, where the spiritual light is emitted, is named as 'Heaven Eye' (Tiānmù, 天目)."[53] It also mentioned in the document, Seventh Bamboo Slips of the Bamboo Bookcase (Yúnjí Qīqiān, 云笈七簽), that: "The space between the two eyebrows is the 'Jade Gate' (Yùmén, 玉門) of Níwán (泥丸)."[54] "Níwán" (泥丸) is a Daoist term, literally meaning "Mud Pill" and implies "the brain" or "Upper Dāntián." The lower center of the Spiritual Valley (Shéngǔ, 神谷) between the two hemispheres of the brain is called "Níwángōng" (泥丸宮) and means "Mud Pill Palace."

2. Observing Vessels
《脈望》

The brain is the Upper Dāntián and is the palace where the Original Shén (Yuánshén) resides. If a person is able to grasp this Original Shén and make it stay at this Original Palace, then the golden Qì (i.e., precious Qì) will rise automatically and the Real Breathing can be stabilized naturally. This is what it means: "If one way is opened, then hundreds of ways will all be opened. When the big gate is opened, then hundreds of gates are all opened."

腦為上田，元神所居之宮，人能握元神，棲于本宮，則金氣自升，真息自定，所謂一竅開而百竅齊開，大關通則百關盡通也。

The brain is considered to be the Upper Dāntián (Shàngdāntián, 上丹田), the residence of the Shén. The Shén resides at the Upper Dāntián since our birth and is thus called "Original Shén" (Yuánshén, 元神). The document, Detailed Outline of Galenical (Běncǎo Gāngmù, 本草綱目) said: "Brain is the residence of the Original Shén."[55] If you are able to condense your Shén and make it stay at its residence, then the Qì in your body will be conserved. The way to keep the Shén at its residence is to keep your mind calm and peaceful, and avoid attraction of human affairs or temptations, and emotional disturbances. When this happens, the Qì storage at the Real Lower Dāntián (Zhēn Xiàdāntián, 真下丹田) will be abundant and can be led upward to nourish the brain and Shén. In addition, the breathing can be slender, soft, and steady. This will result in the opening of obstacles to Qì in the entire body. This is the way of reaching health and longevity.

3. Development of Cāntóngqì
《参同契發揮》

Following the Real Breathing's to-and-fro, allows the Real Qì to ascend and descend, from morning till evening, the Original Shén (Yuánshén) should always reside at the Níwán (Palace).

隨真息之往來，任真氣之升降，自朝至暮，元神常棲于泥丸也。

Real Breathing (Zhēnxí, 真息) means the profound level of "Embryonic Breathing" (Tāixí, 胎息). When you have reached the stage of "Real Breathing," the Qì can circulate smoothly through the entire body without the slightest stagnation. Then you are able to lead it up to nourish your Shén, and down to store it at the Real Lower Dāntián. However, it does not matter how the Qì is circulated and manifested, you must always keep your Shén at its residence so you will not be confused by laymen affairs.

4. Concealed Secret of Féng's Family
《馮氏錦囊》

There is a crux in the body which is named as "Xuánpìn." This place is how the life can be alive by receiving Qì. In fact, this place is the residence of Shén and where the Three Origins (Sānyuán) (Jīng, Qì, and Shén) are gathered. This is the cavity where the essence (Jīng), spirit (Shén), soul (Hún), and vigor (Pò) meet. It is the root where the Golden Elixir (Jīndān) (i.e., Qì) returns and the place where the immortals conceive their Holy Embryo.

身中一竅，名曰玄牝，受氣以生，實為府神，三元所聚，精神魂魄會于此穴，乃金丹還返之根，神仙凝結聖胎之地也。

This document explains the "Spiritual Valley" (Shéngǔ, 神谷) or "Mud Pill Palace" (Níwángōng, 泥丸宮). The Shén resides at this place. When the Shén is gathered and the physical body is nourished by Qì, then there is a physical life. Once this Shén departs from the physical body, then there is death. To nourish this Shén, you must gather the "Three Origins" (Sānyuán, 三元) namely "Jīng" (精) (Essence), "Qì" (氣), and "Shén" (神) (Spirit) at this place. Then the Shén can be raised up to a high level.

"Xuánpìn" (玄牝) has already been explained earlier. "Pò" (魄) is the vital spirit that is supported by vital energy (Qì) when a person is alive. When a person dies, the "Pò" becomes "Hún" (魂) (Soul) meaning the spirit after death. "Jīndān" (金丹) means "Golden Elixir" and implies precious Qì. When the precious Qì is led upward to nourish the Shén, you are able to attain immortality. In Daoist society, there is a song which says: "There is a Shén in every human body. There is a supernatural divine light (Língguāng, 靈光) (which can be developed) in this Shén. This supernatural divine light alone can shine into thousands of valleys. Its Dào of variations is unlimited, and spreads to millions of directions (i.e., ways)."[56] This means once you are able to cultivate your Shén to an enlightened level, this Shén is able to reach everywhere in the universe.

5. Songs of Valley Spirit[3]
谷神歌
(呂祖志・唐・呂岩撰)

Songs of Valley Spirit—1
谷神歌 - 一

I have an interior insubstantial empty valley. When talking about it, it seems it is there, again it seems it is not there. When talking about it, even if it is not there, however, (we) cannot ignore it. When talking about it, even if it is there, however, it cannot be resided in (i.e., occupied physically).
Valley, valley, it is so marvellous. Shén, Shén, it is the real Great Dào. Keep it, protect it, (you) can be on the list of those without death (i.e., longevity). Cultivate and refine it, (you) can be called "an immortal divine" (Xiānrén).

我有一腹空谷虛，言之道有又還無，言之無兮不可舍，言之有兮不可居。
谷兮谷兮太玄妙，神兮神兮真大道，保之守之不死名，修之煉之仙人號。

This song talks about the importance of the "Spiritual Valley" (Shéngǔ, 神谷) and how crucial it is for the cultivation of the "Valley Spirit" (Gǔshén, 谷神) if you wish to reach enlightenment and immortality. This Spiritual Valley is between the two lobes of the brain (Níwángōng, 泥丸宮) that cannot be seen but felt. In this valley the Valley Spirit resides. To reach the Dào of enlightenment, you must feel the existence of the Spiritual Valley and first learn how to keep the Shén there firmly, and then to cultivate it. This is the way to reach immortality. "Xiānrén" (仙人) means "those persons who have reached spiritual immortality (i.e., enlightenment).

Songs of Valley Spirit—2
谷神歌 - 二

When the (Valley) Spirit obtains its singularity (Yī, i.e., simplicity), the Líng (i.e., ingenuity) can be developed. When the (Spiritual) Valley obtains its singularity (i.e., center), the fullness can be achieved. If a person is able to keep this singularity, then from this alone (he) will be able to achieve (his) longevity.
It is not too far (i.e., difficult) to obtain longevity originally. However, it cannot be achieved if (the training) neglects (the training of the physical) body. If trained and the accomplishment is achieved, then the ordinary bones (i.e., normal human physical body) can be changed (into immortality) naturally.

神得一以靈，谷得一以盈，若人能守一，只此自長生。
長生本不遠，離身還不見，煉之功若成，自然凡骨變。

"Yī" (一) here means "one," "singleness," "singularity" or "simplicity." If the Shén is able to condense into a singleness at its residence without dispersion, then the spiritual vibration energy will be strong and powerful. Consequently, you are able to reach "Líng" (靈), which means "ingenuity," "intelligence," "dexterity," and "cleverness." This implies the capability of comprehension, which is the key to enlightenment.

When the Spiritual Valley obtains this concentrated Shén, the coherent resonant energy will be full and strong, and the Qì governed by the Shén will be efficient and effective. This is the key to longevity.

However, in order to obtain your longevity, you must also pay heed to your physical health, and not just mental and spiritual cultivation. The key to longevity is both physical and mental. Only if these two are able to balance each other with a strong foundation, can you then have a long, healthy life. At this point, you should know that Daoists usually pay attention to both physical and mental cultivation. This dual cultivation is called "Xìngmìng Shuāngxiū" (性命雙修) and means "the dual cultivation of temperament and physical life."

Songs of Valley Spirit—3
谷神歌 - 三

If Valley Spirit does not die, (then you have gained) the gate (i.e., crucial key) to Xuánpìn. Exit and enter softly as the Dào is existing within. When (you) cultivate (your Shén) to return it to the insubstantial nihility at midnight, you must know how to use the river transportation to carry (the Qì) to Kūnlún.

> *The dragon is singing and the tiger is also shouting, the wind and the clouds meet together and the old yellow lady is screaming. The fair lady in the fire is shy and charming. Look inward to see the cute baby in the water.*
>
> 谷神不死玄牝門，出入綿綿道若存，修煉還虛夜半子，河車搬載上崑崙。
> 龍又吟、虎又嘯，風雲際會黃婆叫，火中奼女正含嬌，回觀水底嬰兒俏。

As mentioned earlier, "Xuán" (玄) means "Original" (Yuán, 元), and "Pìn" (牝) means mother. Therefore, "Yuánpìn" (玄牝) means the "origin or root of lives" and implies "the key of longevity." In order to keep the Shén at its residence, you must follow the Dào, softly and gently. It will take a great deal of time to learn to keep the Shén at its residence. You must cut off all attractions and emotional disturbances from the outside world. Do this gradually and gently. If you try to force it to happen, the emotional mind will be even more disturbed and the result will be reversed. To lead the Qì upward through the Thrusting Vessel (Chōngmài, 衝脈) (Spinal Cord) to nourish the brain, you must train this at midnight, because the Qì is the strongest in the central energy system at that time.

"Dragon" (Lóng, 龍) and "Tiger" (Hǔ, 虎) mean the Yīn and Yáng Qìs in the body. "Old Yellow Lady" (Huángpó, 黃婆) means the "matchmaker" who brings the Yīn (female) and Yáng (male) together. Through interaction of Yīn and Yáng, the spiritual baby embryo will be conceived. Huángpó can be the mind (Shén) and/or the breathing, which is able to bring the Yīn and Yáng together.

> *The baby (Yīngér) and the shy lady (Chànǚ) meet old yellow lady (Huángpó), the son and the mother meet each other with the same Yì (i.e., mind). In the Golden Palace (Jīndiàn) and Jade Hall (Yùtáng), there are twelve doors. Golden Male (Jīngōng) and Wood Female (Mùmǔ) are just coming.*
> *After passing layers of the important key doors, immediately lock the gate. Inspect cows in the Big Dipper (Dǒuniú) and immediately start the fire. Advance the fire to eliminate Yīn to initiate the sole Yáng. Thousand years of peach has just started to bear fruits.*
>
> 嬰兒奼女見黃婆，兒女相逢兩意合，金殿玉堂門十二，金公木母正來過。
> 重門過后牢關鎖，點撿斗牛先下火，進火消陰始一陽，千歲仙桃初結果。

The baby (Shén) and the shy lady (Qì) are now brought together by the "old yellow lady" (Huángpó, 黃婆) (mind or breathing) and harmonize with each other. Then they are led upward from the Huángtíng (黃庭) to the brain (Upper Dāntián) passing through twelve doors (throat area). The Original Essence and the Shén have therefore been unified. "Yīngér" (嬰兒) means "baby" (son) and implies "the Spiritual Embryo." "Chànǚ" (奼女) (the shy lady, mother) implies "Qì." Therefore, it means the Xīn has been calmed and unified with the Shén at Huángtíng (黃庭). The baby embryo is then conceived. This spiritual embryo is then led upward to the Upper Dāntián.

"Jīndiàn" (金殿) is also called "Jīnshì" (金室). This means "Golden Palace" and implies "lungs." "Yùtáng" (玉堂) means "jade hall" and implies "the palate of the mouth." Twelve doors means the throat area. "Jīngōng" (金公) means "Golden Male" which implies "Original Essence" (Yuánjīng, 元精) and "Mùmǔ" (木母) means "Wood Mother" and implies "liver" (Shén). Liver (Shén) belongs to wood in the Five Elements (Wǔxíng, 五行), which is able to produce the fire which relates to the heart (Xīn, 心). When the Shén and the Xīn are harmonious and unified with each other, the mind can be calmed and the spirit condensed.

After passing through the twelve doors (throat) to the Upper Dāntián, then immediately keep the Spiritual Embryo there. "Dǒuniú" (斗牛) means "Big Dipper", which implies the process of condensing the Shén at the Upper Dāntián. After practicing for a long time, the spiritual embryo can be born. This is the key to longevity (Figure 3-7).

> *The golden bird (Jīnniǎo) flies on the east coast of curved river (Qūjiāng). The jade rabbit (Yùtù) shines with clear light on the west coast. The bird and the rabbit walk to the tip of the mountain. The fair lady in the furnace takes off her blue cloth.*
> *After taking off the blue cloth, the pure clean body is exposed. The baby is then led to the layers of curtain. After ten months of strong and heavy emotion, a boy is born. Say he can live long and will not die.*
> *(I) advise you to practice and to cultivate. If the Valley Spirit does not die, the goal (of immortality) can be achieved. (You) must comprehend (the theory) and carefully adopt those marvellous details. One day, (I) will reach the immortal land (Yíngzhōu) with you.*
>
> 曲江東岸金烏飛，西岸清光玉兔輝，烏兔走歸峰頂上，爐中奼女脫青衣。
> 脫卻青衣露素體，嬰兒引入重幃里，十月情濃產一男，說道長生永不死。
> 勸君煉，勸君修，谷神不死此中求，此中悟取玄微處，與君白日登瀛洲。

"Qūjiāng" (曲江) means "Curved Rivers" and implies "intestines" (Real Lower Dāntián). "Jīnniǎo" (金烏) means "Golden Bird" and implies "Original Spirit" (Yuánshén, 元神). "Yùtù" (玉兔) means "Jade Rabbit" and implies "Original Essence" (Yuánjīng, 元精). Therefore, the first sentence means that the "Original Spirit" and "Original Essence" are unified and both are led upward to the Upper Dāntián. Furnace here means "Upper Dāntián." The lady taking off her blue clothes means to get ready

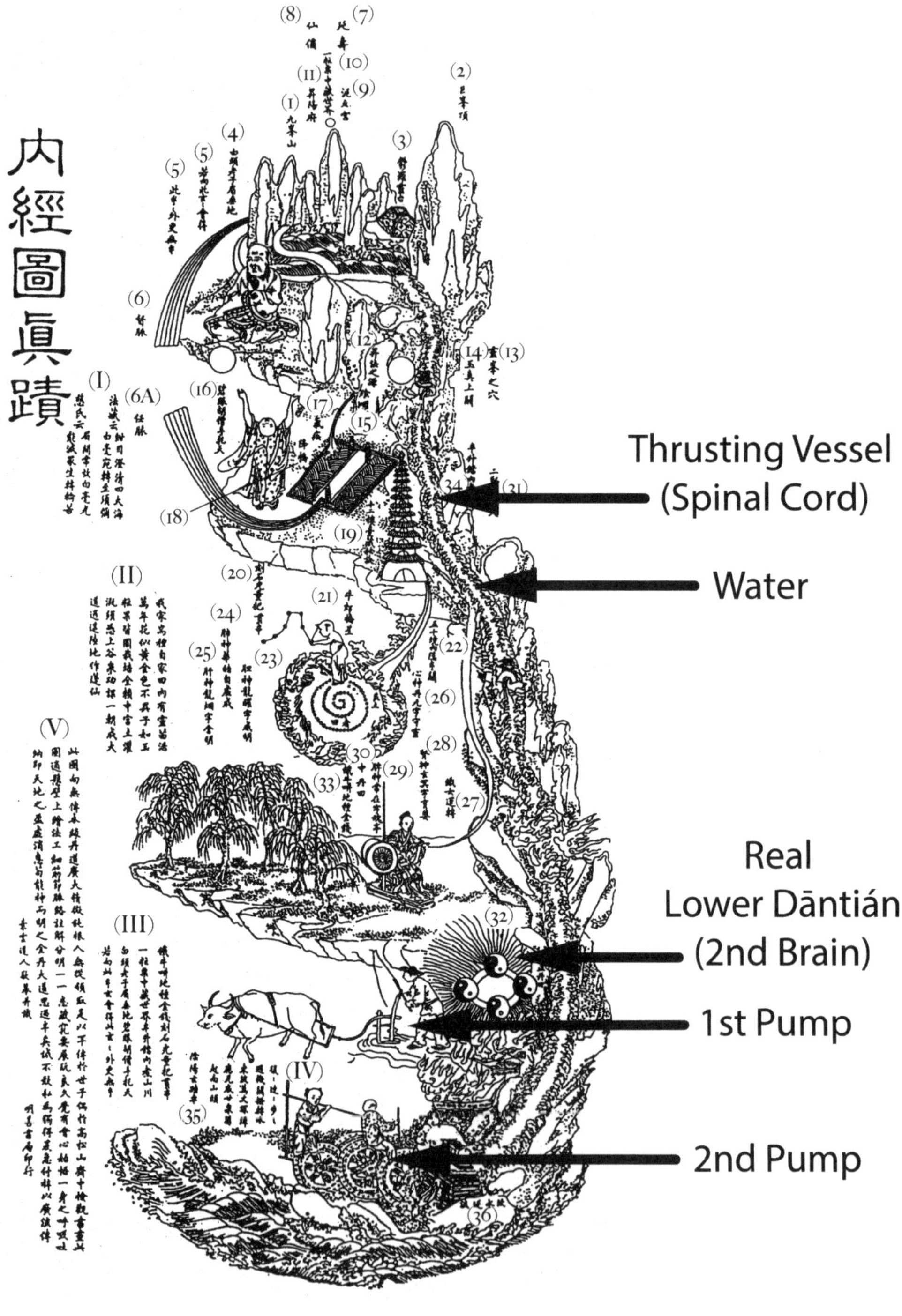

Figure 3-7. Táng Dynasty Inner Energy Illustration

to give birth to the baby. Blue clothes implies the manifestation of the Shén, which is related to the liver. The liver belongs to the color between blue and green in Chinese medicine. That means when the Shén is manifested and implies the birth of the spiritual baby.

The spiritual baby is born after ten months of pregnancy, and kept behind the curtain for nursing. This baby is the beginning of eternal spiritual life. "Yíngzhōu" (瀛洲) is the holy mountain in the east sea where the immortals dwell (in Chinese legend).

6. Thesis of Valley Spirit's Immortality[3]
谷神不死論
(紫清指玄集・宋・白玉蟾撰)

What is the valley? It means the Heaven Valley (Tiāngǔ). What is the Shén? It means the Original Spirit of the entire body. The valley of heaven contains (the capability) of creation and variations, (though) it holds the insubstantial nihility. The valley of the earth contains millions of objects, and holds the mountains and rivers. Humans have the same natural disposition as the heaven and the earth, (therefore we) also have a valley. There is a real singularity conceived in this valley where the Original Spirit (Yuánshén) resides. Thus, there are nine palaces in the head which correspond with the nine heavens above (us). Among them, there is a palace at the center called "Níwán" (i.e., Mud Pill), also called "Huángtíng" (i.e., Yellow Yard), again named "Kūnlún," and additional name 'Tiāngǔ' (i.e., Heaven Valley). The names are numerous. It is the palace where the Original Spirit resides. It is empty as a valley and the Shén is living within. Therefore, (the Shén) is called "Gǔshén" (i.e., Spiritual Valley).

谷者，天谷也。神者，一身之元神也。天之谷，含造化，容虛空；地之谷，容萬物，載山川。人與天地同所稟也，亦有谷焉。其谷藏真一，宅元神，是以頭有九宮，上應九天，中間一宮，謂之泥丸，亦曰黃庭，又名崑崙，又名天谷，其名頗多，乃元神所住之宮，其空如谷，而神居之，故謂之谷神。

The space between the two hemispheres of the brain is called "Heaven Valley" (Tiāngǔ, 天谷). This is because in a human body, the head is considered the heaven while the perineum (Huìyīn, 會陰) is considered the "sea bottom" (Hǎidǐ, 海底). This Heaven Valley has many other names, such as "Spiritual Valley" (Shéngǔ, 神谷), "Yellow Yard" (Huángtíng, 黃庭), "Mud Pill" (Níwán, 泥丸), or "Kūnlún" (崑崙).

It is named "Spiritual Valley" since the Shén resides in this valley. It is named "Yellow Yard" since it is an important place for cultivation. There is another place also called "Yellow Yard" located at the stomach area where the Spiritual Embryo is conceived. It is named "Mud Pill" due to the appearance of the pineal and pituitary glands. It is called "Kūnlún" because Kūnlún is one of the highest mountains in China, close to the sky.

Though the Spiritual Valley is empty and does not contain material objects like the valleys on the earth that contain rivers, trees, and many other objects, the Spiritual Valley has the capability and potential of creation and variation. Daoists believe that there are nine layers of heaven and this means there are nine layers of spiritual cultivation. There is a palace in each layer. The brain also contains nine palaces which correspond with the nine palaces of the heaven. However, among these nine palaces, the center one is the most important. This center is where the Original Spirit (Yuánshén, 元神) resides. Therefore, this central palace is called "Níwángōng" (泥丸宮) and means "Mud Pill Palace." From the scientific point of view, when you concentrate your mind at this place, the function of the pineal and pituitary glands will be activated due to the presence of abundant Qì. This will result in the long-term production of melatonin and growth hormone. These two hormones are the crucial keys to longevity and vitality.

> *When the Shén exists, then live; when the Shén is gone, then die. If (we) connect with the objects (i.e., human affairs) during the daytime and attached by the dreams during the night time, the Shén will not be able to reside at its residence peacefully. Yellow maizes are not yet ripe, the dream is not yet awakened, entire life's glory, splendor, wealth, and rank; hundred years of sorrow, worry, happiness, and joy, isn't it happening just like in a dream? Once (we are) dead, (the life) cannot reverse, (the Shén) roams around and can not return, then life and death are apart, the path between life and death is cut off. From this, (we) can see that if the Shén does not live, a person will not live by himself and if the Shén is dead, a person will also be dead naturally. If the Shén resides at its valley and does not die, how can a person also die? However, the reason that the Valley Spirit (Gǔshén) does not die is because of the Xuánpìn.*
>
> 神存則生，神去則死。日則接于物，夜則接于夢，神不能安其居也。黃粱未熟，南柯未寤，一生之榮辱富貴，百歲之悲憂悅樂，備嘗于一夢之間，使其去而不還，游而不返，則生死路隔，幽明之途絕矣。由是觀之，人不能自生而神生之，人不能自死而神死之。若神居其谷而不死，人安得而死乎？然谷神所以不死者，由玄牝也。

If your mind is always attracted by human affairs and emotions, then your Shén will not be able to stay at its residence. A human life is very short, like a dream. If you waste your time in longing for glory, power, and wealth, and forget how to cultivate your Shén and keep it steady at its residence, you will wake one day and realize that everything you have been longing for is only a dream. In order to have immortality for your Shén, you must keep the Valley Spirit at the Spiritual Valley. This is why Lǎozi said: "The Valley Spirit (Gǔshén) does not die, then it is called 'Xuánpìn' (玄牝). The door (i.e., key) of reaching this 'Xuánpìn' is the root of heaven and earth (i.e., nature). It is very soft and continuous as if it were existing. When it is used, it will not be exhausted."

What is Xuán? It is Yáng and is the heaven. What is Pìn? It is Yīn and is the earth. However, Xuán and Pìn two Qìs all have profound implications. Without meeting those holy men to instruct (you) in the oral secrets, it cannot easily be understood. Inner Classic of Yellow Emperor said: "The Original Shén resides at the Heaven Valley. If (you) protect it, then it (i.e., the cultivation) can be real (i.e., truthful) naturally." This saying implies that there is a heaven valley called "Níwán" in the top section of the body which is the residence of concealed Shén. There is a corresponding valley named "Jiànggōng" (i.e., heart) in the middle section of the body which is the residence of concealed Qì. There is a divine valley called "Guānyuán" (i.e., Key Origin) at the lower section of the body which is the residence of concealed essence.

玄者，陽也，天也；牝者，陰也，地也。然則玄牝二氣，各有深旨，非遇聖人，授以口訣，不可得而知也。《黃帝內經》云：'天谷元神，守之自真。'言人身中上有天谷泥丸，藏神之府也；中有應谷絳宮，藏氣之府也；下有靈谷關元，藏精之府也。

"Xuánpìn" (玄牝) here means the interaction of Yīn and Yáng. When Yīn and Yáng interact with each other, then life will be initiated. Therefore, "Xuánpìn" is the mother of life (i.e., creation and variations). However, it is not easy to understand and learn how to cultivate the Yīn and Yáng Qìs, and allow them to interact with each other. Usually, you will need an experienced teacher to direct you to the correct path personally.

This document mentions that there are three valleys in a human body that you must cultivate. The one in the head is called "Spiritual Valley" (Shéngǔ, 神谷) (Upper Dāntián) where the Valley Spirit resides. There is another one located at the chest area called "Jiànggōng" (絳宮) (Middle Dāntián) that provides you with Post-Birth Qì converted from food and air. There is the third valley called "Guānyuán" (關元) (Lower Dāntián) where the Pre-Birth Qì (Original Qì) is converted from Original Essence (Yuánjīng, 元精). Therefore, this valley conceals the essence of life.

The Heaven Valley is a mysterious palace, is the residence of the Original Shén, is the retention of human natural spiritual disposition, and is the important way of spiritual cultivation. Those holy men follow the important rules of the heaven and the earth, know the origin of variations, protect the Shén and keep it at this mysterious palace, and make the Qì abundantly stored at the residence of Pìn. Shén and Qì mutually interact and this will enable (you) to accomplish the cultivation of the real (Dào) naturally, unified with the Dào, and enter the domain of without death and without life. Therefore, it is said that when the Spiritual Valley does not die, it is called "Xuánpìn." Those holy men know how to apply their cultivation in Xuánpìn, know how to create and vary in a trice. When the Qì of Xuánpìn enters this root (i.e., residence or Real Lower Dāntián), if (you) seal (the breathing) too much, then urgent and if (you) allow it (i.e., breathing) to act freely, then it is out of control. Therefore, what (you) desire is to keep very soft and continuous without any gap or interruption.

天谷，玄宮也，乃元神之室，靈性之所存，是神之要也。聖人則天地之要，知變化之源，神守于玄宮，氣騰于牝府，神氣交感，自然成真，與道為一，而入于不死不生，故曰谷神不死，是謂玄牝也。聖人運用于玄牝之內，造化于恍惚之中，當其玄牝之氣，入乎其根，閉極則失于急，任之則失于蕩，欲其綿綿續續，勿令間斷耳。

"Spiritual Valley" (Shéngǔ, 神谷) is also called "Mud Pill Palace" (Níwángōng, 泥丸宮). The Original Shén (Yuánshén, 元神) residing in this palace is so powerful and marvellous and is the origin of creation and variations. This Shén is related to your mind and thinking, and is the Tàijí (太極) (Grand Ultimate) of the human's heaven and earth (universe or small heaven and earth).

Those persons who obtained the Dào in the past knew how to follow the human Tàijí and natural Tàijí and therefore were able to know the Dào of nature. They knew that the way to unify their Shén with the natural Shén is to keep the Shén at its residence and nourish it with Qì continuously. In this case, the Shén in the human Spiritual Valley and the natural Shén will resonate with each other. This is the way to maintain immortality of the Shén, and is thus called "Xuánpìn" (玄牝), the mother of creation and variations.

The way to keep the Shén at its residence is through correct breathing, being soft as a baby. In order to reach this goal, you must have a baby's heart (pure mind) without external attraction, which allows you to feel internally. Only then can you have soft breathing, as if it were there and as if it were not there (regulated without being regulated.) That is why Lǎozi said: "When concentrating the Qì (air) to reach its softness, can it be as (soft as) a baby?"

What is the meaning of "as if it were existing?" It means maintaining it by following the nature. After maintaining the Shén (at its residence) for a long time, it will be tranquil naturally. After practicing breathing for a long time, it will be stabilized naturally. When the natural disposition (i.e., temperament) has become natural, then it can be used marvelously. In this case, (you) don't have to try hard or force it urgently. Therefore, it is said: "When used, it cannot be exhausted." From this, it can be seen clearly that Xuán and Pìn are the two origins on the top and bottom (of cultivation) and are the correct paths of Qì mother's ascending and descending. Those world people (i.e., laymen) do not know this root and do not study their origin, and say the nose and the mouth are Xuán and Pìn. If the nose and the mouth are Xuán and Pìn, how can they be named the doorways of Xuánpìn? This is all because these people cannot comprehend their marvelousness of training. How can these (theories) be understood if they are not great holy men?

若存者，順其自然而存之，神久自寧，息久自定，性入自然，無為妙用，未嘗至于勤勞迫切，故曰用之不勤。即此而觀，則玄牝為上下二源，氣母升降之正道明矣。世人不窮其根，不究其源，便以鼻為玄，以口為牝。若以鼻口為玄牝，則玄牝之門又將何以名之？此皆不能造其妙，非大聖人安能究是理哉！

This last paragraph talks about Lǎozi's concept of spiritual cultivation. In *Dào Dé Jīng* (道德經), Chapter 6 it is said: "The Valley Spirit (Gǔshén, 谷神) does not die, then it is called 'Xuánpìn.' The key to reaching this 'Xuánpìn' (玄牝) is the root of heaven and earth (nature). It is very soft and continuous as if it were existing. When it is used, it will not be exhausted."[57]

First, this document discusses the meaning of "as if it were existing" (Ruòcún, 若存) it means that you must practice keeping the Shén at its residence (Upper Dāntián), and maintaining and conserving the Qì at the Real Lower Dāntián, until they becomes natural. That means you have reached the stage of "regulating without regulating" (Bùtiáo Értiáo, 不調而調).

Second, it explains that "Xuánpìn" (玄牝) is the interaction of the Shén from the top (Upper Dāntián) and the Qì from the bottom (Real Lower Dāntián), namely the unification and harmonization of the Shén and the Qì. When these two interact with each other, it is the mother of creation and variations, and immortality can then be achieved. Many laymen misunderstand that "Xuánpìn" means the nose and the mouth (breathing), but this is a mistake. Only those who can really comprehend the Dào of cultivation are able to grasp the marvellous trick of the training.

7. Secrets of Applying Qì with Concentrated Shén[3]
《用氣集神訣》
(延陵先生集新舊服氣經・唐・延陵先生集)

Shén is gathered (i.e., condensed) from insubstantial and peaceful (i.e., harmonized and stabilized) with substantial. Shén is wisdom of the Xīn (i.e., emotional mind). When (Xīn) is peaceful without desires, then the Shén can be like a king with harmonious and righteous Qì. Once (you) have reached this stage, then (you) may let it (i.e., Shén) be free without restraints, the longer the better. Keep practicing ceaselessly, so the Qì in the body will reach an extremely peaceful state. This means delight for heaven (nature). If (you are) full of delight for heaven, then live long. When outside the body (i.e., material world) is substantially empty, then it is also (delightful) for heaven. When inside the body is empty and comprehensive (i.e., no emotional bondage or desires), then it is also (delightful) for heaven. After practice for a long long time, then brightness can be derived (i.e., enlightened). All these secrets are understood from internal. After practicing for a long time, then they (i.e., understandings) can be wide and refined. This will match the brightness of the top (i.e., heaven or nature). If bright, then (the Qì) can be developed from essence (Jīng) internally. In such case, the Dào can be reached and this Dào will correspond with Dé (the deed or virtue of nature). The completeness of the Dé is when it is used, it is (the manifestation of) Rén (i.e., benevolence) and when it is divided (i.e., developed or expanded), it is the demonstration of Yì (i.e., righteousness).

神集于虛，而安于實。神，心中知者也。安而無欲，則神王而氣和正。如此之時，則一任所之，唯久彌善。行之不已，體氣至安，謂之樂天，樂天則壽。身外虛空亦天也，身內虛通亦天也，習之久久，乃明生焉。密自內知之，久習彌廣而精，上合于明，明則內發于精，如是乃至于道，道應于德。德之成矣，用而為仁，分而為義。

Shén is insubstantial and cannot be seen. However, the Shén can be felt and condensed into a high spiritual level. Though it is insubstantial, it must nevertheless be harmonized with the material world (i.e., laymen society). The Shén is related to the Wisdom Mind (Yì, 意) and emotional mind (Xīn, 心). However, the emotional mind makes you confused and excited while the Wisdom Mind directs you to focused thinking and decisions. Consequently, Shén can be raised and condensed. When this happens, the emotional mind will be under control and become peaceful and calm. This will result in the harmonization of the Shén and the Qì circulation. This is the stage of "unification of the Shén and the Qì" (Shénqì Xiànghé, 神氣相合). If you practice it often, you will reach a stage of regulating without regulating. In this case, health and longevity can be achieved. In addition, your mind will become neutral and bright, clear and wise, and reach far and wide. Internally, you are wise, and externally you are able to apply the Dào (道) of nature in your actions. This action of nature is called "Dé" (德). When the Dào and Dé are applied in human society, it becomes benevolence (Rén, 仁) and righteousness (Yì, 義).

Essence Qì exits from the head in the daytime and resides at the abdomen (i.e., Real Lower Dāntián) at night. Therefore, (we) should respect (i.e., pay attention to) the head and focus on the abdomen. The colors (i.e., materials) are settled (i.e., existing) externally while respecting the straight (i.e., righteousness) within (the body). Whenever there is an opportunity (i.e., advantage to be taken), there is not (even a slight) thought (of taking it). All in the mind is goodness. This is (the way of using) the Shén and Qì to engage the quality and to harmonize myself into a single body. This is called "Great Smoothness" (Dàshùn). (Consequently) heaven will protect (you) and (you will be) auspicious and without any disadvantage. This is because all the marvellous (demonstrations of nature) have their roots. The Shén's insubstantial nihility, though it stays in (our) Xīn, can connect with its (i.e., natural) system. The Qì firmly concealed in the intestines (Real Lower Dāntián) should be warmly nourished with patience. When (you) live daily, (you) should always close (your) eyes and observe the origin of the Qì internally. Whenever there is an event which causes the Ling's (spiritual mind's) disturbance, then close (your) eyes gladly and observe the Xīn internally. Reject it as if (you are) saying: "My body's Shén and Qì are concealed and developed from my shape, which thus makes me able to reach the Dào." In this case, heaven will endow (you) with auspiciousness. This is because the heaven is the Líng of the insubstantial Qì. If we are able to use it (correctly), then the Dào can be reached to its extremity.

精氣晝出于首，夜栖于腹，當自尊其首，重其腹。色庄于外，敬直于中，應機無想，唯善是與，此神氣事質，合吾一體，謂之大順，天保祐之，吉無不利。凡妙本有所，神在心中之虛，上通其系，氣藴腸中之實，恆宜溫養之。平居常宜閉目內視氣源，每行一事利于生靈，則欣然閉目，內視其心，謝之若曰：‘吾身之神氣，明發于吾形，使吾達道也。’如是則天降之吉。故天者，虛氣之靈，吾能用之，道極于斯矣。

There are Two Poles in your body, one in the head (Upper Dāntián) and the other in the intestines (Real Lower Dāntián). The Real Lower Dāntián is considered to be a 'bio-battery', which provides you with the quantity of Qì (bioelectricity), while Shén resides in the Upper Dāntián, and controls the quality of the Qì manifestation. In the daytime, due to the usage of the brain, the body's Qì is led upward to maintain the brain's function, and when night comes, the Qì returns to its residence (Real Lower Dāntián) for charging. When you cultivate immortality, you must cultivate both the Shén at the top (quality) and the Qì in the Real Lower Dāntián (quantity).

There are many abstractions outside of your body which can cause you emotional disturbance and increase your desires. Whatever thoughts are in your mind and whatever action you are taking, you must be in the goodness of the Dào (道) and Dé (德). If you can do so, you will feel righteous and bright internally. From this righteous feeling, your spirit will naturally be in the state of peace and harmony. This is the way of matching nature, and nature will protect you.

8. Historical Record; Autobiography of Tàishǐgōng 《史記・太史公自序》

How can a person be alive? It is because of (the existence of) the Shén. How can this (Shén) be relied on (depended on for its existence), it is because of the shape (physical body). When the Shén is greatly used, then exhausted. When the shape is greatly labored, then worn out. When the shape and Shén are separated, then die. Those who are dead cannot be revived and those who are separated cannot be returned (reunited). Therefore, those holy men (i.e., persons who have reached the Dào) take it (i.e., spiritual cultivation) very seriously. From this, it can be seen that the Shén is the root of the life while the shape is the tool (i.e., vehicle) of the life.

凡人所生者，神也；所托者，形也。神大用則竭，形大勞則敝，形神離則死，死者不可復生，離者不可復反，故聖人重之。由是觀之，神者，生之本也，形者，生之具也。

According to the Buddhist concept, the spiritual body is the main part of a human, while the physical body is only a vehicle which is used temporarily by the Shén for its cultivation. Therefore, to reach Buddhahood, you must pay more attention to the cultivation of the spiritual body. However, to Daoists, the cultivation of the spiritual body and the healthy condition of the physical body are equally important. This is because it will take many years to cultivate the Shén to reach its enlightenment, and if the physical body is weak and unhealthy, then you will not have a long physical life for spiritual cultivation.

To Buddhist spiritual cultivators, the material world does not exist and there is nothing to be cultivated or considered. In the Buddhist document Altar Classic of Sixth Ancestor (Liùzǔ Tánjīng, c), it is said: "There is no tree in Bodhi originally, and there is also no stand for the shining mirror. If there is nothing at all originally, how can it be dusted?"[58] "Bodhi" means an illuminated or enlightened mind. It is said that Buddha was enlightened under the Bodhi tree. Shining mirror means a pure and clean Shén. When you cultivate your Shén, all the material world disappears. Thus, there is no tree or any mirror stand. If there is no material concept in your mind, how can your mind have the human emotions and desires dusted off.

However, to a Daoist, the material world is as important as the spiritual world, and we must maintain our physical health. In the Daoist document, The Thesis of Nourishing Life (Yǎngshēnglùn, 養生論), it is said: "Uttering and receiving (Tǔnà) (the Qì) through breathing, absorbing the food to nourish the physical body, thus allow the shape (i.e., physical body) and Shén to be mutually harmonized. This means the mutual coordination of external and internal."[59] "Tǔnà" (吐納) which literally means "uttering and receiving," is an ancient Qìgōng term. It means the cultivation of Qì through breathing.

9. The Secrets of Spiritual Applications of All Veracious Holy Embryo

(Guōzhēnrén's Secrets of Embryonic Breathing)[2,3,4]

《諸真聖胎神用訣》

（郭真人胎息訣）

What does the "training" mean? It means to cultivate, to nourish, and to empty. The ears do not hear, the eyes do not see, the nose does not smell, the tongue does not taste, and cease (i.e., to calm) the breathing and stabilize the Xīn (i.e., emotional mind). This method is (to achieve the stage of) "having" from "not having," "nothing" from "something," "color" from "colorless," "empty" from "existing;" consequently, there is "no having" but "having," "something" but "nothing," "colorless" but with "color," "not empty" but "empty." This is the real method of nourishing the Qì and regulating the Shén in Real Embryonic Breathing. It is also said: "When see, I cannot see myself (i.e., forget self), when hear, I cannot hear; separated from various boundaries (i.e., attachments). This is named 'marvellous Dào,' and is the uppermost method."

夫煉者，修也、養也、虛也。耳不聽也，眼不見也，鼻不聞也，舌不味也，息氣定心也。此法從不有中有，不無中無，不色中色，不空中空，非有為有，非無為無，非色為色，非空為空，此乃真胎息養氣調神之法。又云：'視不見我，聽不得聞，離種種邊，名為妙道，此法最為上也。'

"Cultivate" (Xiū, 修) is to cultivate the human temperament so the Shén is able to grow. "Nourish" (Yǎng, 養) means to build up an abundant Qì which can then be used to nourish the physical body and spiritual body. "Empty" (Xū, 虛) implies the emptiness of the human emotions and desires.

In order to reach these three goals, you must get rid of your mind's connection to the outside material and emotional world, and also avoid the temptation of desires from your organs of sense. Therefore, there is no difference between with or without color, whether material exists or not, or whether there is an attempt or not. In all, there is no discrimination of Yīn or Yáng, and this means the state of Wújí (無極) (No Extremity). If you are able to reach this Wújí state, your Embryonic Breathing will be profound.

10. The Secrets of Spiritual Applications of All Veracious Holy Embryo

(Xú Shén Gōng's Secrets of Embryonic Breathing)[2,3,4]

《諸真聖胎神用訣》
（徐神公胎息訣）

What is the Shén? It is the application of insubstantial nihility (Xūwú). What is breathing? It is the application of the Original Qì (Yuánqì). (You should) train to get rid of the bondage of laymen world and become an exceptional person. It does not matter if I gain or lose the treasures or colors (i.e., sensuality), dislike or favor, all being treated the same (i.e., neutral emotional feeling). (In this case, nature) will protect (you) naturally, and the Xīn of Dào (Dàoxīn) (i.e., the will to pursue the Dào) has been achieved. The classic said: "What is the Shén, is actually insubstantial nihility. Once it is used for essence (Jīng), Qì, and Shén, then it is Língtái (i.e., platform of ingenuity) (Upper Dāntián). Those who cultivate their temperament, if they are able to stabilize their breathing, from essence, Qì, and Shén, three things, truly they can obtain longevity, and become the divine renunciation of the world."

夫神者，虛無之用。息者，元氣之用。煉去塵世之境，若是非人，我財色取舍得失，冤親平等如一，自然祐護，道心成矣。經云：〝神者虛無，用之精氣神三者，便是靈台。修性之人，若是息定，精氣神三件可長生不死，必為出世之仙，則不虛矣。〞

To reach immortality, you must learn to cultivate your Shén and Qì. The Shén is insubstantial and cannot be seen, however when it is used, it is marvellous and powerful. To cultivate your Qì, you must know how to accomplish it through correct breathing. In order to cultivate your Shén, you must first stop thinking as a layman, and not be attracted by human emotions, desires, and material satisfaction. If you can see through this and keep your mind in a neutral state, then you are able to preserve and protect your Three Treasures (Sānbǎo, 三寶): essence (Jīng, 精), Qì (氣), and Shén (神). When these three treasures are led upward to meet at the Upper Dāntián, immortality can be achieved.

11. Anthology of Daoist Village
《道鄉集》

What does "to condense" mean? It means "to gather." What is Shén? It is the righteous thought in the Xīn (i.e., emotional mind). What is Xí (i.e., profound breathing)? It is (to induce) the Pre-Heaven Real Qì (i.e., Original Qì). There is no shape and no appearance. It (i.e., Pre-Heaven Qì) is generated at the time of extreme nihility and sincere calmness. Xuè (i.e., cavity, namely Real Lower Dāntián) is the original root of producing this Pre-Heaven Qì. Why (do we) condense (our) Shén at this Qì cavity? It is to place and condense our righteous thought at this Qì cavity and not allow the Shén to be distracted and move away (from the body). When the Shén is condensed, then the fire (i.e., Qì) can be gathered. When the fire is gathered and led downward, the water will rise automatically. This is the important key to fire and water's mutual coordination. It is also the marvellous crucial way to condense the Shén at the Qì cavity. What is Xí? It is breathing. What is Xí-Xí (i.e., Continuous Breathing)? It implies that (the breathing) is very soft and unbroken. What is Guī (i.e., Returning)? It means to reverse the path (of life) and return it (to its origin). What is Gēn (i.e., Root)? It is the root and foundation (of life). Every breath is soft and continuous and returns to this root. This means that the breathing does not separate from the basic foundation of producing the Qì. It is as if it were existing and as if it had been forgotten, and it seems to be there while not being there. This is what it was about "Embryonic Breathing" (practiced) in ancient times. (You) must understand that this breathing follows the natural (way). If the Shén can be condensed at the Qì cavity, then the breathing will also be stabilized at this original root.

夫凝者聚也，神者心中之正念也。息者，先天之真氣也。無形無象，生于虛極靜篤之時，穴即生先天氣之本根。所以凝神氣穴者，即將我心中之正念，凝聚于氣穴，不令神往外馳。神凝則火聚，火聚于下，水自上升，此水火調濟之要訣。亦凝神氣穴之妙諦也。息者，呼吸也。息息者，綿綿不斷之義也。歸者，返回也。根者，基本也。息息歸根，即呼吸不離生氣根本。若存若忘，似有似無，昔所謂胎息者是也。須知此息，本乎自然，神既凝于氣穴，息也定于本根。

This article talks about the mutual unification, coordination, and harmonization of the Shén and the Pre-Heaven Qì (Xiāntiānqì, 先天氣) (Original Qì) at the Real Lower Dāntián. Shén is considered fire (Yáng) while the Pre-Heaven Qì is considered water (Yīn). If you are able to lead your Shén down and unify it with Pre-Heaven Qì, then the mind can be calm and peaceful within your body. Then the Qì can stay at its residence and be stored.

The way to reach this goal is through soft, slender, and continuous breathing, while focusing your Shén at the Real Lower Dāntián. This is the crucial key to Embryonic Breathing, and is also the root of life. From this breathing, the Spiritual Embryo can be conceived.

12. Marvellous Applications of Maintaining the Shape and Cultivating Internal Truth by Great Teacher Dámó 《達磨大師住世留形內真妙用訣》

If (you) don't know how to keep the son and mother (i.e., Shén and Qì) together, then even though the Qì can be stored internally through (the practice of) breathing, nevertheless the Shén is constantly labored (i.e., acting) externally, and can become dirty and confused. Once the Shén is not clean, then the original harmonious Qì will be dispersed gradually and cannot stay (with the Shén). Many Daoists often make this mistake and do not know that the shape and the Shén are main core of practice. If a person does not know how to keep them (i.e., Shén and Qì) internally but keeping them externally, naturally, the residences (of Qì and Shén) will be dangerous and gradually rotten. Furthermore, those non-Daoists (always) labor (their) Shén and fatigue (their) thinking, there is not even a single breath which allows (them) to lead the Qì and Shén to the Qìhǎi (i.e., Real Lower Dāntián). If (they) expect to have longevity, isn't it too far to be reached?

若不知子母相守，氣雖呼吸于內，神常勞役于外，遂使神常穢濁而神不清。神既不清，即元和之氣漸散而不能相守也。道人常用之，而不知根本以形神為主。若人不知守于內而守于外，自然令宅舍虛危，漸見衰壞矣。況非道之人，勞神役思，無一息神氣注于氣海之中，而欲望其長生，豈不遠乎！

The son and the mother imply the Shén and the Qì, which must act like son and mother and never separate from each other. This is called "Shénqì Xiànghé" (神氣相合) and means "the unification or the harmonization of the Shén and Qì." In order to reach this goal, you must first stop the mind's attractions and emotional disturbances from the outside world. Once your mind is attached to them, your Shén will become dirty. Through correct Embryonic Breathing, while you keep your Shén and Qì at the Real Lower Dāntián, you are able to reach the goal of longevity.

13. Chapter of Clear Understanding

(Máo, Rì-Xīn; Sòng Dynasty)

《宋・毛日新；了明篇》

Qì follows Shén and Shén follows Qì, Shén and Qì mutually follow each other and penetrate into Níwán (i.e., Mud Pill). Keep Jīnguān (i.e., Golden Gate) locked and sealed constantly, once (you) have caught the Jīnpǐn (i.e., Golden Product), then (you will increase your) joy internally. Practice diligently and establish (your) strong will. Do not give up this Gōngfū in twelve timings (i.e., twenty-four hours). When the Yīn ends and the Yáng has completed, the Shén will be able to exit from the body. When this Gōng has been accomplished, (your) name will be on the list of immortality.

氣隨神，神隨氣，神氣相隨，透入泥丸裡。長把金關牢鎖閉，捉得金品，暗地添歡喜。下辛勤，須發志，十二時中，莫把功夫棄。陰盡陽全神出體，功行成時，名列神仙位。

This poetry talks about the mutual dependency of the Shén and the Qì. Once the Shén and the Qì can be led upward to the Níwángōng (泥丸宮) (Upper Dāntián), then you should immediately keep it there firmly. "Jīnguān" (金關) means "Golden Gate," which implies "Upper Dāntián." "Jīnpǐn" (金品) means "Golden Material" and implies "Spiritual Embryo." "Shíèrshí" (十二時) means "twelve timings" which are the traditional Chinese divisions for one a day.

14. The Complete Book of Principal Contents of Human Life and Temperament

(Mr. Huànzhēn's Secret of Embryonic Breathing)[2]

《性命圭旨全書》

（幻真先生胎息訣）

It is said that human's Original Shén is hidden in the Qì cavity. It is just like millions of objects hidden in the Kūn earth. The Shén enters the earth just like the heaven's Qì descends and reaches down to the earth. When Qì and Shén are combined, it is as the Dào of the earth has been supported by the heaven.

謂人之元神，藏于氣穴，猶萬物藏于坤土。神入地中，猶天氣降而至予地。氣與神合，猶地道之承于天。

Original Shén (Yuánshén, 元神) means the Shén which came with you when you were born. This Shén is concealed at its residence (Upper Dāntián) originally. When this Shén descends into the Real Lower Dāntián (Qì cavity) (Qìxuè, 氣穴), it will be just like the heaven's Qì descending to the earth (Kūntǔ, 坤土). When this happens, the Shén and the Qì are unified and harmonized with each other. This is the key to life and longevity. "Kūn" (坤) represents the earth in the Eight Trigrams, that is why it is called "Kūntǔ" (坤土).

15. Ten Books of Cultivating Truth; Short Cut of Miscellaneous Writing
《修真十書・雜著捷徑》

Qì is nourished by Qì, and Qì then meets Shén. Shén and Qì are not separated, then it is the cultivation of truth (i.e., true cultivation). The son does not leave the mother and the mother will not let the son go. When the son and mother stay together, then live long without dying.

氣養于氣，氣會于神，神氣不散，是為修真。子不離母，母不放子，子母共守，長生不死。

In order to build up the Qì to an abundant level at the Real Lower Dāntián (Zhēn Xiàdāntián, 真下丹田), you must know where to find the extra Qì and how to store it in the Real Lower Dāntián. You must also know how to keep your Shén there. When the Shén and the Qì can be unified and harmonized with each other, the Spiritual Embryo (Shèngtāi, 聖胎) can be conceived. The Shén and the Qì are just like the son and the mother who will not part from each other. This is the way of reaching longevity.

3.7 Methods of Embryonic Breathing (Tāixífǎ, 胎息法)

1. Embryonic Breathing Inscription[2,3]
《胎息銘》

Thirty-six swallowings, each one must be treated as first priority (i.e., most important). When uttering (i.e., exhaling), it should be extremely slender and when receiving (i.e., inhaling), it should be very soft and continuous. It does not matter whether (you are) sitting, lying down, or standing, all should be done naturally. Abstain (yourself) from noise and disturbance, avoid eating meat or fish. Though it is given the name "Embryonic Breathing," it actually is the (training of) internal elixir. It is used not only for treating sickness, but also for longevity. After (you have) practiced for a long time, (your) name will be on the top list of immortality.

三十六咽，一咽為先。吐為細細，納為綿綿。坐臥亦爾，行立坦然。戒于喧雜，忌以腥羶。假名胎息，實為內丹。非只治病，決定延年。久久行之，名列上仙。

This document emphasizes the importance of swallowing saliva during Embryonic Breathing meditation. When you meditate, the tongue should touch the palate of the mouth to connect the Yīn Conception Vessel (Rènmài, 任脈) and the Yáng Governing Vessel (Dūmài, 督脈). Then saliva (heavenly water) will be generated. The head is considered the heaven (Tiānlínggài, 天靈蓋) while the groin area is considered to be the sea-bottom (Hǎidǐ, 海底). The saliva generated in the mouth is thus called "heavenly water" (Tiānchíshuǐ, 天池水).

Whenever the saliva is full in the mouth and starts to bother you, you should swallow it. First, you inhale and then swallow, and immediately follow with the exhalation while leading the swallowed saliva to the Real Lower Dāntián (Zhēn Xiàdāntián, 真下丹田). Naturally, your saliva will never reach the abdominal area. However, the mind leads the Qì down to return to the Real Lower Dāntián.

In order to generate saliva, your breathing must be soft, slender, and calm. Your body must also be in an extremely relaxed state. If your breathing is fast, the Qì will easily be manifested into external physical activity, which can prevent you from storing the Qì at the Real Lower Dāntián. You should meditate until you have accumulated thirty-six mouthfuls of saliva and swallowed them. If you are able to do so, you will be able to reach health and longevity. Naturally, when you practice Embryonic Breathing, you must select a quiet and peaceful place so your mind can enter a profound meditative state. This is the crucial key to Embryonic Breathing meditation.

2. Interpretation of Embryonic Breathing Inscription

(Eight Notes of Life Abidance)
(Gāo, Lián, Míng Dynasty)[3]

《胎息銘解》
《遵生八箋》
(明・高濂撰)

Gāozi said: "The secret of Embryonic Breathing mentioned earlier is the same as Lǐzhēnrén's sixteen-words-secret. However, this (practice) must be done after Zǐ (11 p.m.–1 a.m.) at the time of Chǒu (1–3 a.m.) or Yín (3–5 a.m.). This is because it is too cold at the Zǐ during winter. During summer time, Wǔ (11 a.m.–1 p.m.) is also too hot (for practice). Therefore, use Yín (3–5 a.m.) in winter time and Yǒu (5–7 p.m.) in summertime. These requirements are only for beginning. After practicing for a long time, whenever (you) sit down, it is the right Zǐ and Wǔ (timing). It is not necessary to restrict the set time (for practice any more). At the beginning (of practice, the hands are) held to firm (Wògù) (the mind), bend (your) legs and use the heels to press the root of the jade stem (i.e., penis) to firm the Qì of the essence. Sitting in this position with crossed legs, and hands in place, (use the mind) to transport the Qì. (You) must follow this exposition. One swallowing and one uttering (i.e., breath), all from the nose. The sound generated (from breathing) must be slender (i.e., weak) and not allowed to be heard by the ears. After thirty-six swallowings, extend the four limbs comfortably. Take in the clean air through the nose, and do not lead it down the throat. Simply raise up (your) head and lead (the Qì) to the entire body and four limbs. Lead (the Qì) followed by the gradual and slow extending motion of the arms and legs. Whenever the Qì in the abdominal area becomes stagnant, (you should) also not allow it to reach the throat and exit through the mouth. Again, raise the head up and lead the Qì to circulate through the entire body with the extension of the arms and legs. During the practice, if (you) suddenly feel the Qì circulating upward, (you) should also use the same way to lead. If (you) have extra time and leisure, then also practice Lízhēnrén's sixteen words of Táng Dynasty. In this case, (you) will not be hungry or thirsty. It seems as (you) have just taken a meal. (You) should not get tired and stop. After (you) have practiced for a long time, the achievement is hard to be described in words."

高子曰：〝前胎息訣與后李真人一十六字訣相同。但此條每于半夜子后，或丑、寅時候，冬月恐子時嚴寒，夏月恐午時太熱，故冬以寅時，夏以酉時。初起如此，習久坐下即是子午，何必固時。初起握固，以腳后跟曲轉，頂住玉莖柯根，使精氣固定，手趺足盤，以行其氣。務依此銘，一咽一吐，皆以鼻竅中出入，出聲宜細，不令有聲聞之于耳。三十六咽數畢，舒伸四肢，鼻引清氣，亦勿咽入喉中，只昂頭引向遍體四肢，以手足徐徐伸縮而導引之。凡腹中氣轉噦上，亦勿使之直放口中出，亦用昂頭徐徐舒伸手足導而引之，使氣遍轉四肢。凡行持間忽遇此氣轉動上達，皆如此以導之。餘則日得空閒，即以唐・李真人十六字行之。自然不飢不渴，如嘗飲食一般。不可厭倦間斷，久久行之，功不盡述。〞

Li, Zhen-Ren's sixteen words were translated and commented on earlier. These sixteen words are: "Once inhaling, immediately lift up (the perineum) to return the Qì to the navel (Lower Dāntián); once lifting, immediately swallow (to allow) the water and fire to meet." This is the method of swallowing saliva with the coordination of the perineum (Huìyīn, 會陰). Please refer to the earlier explanation of these sixteen words.

Concerning the timing of practicing Embryonic Breathing, many documents explain that the best time is midnight (Zǐ, 子) and also noon (Wǔ, 午). This is because the Qì is strongest in the Thrusting Vessel (Chōngmài, 衝脈) (Spinal Cord) at midnight and therefore, it is the most effective time to lead the Qì to the center and store it there. The reason for practicing at noontime is that your body is then in its most Yáng state, and you will not need too much Qì to maintain the strength of the Guardian Qì (Wèiqì, 衛氣) for your immune system. This is the best time to store the extra Qì at the Real Lower Dāntián.

However, according to this document, beginners should not use these two times, due to the body's state and the environment's Qì status, being extreme Yīn (midnight) and extreme Yáng (noon). It will be harder for beginners to adopt these times and effectively store the Qì at the Real Lower Dāntián. This document suggests that the best time for beginners should be Chǒu (1–3 a.m.) or Yín (3–5 a.m.) in wintertime and Yǒu (5–7 p.m.) in summertime. As a matter of fact, once you have grasped the key to practice, you may practice Embryonic Breathing at any time.

The posture of meditation is to hold the hands in front of the abdominal area and to firm the mind there. This exercise is called "Wògù" (握固) and means "to hold and firm." In *Dào Dé Jīng* (道德經), Chapter 55, it is said: "When the bones are weak and tendons are soft, (one) should Wògù."[60] When you hold your hands at the abdominal area, you are firming your mind at the abdominal area, consequently, the Qì will stay in its residence and be conserved. Only when the Qì can be firmly stored at the Real Lower Dāntián, can the physical body be developed and conditioned.

In Buddhist society, "Wògù" is also called "Shǒuyìn" (手印) which means "hands' stamp." Stamp here means to "press against." According to Buddhist documents, there are two functions of holding stamps: 1. To assist the mind to stay at the abdominal area which allows you to calm and meditate; 2. After the mind is able to stay at the abdominal area, it can be used to maintain the mind and Shén at the breathing. Consequently, the achievement of meditation can reach its highest level. This is the goal of Buddhahood.[61]

The methods of holding the hands are many. In the document, Thesis on the Origins and Symptoms of Various Diseases (Zhūbìng Yuánhòulùn, 諸病源候論), it says: "What is Wògù? Four fingers of both hands hold the thumb inside individually."[62] That means to use four fingers of each hand to hold the thumb at the center of the palm and keep them in front of the abdominal area. However, another document, Required Anthology of Reaching the Dao's Entrance (Dàomén Tōngjiào Bìyòngjí, 道門通教必用集) said: "Wògù is to use the thumb to press the middle joint of the middle finger. Four fingers are bending toward the palm center."[63] From this, you can see that there are many possible ways of holding the hands in front of the abdominal area. From my personal experience, the best way is to lay both hands comfortably and naturally over each other right in front of the abdominal area. As to which hand should be on the top and which should be on the bottom, it depends on your natural feeling. The most comfortable one is the correct one for you. If you force yourself to change to the other way, your mind and central feeling will be distorted and affected.

When you meditate, you should cross your legs and sit. However, if you experience numbness of the legs or an uncomfortable feeling, this will affect your meditative mind. Then you may meditate in any comfortable posture you like. You should understand that when you practice Embryonic Breathing, there is no problem with any kind of posture, since you are simply storing the Qì at its residence. However, if you practice using the mind to lead the Qì for circulation, such as Small Cyclic Heaven and Grand Cyclic Heaven meditation, then the specific posture becomes crucial. The wrong posture can cause serious problems or dangers.

This document also mentions that right after your meditation, you should extend your four limbs and stretch your torso. This is to prevent the Qì circulation from becoming stagnant due to the long sitting position. When you do this, extend your limbs while using your mind to lead the Qì to the limbs.

3. The Secrets of Spiritual Applications of All Veracious Holy Embryo (Lǐzhēnrén's Secrets of Embryonic Breathing)[2,3,4]

《諸真聖胎神用訣》
（李真人胎息訣）

Those who practice the real Qì from Embryonic Breathing should enter a quiet room, burn incense, face the wall, sit down with crossed legs facing east south, the Xīn (i.e., emotional mind) does not have any worry, the Yì (i.e., Wisdom Mind) does not have any thinking, keep the Shén clear and stabilize the breathing, always observe (i.e., pay attention to) the entire body, then (the Qì) will circulate smoothly and fluidly. Those learners (i.e., beginners) must not seal the breathing completely. If (you) seal the breathing entirely, then the Shén can be damaged (i.e., fatigued mentally). Just gauge the length of the breathing by yourself, allow the air to enter and exit (the nose), do not make the sound audible by your own ears. In this case, it will be marvellous. If (you) always regulate this breathing and have reached the stage of no exit and no entrance (of the air), then (the Shén) will be able to stay at the Real Lower Dāntián firmly. Staying means the 'Real Holy Embryo' (is conceived) and the cultivation of the Dào can surely be achieved.

夫胎息真氣者，入于一靜室，焚香面壁，東南結跏趺坐，心無掛念，意無所思，澄神定息，常于遍身觀之，自然通暢。諸學之人，不得全閉定氣，全閉則傷神。但量自家息之長短，放氣出入，不得自耳聞之，如此則妙也。若常常調息，不出不入，久而在于丹田固守，在之者，名為真胎也，道必成矣。

This document mentions a few things about practicing Embryonic Breathing. First, you must find a quiet room and avoid any disturbance from outside. Second, you should burn incense. Ancient Daoists had a common habit of burning incense when they meditated. They believed this would help them calm down their mind. In addition, burning incense was one of the ways of measuring the duration of meditation.

Third, when you meditate, you should face either east (daytime) or south (nighttime) so you are able to absorb the natural Qì offered by the sun and by the earth's magnetic field. Fourth, your Xīn and Yì must be calm and neutral. Nothing bothers you. Fifth, you should always pay attention to the body and feel the Qì status in the body.

If you are not able to feel any stagnation of the Qì, then you allow the Qì to be led and circulated smoothly and naturally.

When you store the Qì at the Real Lower Dāntián, you should learn to extend your breathing gradually and slowly. You should not hold your breath, as this will make you tense and will disturb your mind and Shén. After you have practiced for a long time, you will feel as if you were breathing, and yet as if you were not. In this case, you will have reached a profound meditative state of "regulating of no regulating." The mind and the Shén are able to stay at the Real Lower Dāntián. Then you have found the key to Embryonic Breathing.

4. The Secrets of Spiritual Applications of All Veracious Holy Embryo

(Bàopǔzi's Secrets of Embryonic Breathing)[2,3,4]

《諸真聖胎神用訣》

（抱朴子胎息訣）

Those who cultivate human temperament must practice the stabilization of the breathing. What is stabilized breathing? It means: righteous, peaceful, smooth, return (to the root), tamed (i.e., controlled), tranquil, and calm breathing. If (you) are always able to do so in (your) four living manners (Sìwēiyí) (i.e., walking, residing, sitting, and lying) and catch the secret to enter the Real Dào (Zhēndào), the mind is not distracted by surrounding environments, empty the Xīn and solid abdomen (i.e., full Qì in the Lower Dāntián), then it is the most marvellous. When the breathing is clarified, the Xīn will be stabilized; when the Xīn is stabilized, then the Qì will be quiet; when the Qì is quiet, then the Shén will be calm; when the Shén is calm, then the surrounding environment is empty (i.e., emptiness of material world); when the surrounding environment is empty, then (everything is) quiet and nothing exists (i.e., nothingness of the mind); when quiet and nothing is existing, then clear and calm; when it is clear and calm, the Dào is generated; when the Dào is generated, then it becomes natural; when it has become natural, then free and unfettered. Once (you are) free and unfettered, then this is no limitation (of cultivation) and everything can be achieved as you wish, which can therefore result in immortality. The Five Elements (Wǔxíng) will all gather, the Six Qì (Liùqì) will be unified and harmonized, the Eight Trigrams (Bāguà) will match accordingly; this will result in the formation of internal elixir and the physical body will never be damaged.

凡修性之人，須要定息。息者，正也、安也、順也、歸也、伏也、寧也、靜也。若四威儀中，常作如是，訣入真道，勿著諸境，虛心實腹，最為妙也。但澄息心定，心定則氣寂，氣寂則神靜，神靜則境空，境空則寂滅，寂滅則無事，無事則清靜，清靜則道生，道生則自然，自然則逍遙。既入逍遙，則無量自在，得做神仙。自然五行總聚，六氣和合，八卦配偶，成于內丹，身形永劫不壞矣。

"Xí" (息) literally means "to cease" or "to calm." However, in Qìgōng society, Xi also often means "breathing." Therefore, it often confuses Qìgōng beginners. "Cease" means to stop thinking about your breathing (Zhǐxí, 止息). An ancient Daoist named Lǐ, Qīng-Ān (李清庵) said: "Regulating breathing means to regulate the breathing until (you) stop."[64]

This document emphasizes the stabilization of the breathing. In order to reach this goal, the breathing must be regulated until it is righteous, peaceful, smooth, rooted, tamed (i.e., controlled), tranquil, and calm. When this happens, the physical body will be relaxed, the emotional mind calm, and the Qì can circulate smoothly and naturally. "Rooted" here means to return to the original breathing behavior of a newborn child.

"Sìwēiyí" (四威儀) means "four solemn living manners" which include walking, residing, sitting, and lying.[65] If you are able to regulate your breathing until it has reached the stage of no-regulating in your daily life, then you have established a powerful habit in your life through correct breathing manner. Furthermore, if you are able to stabilize and empty your Xīn (i.e., emotional mind) and fill up the Qì in your Real Lower Dāntián, then it will be the most marvellous cultivation for your life.

When the breathing is regulated, the Xīn will be calm and stabilized. Only then will the Qì not be excited. Consequently, the Shén can be centered and kept at its residence, and you have established the most important spiritual cultivation for your enlightenment. When the Shén is centered, you will not be attracted by daily human affairs. This is the path to immortality.

"Wǔxíng" (五行) means "Five Elements" namely "Jīn" (金) (Metal), "Mù" (木) (Wood), "Shuǐ" (水) (Water), "Huǒ" (火) (Fire), and "Tǔ" (土) (Earth). These Five Elements correspond with the five internal Yīn organs: lungs, liver, kidneys, heart, and spleen. Therefore, Five Elements here means the unification and harmonization of the five organs' Qì. "Liùqì" (六氣) means "Six Qìs" including the body's Qì, blood, saliva, liquid, essence, and meridians. To some people, "Liùqì" also means the six different climates including wind, heat, damp, fire, dry, and cold.[66]

5. Three Importances of Conserving the Life
(Yuán, Huáng, Míng Dynasty)[2,3]
《攝生三要》
(明・袁黄)

At the beginning, seal a mouth full of air (i.e., stop breathing after inhalation), use the navel to breathe, count till eighty-one or one hundred and twenty, then let the air out through the mouth. This breath should be extremely slender and reach a stage that (if) there is a feather placed right in front of the mouth and nose, it will not be moved. Practice gradually and also gradually increase (the number of counting). (If) the counting can reach to a thousand, then the old can be converted into young each day... However, if (you) just know how to seal the air, and without knowing Embryonic Breathing, then it is useless.

初閉氣一口，以臍呼吸，數之至八十一，或一百二十，乃以口吐氣出之，當令極細，以鴻毛著予口鼻之上，吐氣而鴻毛不動為度。漸習漸增，數之久可至千，則老者更少，日還一日矣。．．．．但知閉氣，不知胎息，無益也。

The key method of Embryonic Breathing is to keep the mind steady at the Real Lower Dāntián, and the physical body calm to their extreme states. Then the oxygen consumption can diminish significantly. Through the correct navel breathing method (Embryonic Breathing), the Spiritual Embryo can be formalized.

Theoretically, after your inhalation, if you hold your breath for just a few seconds, you are condensing the Qì inward toward the center of your body. The longer you are able to hold without tightening your physical body and disturbing your mind, the more efficiently the Qì can be stored at the Real Lower Dāntián. However, it is not easy to hold the breath for a long time. It will take a lot of practice with the correct method. We will discuss the breathing methods more specifically later in this book.

When this document mentions using the navel to breathe, it means "abdominal breathing." The document Three Importances of Conserving the Life (Shèshēng Sānyào, 攝生三要), says that: "(You) must think (i.e., imagine) that the Qì exits and enters from the navel. (You) must regulate it until the breathing is extremely slender. Then, (it seems you) do not use the mouth and nose, but you use the navel for (your) breathing as if (you) are the fetus in the womb."[67] Many people misunderstand that we can exchange oxygen and carbon dioxide through the navel after birth. They are wrong and try to comprehend the document literally, instead of achieving understanding through practice. In fact, this document emphasizes the importance of abdominal breathing (navel breathing) until the breathing is so soft and slender. Then it seems there is no air exiting or entering from the nose or mouth. It does not mean you should actually stop your breathing completely, as you would die due to the lack of oxygen.

6. Observing Vessels[2]
《脈望》

What is "Sealing the Breath"? (Bìqì) does not mean to hold the breath. It means that the Shén is steady and the Qì is harmonious, stop thinking and forget about worry, allow the nose breathing to be natural, smooth, and slender, as if it is there and as if it is not there.

閉氣者，非閉噎其氣也，乃神定氣和，絕思忘慮，便鼻息悠悠，若有若無。

This short document has clearly pointed out that "sealing the breathing" does not mean stopping the respiration. It means when your Shén has been stabilized and kept at its residence (Upper Dāntián), then the Qì circulation will be harmonious, and the mind will be clear without worry. It is said, in the document The Righteous Rules of Heavenly Immortality (Tiānxiān Zhènglǐ, 天仙正理), that: "Though it is named as 'sealing the breathing,' (actually) it means there is a complete emptiness (of the mind) internally just like the nothingness of the Tàixū."[68] "Tàixū" (太虛) means "Grand Emptiness" and implies the great nature of the universe.

7. The Complete Book of Principal Contents of Human Life and Temperament

(Wáng, Fāng-Píng's Secrets of Embryonic Breathing)[2]

《性命圭旨全書》
（王方平胎息訣）

Those people who follow the Dào must pay attention to the four timings: Zǐ (11–1 a.m.), Wǔ (11–1 p.m.), Mǎo (5–7 a.m.), and Yǒu (5–7 p.m.). These are the gates of Yīn and Yáng's exit and entrance. Stabilize the Xīn and do not be moved (i.e., calm down the mind) is called "Chán" (i.e., meditation). The Shén is communicative and capable of reaching millions of variations, this is called "Líng" (i.e., Supernatural Spirituality). The intelligent mind is able to handle millions of events thoughtfully, this is called "Huì" (i.e., Wisdom). The origin of the Dào is harmonious and peaceful, this is called "Xiū" (i.e., Cultivation). The real Qì has returned to its origin, this is called "Liàn" (i.e., Refine or Train). The dragon and tiger mutually interact with each other, this is called "Dān" (i.e., Elixir). When the three Original Qìs have unified, it is called "Liǎo" (i.e., End or Completed). Those who have a strong will in pursuing the Dào know these origins and thus cultivate their human temperament by following the methods. Naturally, they are able to enter the Great Dào (Dàdào) of longevity."

奉道之士，須審子午卯酉四時，乃是陰陽出入之門戶。定心不動，謂之曰禪。神通萬變，謂之曰靈。智周萬事，謂之曰慧。道元和氣，謂之曰修。真氣歸元，謂之曰煉。龍虎相交，謂之曰丹。三元同氣，謂之曰了。有志于道者，知此根源，依法修性，自可入于長生大道矣。

This document talks about the four proper times for meditation. They are: Zǐ (子) (11–1 a.m., midnight), Wǔ (午) (11–1 p.m., noon), Mǎo (卯) (5–7 a.m., dawn), and Yǒu (酉) (5–7 p.m., dusk). These four times are when Yīn and Yáng change in nature. Therefore, the Qì circulation in your body will also vary accordingly. It is believed by many Qìgōng practitioners that if you meditate at these four times, you are able to effectively remove possible Qì stagnation from the body.

"Chán" (禪) is a Buddhist term for "meditation" and means to regulate the Xīn until it is calm and steady. "Líng" (靈) means "Supernatural Inspiration," which allows you to comprehend and understand the changes or variations of nature. "Huì" (慧) means "Intelligence" or "Wisdom" through pondering, analyzing, and comprehension so you are able to handle millions of events without being confused. "Xiū" (修) (to cultivate) means to cultivate the mind and Shén so you are able to trace back to the origin of the Dào. Once you are able to do so, you will be able to harmonize with nature and find the origin of life. "Liàn" (煉) means "to refine" or "to purify" the spirit and keep it at its residence. When this happens, the Qì will be able to stay there (Real Lower Dāntián) through Embryonic Breathing. This will result in the conception of the Spiritual Embryo (Elixir). Later, this Spiritual Embryo is led upward through the Thrusting Vessel (Chōngmài, 衝脈) (spinal cord) to the brain for enlightenment. This process means "Liǎo" (了) and implies "the end" or "the completion" of the cultivation. Then the "three Qì's" (Essence, Qì, and spirit) will all return to their origins (Sānqì Guīyuán, 三氣歸元).

8. The Secrets of Spiritual Applications of All Veracious Holy Embryo

(Tiāntái Daoist's Secrets of Embryonic Breathing)[2,3,4]

《諸真聖胎神用訣》

（天台道者胎息訣）

Whoever wishes to cultivate and train (the Dào) should maintain (his training) all the time (i.e., constantly). (He) must be able to endure the humiliation and reject the evil thoughts with a sole mind (i.e., firmed mind). Keep (his) sincere mind perseverant and strong so as to transport the heart Qì (i.e., Fire Qì) and kidneys Qì (i.e., water Qì) up and down, to and fro, thus interacting at the Central Palace (Zhōnggōng). The whole Shén must not be dispersed and the Original Qì (Yuánqì) must be nourished. In this case, the Dānshā (i.e., Elixir) and the Huángyá (i.e., Real Yáng) will be sprouted naturally. The root will be deep and the stalk will be firmed. Always keep the breathing soft and slender, so as to reach longevity. In this case, (you) have transcended the laymen society and gained the Dào.

凡人修煉，常行平等，忍辱一屏，邪心所起，真心志堅，運心腎二氣，上下往來，交媾于中宮。諸神不散，溫養元氣，丹砂黃芽自出，深根固蒂，永息綿綿，久而長生，出世得道矣。

This article first points out that in order to reach the goal of spiritual cultivation, you must be patient, consistent, and not be disturbed by the dirty emotional mind. In order to produce the Internal Elixir (Nèidān, 內丹), you must transport the heart Qì (i.e., Post-Heaven Qì or Fire Qì) downward from the Middle Dāntián and the kidneys' Qì (i.e., Pre-Heaven Qì or Water Qì) upward from the Real Lower Dāntián so they can meet at Zhōnggōng (中宮) (Huángtíng, 黃庭) (inner navel area) and interact with each other. If you are able to keep your Shén there, the elixir or Spiritual Embryo will be conceived there naturally. This up-and-down transportation of Qì is commonly called "Kǎn-Lí" (坎離) and means "water-fire."

In the document, Observing Vessels (Màiwàng, 脈望), it is said: "The kidneys' Qì gets together with the heart's Qì. (When) the Qì (is refined and) has reached its extremity, the liquid (i.e., refined mixed material) will be produced. There is a righteous Yáng Qì which is matching with the real Yīn Qì within, and this is called the intercourse of the dragon (Lóng, 龍) and tiger (Hǔ, 虎). After many days (of cultivation), there is a material conceived the size of a grain of rice. This is called 'Golden Elixir Great Herb' (Jīndān Dàyào, 金丹大藥)."[69] The document, Thesis of Zhōnglǚ's Preaching in Dào (Zhōnglǚ Chuándào Lùn, 鍾呂傳道論), said: "At the beginning, model the heaven's rule and function, use the Yīn and Yáng's ascent and descent theory, make the real fire (from heart) and real water (from kidneys) unified as one. Refine it into the Great Herb (Dàyào, 大藥) and keep at the Dāntián forever."[70] *The Complete Book of Principal Contents of Human Life and Temperament* (*Xìngmìng Guīzhǐ Quánshū*, 性命圭旨全書) said: "(When) there is an intercourse of the heaven's Yáng and the earth's Yīn, then millions of lives are born. Our bodies use this Yīn and Yáng and makes them intercourse so the Great Herb (Dàyào, 大藥) can be produced. This is no different from the production of millions of objects by heaven and earth. All are just originated from Yīn and Yáng two Qìs, one gives and one derives (i.e., mutual interaction)."[71]

9. Seventh Bamboo Slips of the Bamboo Bookcase, Internal Elixir (Lǎojūn's Embryonic Breathing)[2,3]

《云笈七簽・內丹》
（老君胎息法）

Lǎojūn (i.e., Lǎozi) said: "(The key to) man's immortality is in the Embryonic Breathing." At midnight and before noon, stretch and extend the legs and arms, bend the feet and cough. After two or three times of respiration, then immediately sit (to meditate). Hold the hands firmly (Wògù) and restrain (your) Xīn at the place under the navel. Use Yì to imagine there is a man's shadow about two or three inches long and use the long inhalation to lead it into the mouth and immediately seal (the breathing). Seal the breath but do not swallow or let it leave the mouth. Then condense the Qì under the navel into a small spot about the size of a grain of rice. After the number has been counted, then inhale as before. At the beginning, (you) may count only thirty-two spots (i.e., times) and gradually increase to hundreds. If (you) are able to count to several thousands, then this is a 'Small Embryonic Breathing' which is the method of avoiding aging (i.e., of longevity).

老君曰：〝人之不死，在于胎息矣。〞夜半時，日中前，自舒展腳手，拗腳咳嗽。長出氣三兩度，即坐握固，攝心臍下，意想影人長三、二寸，以息長吸，引來入口中，即閉，閉定勿咽之，亦勿令出口。即于臍下合氣作小點子，下之米大，如下數已盡，卻返吸如前。初可數得三十、二十點子，漸可數百。若能至數千點子，此小胎息，為長生卻老之術。

Lǎozi in *Dào Dé Jīng* (道德經), Chapter 16, said: "Approaching the nihility (i.e., nothingness or emptiness) to its extremity and maintaining the calmness with sincerity." This is the crucial key to Embryonic Breathing. From correct Embryonic Breathing, we will be able to return ourselves to the root (i.e., origin of life), and this means 'calmness.' When we are calm, then it means "repetition of a life." According to Daoist society, this implies the birth of the Spiritual Embryo. When life repeats, it means "constant natural routine" and therefore the Dào. If it is the Dào, then it can be long, and the death of the body will not be near. Thus, longevity can be attained.

This document mentions that the time of practicing Embryonic Breathing should be at midnight and noon. First loosen up your body and clear your throat. Test yourself for a couple of breaths and see if everything is as smooth and as natural as you wish. You must be in a comfortable position both physically and mentally. Hold your hands right in front of the abdominal area and also bring your mind there. If you have difficulty keeping your mind there, then imagine there is a human shadow there, so you can pay attention to the activity of this shadow. In this case, your mind will not wander and be distracted by the surrounding environment.

First inhale deeply and lead the Qì down to the abdominal area (i.e., Real Lower Dāntián) and then hold the breath. Count the number inside your mind. You may count only a few at the beginning. However, after you have practiced for a long time, you will be able to count more. That implies your body and mind are extremely relaxed and calm. Then you will find the root of life and re-establish a new life (i.e., Spiritual Embryo).

10. The Secrets of Spiritual Applications of All Veracious Holy Embryo

(Dámó Chán Teacher's Secrets of Embryonic Breathing)[2,3]

《諸真聖胎神用訣》

（達磨禪師胎息訣）

What is the training of Embryonic Breathing? It is the training of Qì and the stabilization of Xīn. If (you) can always accord the breathing with (your) Xīn, then (Xīn) will not affiliate with millions of objects. If the Qì is not stabilized, then the Chán (i.e., meditation) will also be empty. If the Qì can be stabilized, then the color body (i.e., physical body) will not be sick and the Chán and Dào are both peaceful. Those who wish to cultivate their human temperament, if the Xīn is unrestrained, resulting in the loss or divergence of Original Qì (Yuánqì), then how can the Dào be accomplished? Ancient people said: 'When Qì is stabilized, the Xīn will be steady. When Qì is condensed, the Xīn is calm. This is the crucial key to reaching the Great Dào' (Dàdào). This is also named as 'Returning the Elixir' (Fǎndān). Daoists do not have such everyday worries, so it can be named as 'real stabilization in observing the Chán.' Therefore, those virtuous and holy persons in the past three generations all used these secret keys to cultivate their human temperaments. It is called "Dual Cultivation of Chán and Dìng."

夫煉胎息者，煉氣定心是也。常息于心輪，則不著萬物，氣若不定，禪亦空也。氣若定，則色身無病，禪道雙安。修性之人，因不守心，元氣失了不收，道怎成矣？古人云：'氣定心定，氣凝心靜，是大道之要。'又名：'返丹。'道人無諸掛念，日日如斯，則名真定禪觀。故三世賢聖，修性皆在此訣，名為禪定雙修也。

"Chán" (禪) is a Buddhist term for meditation. Through this meditation, one is able to comprehend the meaning of life and also the relationship between human and nature. The final goal is to reach Buddhahood so the Shén can survive independently without the physical body. This means eternal spiritual life.

To reach this goal, you must first stabilize your Xīn (心) (emotional mind), and not be attracted by the external environment. This training is called "Dìng" (定) and means the stabilization of the physical and mental bodies. The crucial key to reaching this goal is through correct Embryonic Breathing.

"Dān" (丹) means "elixir" and "Fǎn" (返) means "return." Therefore, "Fǎndān" means to return the elixir to its origin, maintaining the Qì (elixir) at its residence so it will not be lost.

This document explains that in order to reach enlightenment or Buddhahood, you must train your Qì and stabilize your Xīn. The way to do so is through breathing. When the breathing can be regulated correctly, the Xīn will be restrained and the Shén will remain at its residence. Only then can you refine it and reach the goal of enlightenment.

11. The Secrets of Spiritual Applications of All Veracious Holy Embryo (Liúzhēnrén's Secret of Embryonic Breathing)[2,3]

《諸真聖胎神用訣》

（劉真人胎息訣）

If (one) wishes to practice the Original Dào (i.e., True Dào) of Embryonic Breathing, Xīn must not kill, must not have desire, must not rob, steal, or be evil, must not be absurd, act insane, or be crazy. Then the mind will naturally be bright and clear. (He) should always abstain from meat, wine, etc., slenderly regulate the Real Breathing (Zhēnxí, Embryonic Breathing), and observe and shine (i.e., cleanse) entire self (physical and mental) body. (When this happens) the body and mind are clear and quiet. This is the Daoist with longevity. If the metal sinks (to the bottom) (i.e., firmed and rooted) and the treasure objects (i.e., three treasures) are strong and hard (i.e., well protected), Six Doors (Liùmén) are not opened, then evil Qì cannot enter. Hence, the entire body will not be sick. (However) if the Six Doors are not closed and all treasures are stolen, then sickness will be initiated, and the Dào cannot be accomplished. It is praised as: 'The Real Qì within the Xīn is the heavenly essence (i.e., essential key). This is the way to offer (you) a clear Shén and clean Qì which is shining like a mirror. If (one) follows this Great Dào and uses it marvelously, the mind will be clean and calm and the Qì will give birth to divine Shén. One to and one fro, do not stop even momentarily, there is no place at the top and the bottom not being cultivated. Thus the creation and variation (i.e., refinement of spiritual and physical body) can be completed. The Shén is calm and the Qì is clear without contamination, and this will result in steady breathing and the cultivation (of the Dào) will naturally be effective.' Those who study (the Dào) in the future, if (they) do not study its origin, then absurd thoughts cannot be stopped, nor can those initiated and ceased be stopped. Consequently, (the mind) leaves, following surrounding objects, and how can (they) then achieve the goal of Embryonic Breathing?

若修胎息元道之法，心不殺、不欲、不盜、不偷、不邪、不妄、不顛、不狂，心自明朗。常守齋戒，真息常調，觀照遍身世界，身心清靜，乃是長生道人。若金沉寶貝堅實，六門不開，邪氣不入，一身無病患。若六門不閉，盜盡金寶，人生疾也，道自不成矣。頌曰：'心中真氣是天英，正是神清氣鏡明，大道若依玄妙用，心中清靜氣生靈。一去一來不暫停，上下無休造化成，神靜氣澄無事染，這回息住自然靈。' 后學之者，不習元道，妄念不停，生滅不息，隨他物去了，怎成胎息也。

To accomplish Embryonic Breathing, you must first regulate your mind. Do not be evil and contaminated by surrounding objects, or generate desires. You should keep away from eating meat (i.e., stop killing) which can generate violent and aggressive emotions. You should also close "Liùmén" (六門, Six Doors), isolating your mind from outside temptations. The six doors are the eyes, ears, mouth, and nose.

The key to cultivating the Real Qì by regulating the Xīn inside the body is not a hard task. Simply keep the mind and Shén clean, then your breathing will naturally be deep and natural, and the spiritual divine will be generated.

12. The Secrets of Spiritual Applications of All Veracious Holy Embryo (Héxiāngū's Secret of Embryonic Breathing)[2,3]

《諸真聖胎神用訣》

（何仙姑胎息訣）

To train means to cultivate; to breathe means (to regulate) the Qì, (to condense) the Shén, and (to preserve) the essence. The origin of the Qì converted from breathing is a clean and calm Real Qì. Use (the self internal) observation (i.e., self internal feeling) and lead it out and in to the Dāntián slenderly. If (one) knows this, (he) will be able to tame the dragon and tiger automatically. If the Xīn (i.e., emotional mind) is not lured, the Shén does not contemplate, the Qì is not (disturbed by) desires, this is called 'Great Steadiness' (Dàdìng). If (one's) Real Qì is able to reside in the shape and material (i.e., physical body), then (he) will be in the position of immortality with unlimited variations and can be called a 'Truthful Person'

(Zhēnrén). What is Embryonic Breathing? (One) must retain the Shén (Cúnshén) and stabilize the Yì (Dìngyì). What are the three importances which should be embraced and kept? (They) are essence, Qì, and Shén. Those who cultivate the human temperament must always keep these three importances at 6 a.m., then the treasures will be gathered automatically. The country (i.e., body) is rich and the people (i.e., Qì) are peaceful, the mind-king is free, the Shén is harmonious and pleasant; fewer sickness, fewer worries, the body is light and easy, and the ears and eyes are sharp and bright. This is the real path for those who cultivate the truth. If (you) practice these methods three to five years, the heaven will protect (you), the divine nature will guard (you), and general people will love and respect (you). After a long time, (you) will gain the Dào automatically.

夫煉者，修也；息者，氣也、神也、精也。息氣本源者，清靜真氣也。觀入丹田，細細出入，知此者龍虎自伏。若心無動，神無思，氣無欲，則名曰太定。真氣存于形質，真仙之位，變化無窮，號曰真人矣。夫胎息者，須存神定意。抱守三關者，精氣神也。凡修行之人，須每于六時，常抱守三法，則自然有寶聚也。國富民安，心王自在，乃神和暢，少病也、少惱也、身體輕便也、耳目聰明也，是修真之人，真道徑路。若三五年間，常行此法，天護祐，神加持，凡人愛敬，久而自然得道矣。

Commonly, dragon (Lóng, 龍) and tiger (Hǔ, 虎) are used to represent Yīn and Yáng's interaction in Chinese Qìgōng society. It is believed that in order to conceive a Spiritual Embryo, you must know how to lead the Fire Qì downwards from the Middle Dāntián, and the water Qì upwards from the Lower Dāntián. Then Yīn and Yáng will interact at the Huángtíng (黄庭) (inner area behind the navel) and the Spiritual Embryo can be conceived.

In order to reach this goal, you must lead the Qì to the Huángtíng through correct Embryonic Breathing. Your mind must be in an extremely calm and meditative state, giving you deep internal feeling (Nèiguān, 內觀). "Nèiguān" means to observe your inner self through feeling. To train this deep feeling will take time and a lot of practice and it is thus called "Nèishì Gōngfū" (內視功夫) (Gōngfū of internal vision). At this point, you should know clearly that feeling is a language between your mind and body. Without it, your mind will not be able to recognize the place and lead the Qì there. To reach it, your mind must be calm and profound, and you must bring your mind and Shén back to your body through Embryonic Breathing.

"Cúnshén" (存神) means "to retain the Shén" at its residence. It is said in Daoist society: "Cúnshén means there is no new thinking initiated or thought remaining. It only means to condense the Shén at a point without allowing it to be dispersed and lost."[72]

In Chinese Qìgōng society, the physical body is commonly analogized to a country, Qì to people, and the mind to the king. This analogy often gives a practitioner a better idea of how the mind is able to lead the Qì.

13. The Secrets of Spiritual Applications of All Veracious Holy Embryo

(Zhāngtiānshī's Secret of Embryonic Breathing)[2,3,4]

《諸真聖胎神用訣》

（張天師胎息訣）

The Original Qì (Yuánqì) does not have shape (i.e., cannot be seen), the Real Xīn (i.e., emotional mind) does not have standard rules (i.e., changes all the time), and Great Dào (Dàdào) cannot be traced. Only the practice method of regulating breathing contains the Real Dào (Zhēndào). It is said: 'The Xīn is calm, the Qì is stable, and the Shén is retained.' Those who cultivate the Dào, if (they) are able to follow the method of practicing Great Elixir (Dàdān) to reach the Original Dào (Yuándào), then (the mind) will be clean and insubstantial, extremely calm, without worries and the Yì is forgotten, empty and quiet with nothingness, and millions of methods are not traceable. This is the real cultivation of Embryonic Breathing. In this case, there is no doubt (that one is able to) become an immortal.

夫元氣無形，真心無法，大道無跡。唯煉息一法，乃含真道。又云：'心定氣定神定。' 凡修道流，若合大丹元道，清虛寂靜，絕慮忘意，空靜無物，萬法無蹤，真修胎息也，成仙無疑也。

Original Qì cannot be seen but only felt through the mind. The emotional mind varies from individual to individual, place to place, and from time to time. Therefore, there are no standard rules to restrain it or control it. To cultivate the invisible Dào, you must calm down your Xīn and comprehend it. Without a clear and controllable Xīn, the mind will be confused and the Shén dispersed. Then the goal of reaching the Great Dào (Dàdào, 大道) will be impossible.

The best way is through regulating your breathing; then the mind can be calm, and without any worry from human affairs. Then the Yì (意) can lead the Qì upwards to nourish the Shén, and you have achieved the goal of Great Elixir (Dàdān, 大丹), the way of Original Dào (Yuándào, 元道). Then both Xīn and Yì will disappear, and everything is empty in the mind. This is the achievement of Embryonic Breathing.

14. The Secrets of Spiritual Applications of All Veracious Holy Embryo

(Guǐgǔzi's Secret of Embryonic Breathing)[2,3,4]

《諸真聖胎神用訣》

（鬼谷子胎息訣）

Those who cultivate the Dào must return to their origins (i.e., original natural being), go back to (their original) purity, and harmonize with the Real Qì (Zhēnqì) internally. Consequently, the Dào can be returned, and through (natural influences of) Four Phases (Sìxiàng), Five Elements (Wǔxíng), Six Qìs (Liùqì),

Seven Origins (Qīyuán), and Eight Trigrams (Bāguà), the Essence, the Qì, and the Shén can be formalized into shape and substance (i.e., human form). This is gaining the substantial from the insubstantial, make something from nothingness, where the Real Elixir (Zhēndān) is secreted. Therefore, to train the Xīn into Shén, to train essence into shape, and train Qì for life are the training of Qì in its ascent and descent of Yīn and Yáng. What is the origin of Qì? It is the root of life. Therefore, it is a Great Dào if (you) cultivate these three methods.

凡修道之人，返本還純，內合真氣。故道返則四象、五行、六氣、七元、八卦，而煉精、氣、神，成其形質，則是虛中取實，無中取有，而內秘真丹也。故煉心為神，煉精為形，煉氣為命，此是陰陽升降之氣也。氣源者，命之根也。故修三法，則大道也。

"Sìxiàng" (四象) means "Four Phases," which derived from Yīn and Yáng. "Wǔxíng" (五行) means "Five Elements" namely metal (Jīn, 金), wood (Mù, 木), water (Shuǐ, 水), fire (Huǒ, 火), and earth (Tǔ, 土). "Liùqì" (六氣) means the Qì existing in air, blood, saliva, liquid, essence, and vessels. "Qīyuán" (七元) means "Seven Origins" and implies the original function of the seven orifices of eyes, nose, mouth, and ears which are related to the five internal organs; liver, lungs, heart, spleen, and kidneys. Qīyuán also means the original Qì level of the five internal organs. "Bāguà" means "Eight Trigrams" and implies heaven, earth, lake, mountain, wind, water, fire, and thunder—all natural energy.

This document points out that in order to reach the Dào, you must return your self-being to its original purity. To reach it, you must coordinate and harmonize the natural energy, and also the energy circulating within the body. Then refine the mind so the Shén can be condensed, refine the essence so the physical body can be strong and healthy, and refine the Qì so the life force is powerful and abundant. These three things are the keys to reaching the Dào.

15. The Secrets of Spiritual Applications of All Veracious Holy Embryo

(Yellow Emperor's Secrets of Embryonic Breathing)[2,3,4]

《諸真聖胎神用訣》

（黃帝胎息訣）

Those who cultivate the Dào should always observe themselves internally, get rid of the Three Corpses (Sānshī), and the Six Emotions (Liùqíng), return to internal so as to keep (i.e., protect) the three (treasures) (i.e., Jīng, Qì, and Shén). The Xīn and Shén are kept at their residences, the Qì is condensed without dispersion, and the Shén is cheerful. The techniques of cultivating the Qì, training the shape (i.e., physical body), and maintaining human temperament, should not be forgotten. This is the key to real Embryonic Breathing and the key training of the Great Herb (Dàyào).

凡修道者，常行內觀。遣去三尸，出于六情。返內存三，心神守宮。氣閉不散，諸神歡暢。養氣、煉形、存性，此三法不可棄。是真一胎息也，玄關大藥也。

"Sānshī" (三尸) means "Three Corpses" and are the three desires which could lead to your death. Three desires are the temptations of money, taste (food), and sex. "Liùqíng" (六情) means "Six Emotions" and implies the six emotional desires derived from the pleasures of eyes, ears, nose, tongue, body, and mind.

If you are able to keep your mind absorbed internally, and keep away from all emotional attractions and temptations, then the emotional mind can be calm, and Shén can stay at its residence. Then Qì can be led to its residence (Real Lower Dāntián) and preserved. When the Shén and the Qì are harmonized with each other, then the Spiritual Embryo can be conceived.

There are three important cultivations to reach this goal: nourishing the Qì, training the physical body, and refining the human temperament. Nourishing the Qì means to build up the Qì at the Real Lower Dāntián to an abundant level, so it can be used to rebuild the physical body and strengthen the immune system. However, the most important of all is to refine your Shén through the cultivation of human temperament.

16. The Secrets of Spiritual Applications of All Veracious Holy Embryo
(Cáoxiāngū's Secrets of Embryonic Breathing) [3,4]

《諸真聖胎神用訣》
(曹仙姑胎息訣)

Furthermore, Embryonic Breathing cannot be done through stratagem (i.e., trick). If it could be done (with trick), then it would be far away from the Dào. Human life must rely on the existence of Shén, and when Qì stays, the Dào (of life) can exist. Shén and Qì, these two must rely on each other so (life) can be achieved. Those whose temperament and physical life are weak, after comprehending this spiritual (practice) can then be bright and shining (i.e., enlightened), harmonious, circulating cyclically (i.e., continuously), softly, and fluently. Consequently, the Shén is peaceful and the Qì circulation unobstructed. When the Qì circulation is unobstructed, the blood circulation will be harmonious, and the bones will be strong. Then the bone marrow will be full, and (the Qì stored at) the abdomen will be abundant. Then the lower section of the body will be solid, and walking and stepping will be light and invigorated. The movements will not be tired, and the four limbs will be healthy and strong. This is just like a country that has strong boundaries to keep it safe and tranquil. When the Qì and blood are harmonious and circulate abundantly, it is like a country that has plentiful financial reserves. As if a family is rich, the Shén and aspiration are harmonious and delighted, the color of the face (i.e., facial appearance) is cheerful, walking like dancing, all of these imply the approaching of the immortal Dào. Therefore, it is said: "Today's people are always longing for Buddhism and Daoism. All they wish is to get rid of disasters and avoid calamities. If they were able to build up a strong will (for cultivation) and get rid of absurd ways, this would gradually allow them to reach the understanding of human life. If (they can) do it, then Embryonic Breathing can be achieved."

且胎息者，非方術之所能為。為者，則失道遠矣。且人之生也，須以神存，氣留道生。神與氣兩者，相須乃成。性命虛者，通靈而光明，和者周流而柔潤。神安則氣暢，氣暢則血融，血融則骨強，骨強則髓滿，髓滿則腹盈，腹盈則下實，下實則行步輕健，行步輕健則動作不疲，四肢康強。猶國之封域平泰。氣血和盛，猷國之府庫充實。譬人家富，神志和悅，顏色自怡，行步歌舞，仙道近矣。故曰：'今人念佛念道，只要除災救禍，不如志念除妄，還好麼達人觀。斯而行之，自成胎息者矣。'

Attaining Embryonic Breathing is not a trick but a method. If it were a trick, it would be easy. However, it is a method, and will take time and effort to practice and make it work. If it could be done as a trick, then the Dào would have been lost.

This document specifies the key points of practice and also its benefits. 1. Retain the Shén peacefully at its residence, 2. Maintain the Qì at the Real Lower Dāntián, and 3. Shén and Qì harmonize with each other. Actually, these are the same crucial points all other documents have emphasized.

17. The Secrets of Spiritual Applications of All Veracious Holy Embryo

(Yuán, Tiān-Gāng's Secrets of Embryonic Breathing)[2,3,4]

《諸真聖胎神用訣》

（袁天綱胎息訣）

What is Yīn and Yáng, it is actually the Real Qì (Zhēnqì) of the heaven and the earth (i.e., nature). One Yīn and one Yáng, (thus) millions of objects (lives) are born. Human Qì is the Qì (i.e., air) of breathing. Heaven (Great Nature) Qì (i.e., natural energy) is that which derives the winter and summer (i.e., four seasons). It is also said: "These two things (Yīn and Yáng) are able to change the Qì of the four seasons and are the Wùjǐ (Ten Celestial Stems) which conceal the Real Qì (of nature)." "The Spring arrives at Xùn which is able to bear and bloom millions of objects; the Summer arrives at Kūn which is able to grow and raise millions of objects; the Fall arrives at Qián which is able to ripen millions of objects; and the Winter arrives at Gěn which is able to conceal millions of objects." All of these result from the Yīn and Yáng's deified applications of appearance and disappearance (i.e., existence), and rising and falling. Consequently, water is generated from Yángqì and bears wood, while fire is initiated from Yīnqì and bears metal. Yáng is initiated at Zǐ (11 p.m.–1 a.m.) and emerges at Mǎo (5–7 a.m.), Yīn begins at Wǔ (11 a.m.–1 p.m..) and enters (i.e., grows stronger) at Yǒu (5–7 p.m.). These four crucial timings are the key doors of heaven and earth (i.e., nature). Those who wish to reach the Great Dào must know how to absorb the righteous Qì of these four timings. During cultivation, active breathing belongs to Yīn, while stabilized breathing belongs to Yáng. During the practice, (you) must have a steady Xīn and a strong will, stabilized Shén and calm breathing. Then the dragon and the tiger will meet to conceive the Holy Embryo. This is called the Embryonic Breathing of the Real Person (Zhēnrén) (i.e., one who has reached the Dào).

夫陰陽者，天地之真氣，一陰一陽，生育萬物，在人為呼吸之氣，在天為寒暑之氣。又云：'此兩者能改移四時之氣，此乃戊己包藏真氣。' 云春至在巽，能發生萬物；夏至在坤，能長養萬物；秋至在乾，能成熟萬物；冬至在艮，能含藏萬物。' 此皆陰陽出沒升降神用，故陽氣出水盛木，陰氣出火盛金。陽生于子出乎卯，陰生于午入乎酉。此四仲之辰，皆是天地之門戶也。凡大道者，必取四時之正氣。凡修行動息為陰，定息為陽。凡作時須得心定力定，神定息定，龍親虎會，結就聖胎，名曰真人胎息也。

"Wù" (戊) and "Jǐ" (己) are two of The Ten Celestial Stems (Shítiāngān, 十天干). Chinese use The Ten Celestial Stems together with Twelve Terrestrial Branches (Shíèr Dìzhī, 十二地支) to form a cycle of sixty. From this, they distinguish the different natural cycles of the year. Wù-jǐ implies the natural timings.

"Xùn" (巽), "Kūn" (坤), "Qián" (乾), and "Gěn" (艮) are the four terms of The Eight Trigrams (Bāguà, 八卦) used to represent different seasons. "Zǐ" (子), "Mǎo" (卯), "Wǔ" (午), and "Yǒu" (酉) are the four periods of the Twelve Terrestrial Branches used to represent different times of day. During cultivation, the active breathing belongs to Yīn, since the body will be more tense and thus consume more Qì. This will result in the weakening of the stored Qì. However, if you have a regulated stabilized breathing, the Qì at the Real Dāntián can be stored to an abundant level, and this belongs to Yáng.

In order to achieve spiritual cultivation effectively, you must coordinate with the times of the year and the day, to be in harmony with nature and gain great benefit from it.

3.8 Other Related Documents 其他有關文獻

1. The Secret of Cultivating Original Qì Internally by Mr. Huànzhēn[2] 《幻真先生內服元氣訣》

If there is a sudden uncomfortable feeling in cultivation or an occasional sickness, then immediately go to a secret room. Follow the method of breathing to cultivate the Qì. After the Qì becomes abundant, then stop and regulate it (smoothly) and swallow it (i.e., lead it down to the Lower Dāntián with saliva). Think of the place where there is pain, seal (your) breath and place (your) whole mind there, use the Yì to attack (the sick place). When inhalation has reached its limit, then expel it.

After complete (exhalation), again swallow. Continue and follow the same method to attack. When the breathing becomes urgent, then stop. After breathing has been regulated, again attack. It may take twenty to fifty times, attack the painful place until sweat, and turn into red color, then stop. If there is no improvement, then practice it every midnight or early morning. Practice day and night and use the Yì to attack. It does not matter if the sickness is at the head, face, hand, or feet, just attack wherever there is a problem.

忽有修養乖宜，偶生疾患，宜速于密室，依服氣法，布足訖則調氣咽之，念所苦之處，閉氣想注，以意攻之。氣極則吐之，訖，復咽。相繼依前攻之，氣急則止，氣調復攻，或二十至五十，攻覺所苦處，汗出通潤即止。如未損，即每日夜半，或五更晝日頻作，以意攻及。若病在頭面、手足，但有疾之處則攻之。

The sicknesses here refer to common uncomfortable feelings or injury. For example, the beginning of catching cold, joint pain, internal pain caused from Qì and blood stagnation, or some minor injuries. Normally, these problems can be removed or corrected through meditation.

The first step in self-healing through meditation is to build up the Qì storage to an abundant level in the Lower Dāntián through abdominal breathing, or in the Real Lower Dāntián by Embryonic Breathing. Then inhale smoothly and slenderly and swallow (Yàn, 咽) the saliva, while using your Yì to lead the Qì to the painful place. Hold the breath until it reaches its limit, then exhale slowly and use the mind to lead the Qì away from the painful place. Repeat this process continuously. If you feel breathing has become urgent, then return to normal breathing until it is comfortable. After recovery from the urgent breathing, repeat the entire process again. You may have to do it for twenty to fifty times. It does not matter, keep doing it until the painful place starts to sweat or the skin color turns pink, then you should stop. If it does not help to ease the pain, then repeat every day and night until the pain has been removed.

2. The Important Secret Song of Embryonic Breathing[2]
《胎息秘要歌訣》

If the body gets sick suddenly or there is abnormal irregularity (i.e., uncomfortable feeling) or injury, condense (your) Yì and return (yourself) to a leisure room (i.e., separate and secret room). Strip the body and lie down on the bed. Face up as sleeping and hold firm (i.e., place both your hands at the abdominal area). Bite (your) teeth and burn incense. After swallowing thirty-six times, the Qì in the (Lower) Dāntián has passed the normal stage (of storing). Follow the Xīn to lead (the Qì) continuously. It is best to lead it to the injured place. It is adequate when it sweats. This will spare the effort in searching for medical prescriptions.

忽然身染疾，非理有損傷。斂意歸閒室，脫身臥本床。仰眠兼握固，
扣齒與焚香。三十六咽足，丹田氣越常。隨心連引導，損處最為良。
汗出以為度，省求廣利方。

To place the hands at the Lower Dāntián area is called "Hold to Firm" (Wògù, 握固). The mind will be firmed at the Lower Dāntián area and the Qì can be stored efficiently. Biting the teeth (Kòuchǐ, 扣齒) is used to wake up the brain and raise up the Shén. Burning incense (Fénxiāng, 焚香) is to help you calm down the mind. All other descriptions of the training methods are the same as in the previous document.

The above two documents, describing self-healing using meditation, are translated for your reference. The most important way to reach successful healing is through practice and accumulating experience. From constant practice and continuous pondering, you will soon grasp the secret key to healing.

References

1. *Dào Dé Jīng and Qìgōng* (道德經與氣功), by Dīng, Xīn-Bǎi (丁辛百) and Pān, Míng-Huán (潘明環), 安徽科學技術出版社, Ānhuī, China 1996.
2. *Chinese Qìgōng Dictionary* (中國氣功辭典), by Lǚ, Guāng-Róng (呂光榮), 人民衛生出版社, Běijīng, China, 1988.
3. *The Great Completion of Chinese Qìgōng* (中國氣功大成), by Fāng, Chūn-Yáng (方春陽), 吉林科學技術出版社, Jílín, China, 1989.
4. *The Study of Practical Chinese Medical Qìgōng* (實用中醫氣功學), by Mǎ, Jì-Rén (馬濟人), 上海科學技術出版社, Shànghǎi, China, 1992.
5. *The Complete Book of Nourishing the Life in Chinese Daoist Qìgōng* (中國道教氣功養生大全), by Lǐ, Yuǎn-Guó (李遠國), 四川辭書出版社, Chéngdū, Sìchuān, China, 1991.
6. *The Great Completion of Chinese Life Nourishing* (中國養生大成), by Fāng, Chūn-Yáng (方春陽), 吉林科學技術出版社, Jílín, China, 1992.
7. *Important Collection of Concealed Daoist Qìgōng* (道藏氣功要集), by Hóng, Pī-Mó (洪丕謨), 上海書店, Shànghǎi, China, 1991.
8. 《性命圭旨全書・亨集》：〝專氣致柔神久留，往來真息自悠悠。綿綿迤邐歸元氣，不汲靈泉常自流。〞
9. 〝吐唯細細，納唯綿綿〞
10. 《道言淺近》：〝調息要調真息息〞，〝凝神調息，只要心平氣和。〞
11. 《性命圭旨全書・蟄藏氣穴，眾妙歸根》：〝調息要調真息息，煉神須煉不神神。〞
12. "Complex and Hidden Brain in the Gut Makes Stomachaches and Butterflies," by Sandra Blakeslee, *The New York Times*, Science, January 23, 1996.
13. *The Second Brain: The Scientific Basis of Gut Instinct and a Groundbreaking New Understanding of Nervous Disorders of the Stomach and Intestine*, Michael D. Gershon, New York: Harper Collins Publications, 1998.

14. 行氣如九曲珠，無微不到。

15. 《胎息經注》：〝臍下三寸為氣海，亦為下丹田，亦為玄牝。蓋玄者，水也；牝者，母也。．．．．修道者，常伏其氣于臍下，守其神于身內，神氣相合而生玄胎。玄胎既結，乃自生身，即為內丹。〞

16. 《馮氏錦囊》：〝身中一竅，名曰玄牝，受之以生，實為府神，三元所聚，精神魂魄會于此穴，乃金丹還返之根，神仙凝結聖胎之地也。〞

17. 《道德經・六章》：〝谷神不死，是謂玄牝；玄牝之門，是謂天地根。綿綿若存，用之不盡。〞

18. 《道德經・一章》：〝道、可道，非、常道。〞

19. 《道德經・二十五章》：〝有物混成，先天地生；寂兮寥兮，獨立而不改，周行而不殆；可以為天下母。吾不知其名，字之曰道，強為之名曰大。〞

20. 《黃庭內景經・梁丘子注》：〝五牙者，五行之生氣，以配五臟。〞

21. 《黃庭經講義》：〝黃，乃土色，土位中央。庭，乃階前空也。名為黃庭，即表中空之義。〞〝臍內空處，即黃庭也。〞

22. 《道德經・十章》：〝載營魄抱一，能無離乎？〞

23. 〝跳出三界外，不在五行中。〞

24. 真一者，指身體陰陽合二而一。

25. 《存神固氣論》：〝人能將自己天真，安於天谷之內，乃守真一之道也。〞

26. 〝胎息者，守真一之道，即神息相依，神凝氣定。〞

27. 《脈望》：〝能守真一，息不往來。〞又曰：〝能守真一，則真氣自凝，陽神自聚。〞

28. 《抱朴子內篇・地真卷》：〝在人兩眉間，卻行一寸為明堂，二寸為洞房，三寸為上丹田也。〞

29. 《東醫保鑒》引《仙經》曰：〝腦為髓海，上丹田・・・藏神之府也。〞

30. 《抱朴子內篇・地真卷》：〝心下絳宮、金闕，中丹田也。〞

31. 《東醫保鑒》引《仙經》曰：〝心為絳宮，中丹田・・・藏氣之府也。〞

32. *The Body Electric*, by Robert O. Becker, M.D. and Gary Selden, Quill, William Morrow, New York, 1985.

33. 《東醫保鑒》引《仙經》曰：〝臍下三寸為下丹田・・・藏精之府也。〞

34. 《云笈七籤卷十八・老子中經》曰：〝丹田者，人之根也，精神之所藏也，五氣之元也，赤子之府，男子以藏精，女子以藏水，主生子，合和陰陽之門戶也。在臍下三寸，附著脊膂，兩腎根也。〞

35. 王錄識餘云：〝銅人針灸圖，載臟腑一身俞穴有玉環，余不知玉環是何物。〞張紫陽玉清金華祕文，論神仙結丹處曰：〝心上腎下，脾左肝右，生門在前，密戶居後，其連如環，其白如棉，方圓徑寸，密裹一身之精粹，此即玉環。〞

36. 《黃庭外景經・石和陽註》：〝命門之上，有玄關二竅，左玄右牝，中虛一處，名曰黃庭。〞

37. 《道鄉集》：〝何謂文火？若守若存，勿亡勿助。〞〝吐唯細細，納唯綿綿〞

38.《道德經・十六章》：〝致虛極，守靜篤。〞

39.《慧苑音義・上》：〝禪那，此云靜心思慮也。舊翻為思維修者，略也。〞

40. 眼觀鼻，鼻觀心。

41. 大定：〝佛心澄明，謂之大定。〞指腦神安靜，形體放鬆，神形相對協調與穩定。

42.《道德經・一章》：〝常無，欲以觀其妙。常有，欲以觀其徼。〞

43.《同指要鈔》：〝一代教門，皆以觀心為要。〞

44.《道德經・十六章》：〝致虛極，守靜篤；萬物并作，吾以觀其復。夫物芸芸，各復歸其根。歸根曰靜，靜曰復命。〞

45.〔三觀〕：一・空觀：觀諸法之空諦。二・假觀：觀諸法之假。三・中觀：一觀諸法亦非空，亦非假，即中也。二觀諸法亦空亦假，即是中，謂為雙照之觀。

46. 即覺或智之意。如覺悟、覺察、覺知諸法之事理，而了了分明。如睡夢之寤，謂之覺悟。覺察煩惱，使不為害，如世人之覺之為賊者，故云覺察。

47. 佛在靈山莫遠求，靈山只在汝心頭。人人有個靈山塔，好向靈山塔下修。

48.《性命圭旨全書・涵養本源，救護命寶》：〝學道先須學自心，自心深處最難尋。若還尋到無尋處，方悟凡心即佛心。〞指覺悟之心。

49.《性命圭旨全書・王子喬胎息訣》：〝子、午、卯、酉四時，乃是陰陽出入之門戶。〞

50. 活子時：〝習煉氣功中，形神安靜，凝神入氣穴，覺丹田氣動，陰陽生發之時。〞

51.《脈望》：〝下手立丹基，休向子午推，靜中才一動，便是癸生時，謂之活子時。〞

52. 〝指造化生育萬物之根本，亦即天地萬物之母，即道之別稱也。〞

53.《武當修真圖》：〝明堂下，兩眉連線中點上方。有神光出，而曰天目。〞

54.《云笈七簽》：〝兩眉間為泥丸之玉門。〞

55.《本草綱目》：〝腦為元神之府。〞

56. 〝人人身中有一神，一神中有一靈光，靈光獨耀超千谷，道化無窮徹萬方。〞

57.《道德經・六章》：〝谷神不死，是謂玄牝。玄牝之門，是謂天地根，綿綿若存，用之不勤。〞

58.《六祖壇經》：〝菩提本無樹，明鏡亦非台，本來無一物，何處惹塵埃。〞

59.《養生論》：〝呼吸吐納，服食養身，使形神相親，表裡既濟也。〞

60.《道德經・五十五》：〝骨弱筋柔而握固。〞

61. 指行佛家氣功時，手的姿勢。其作用有二：一精神思維活動專注于手印，持之以恆，獲得禪定。二調節手形成印後，精神思維活動專注于呼吸，達到最高境界，〝即身成佛。

62.《諸病源候論・風身體手足不隨候》：〝握固者，以兩手各自以四指把手姆指。〞

63.《道門通教必用集》：〝握固以大指掐中指指節，四指齊收于心。〞

64. 調息要調無息息。

65. 《菩薩善戒經》：〝威儀苦者，名身四威儀。一者行，二者住，三者坐，四者臥。菩薩苦行苦坐，晝夜常調惡業之心。忍行坐苦，非時不臥，非時不住。所住內外，若床若地，若草若葉。于此四處，常念供養佛法僧寶。〞

66. 六氣：人體氣，血，津，液，精，脈等六種物質。或風，熱（暑），濕，火，燥，寒六種氣候。

67. 《攝生三要》：〝須想其氣，出從臍出，入從臍滅。調得極細，然後不用口鼻，但以臍呼吸，如在胞胎之中。〞指應用腹肌鼓凹作為氣體變換的動力。呼吸的樞機在臍，口鼻僅是呼吸之氣出入的通道。

68. 《天仙正理・伏氣直論》：〝托名閉息者，而內則空空如太虛之無物。〞

69. 《脈望》：〝腎氣投心氣，氣極生液，液中有正陽之氣，配合真一之水，名曰龍虎交媾，日得黍米之大，名曰金丹大藥。〞

70. 《鍾呂傳道論・論日月》：〝始也效法天機，用陰陽升降之理，使真水真火合而為一，煉成大藥，永鎮丹田。〞

71. 《性命圭旨全書・天人合發，采藥歸壺》：〝天地以此陰陽交媾而生萬物，吾身以此陰陽交媾而生大藥，與天地萬物不異，總是陰陽二氣一施一化。〞

72. 若夫存神，則無所想。不過將神凝聚于一點，不使散漏之謂也。

CHAPTER 4

Summaries from Ancient Documents

4.1 INTRODUCTION (JIÈSHÀO, 介紹)

I would like to summarize a few general points from the documents translated and commented upon in the last chapter.

1. Many documents discuss the same things and emphasize the same practices, though the years of writing were different.
2. These ancient documents can only offer you some references and experiences. It is up to you to make a wise and clear judgment. Each document is like a road sign or map to the garden of Embryonic Breathing. Some of them are considered very important and crucial, some less so, and some others may lead you to the wrong path.
3. I have covered almost all of the available documents related to Embryonic Breathing in the previous chapter. Due to my limited knowledge and experience, there are some places which may be beyond my understanding. I hope those who have a deeper Qìgōng experience will fill up these voids.
4. Again, I would like to point out that it is not easy to translate these ancient documents. I have tried to translate them as close to the meaning as possible. Often, if you translate it word by word, the actual meaning will be distorted or lost.

In the next section, from my personal understanding, I would like to draw conclusions from the important concepts in the ancient documents. I hope this chapter will offer you a clear idea, both for understanding and for practice. This will provide you with a good foundation for your practice, which we will discuss in Part III of this book.

4.2 Summaries of Important Points (Yàodiǎn Zǒngjié, 要點總結)

In this section, first I would like to review the body's energy structure briefly, which was already discussed in Chapter 2. If you still have questions concerning this brief summary, you should refer back to Chapter 2. Without this theoretical foundation, many of the summaries concluded from ancient documents will not make sense. After we have concluded those important theoretical and training points, we will list the benefits of Embryonic Breathing.

Two Qì Poles in a Human Body (Rénshēn Liǎngyí, 人身兩儀). As discussed in Chapter 2, we have three Dāntiáns. The top (Upper Dāntián) and the bottom (Real Lower Dāntián) ones establish a two-pole system which thus constitutes a human central energy line. These Two Poles, one Yīn and one Yáng, synchronize and harmonize with each other. They are just like the Poles of a magnet which cannot be separated. The Real Lower Dāntián (Human Gut or second brain) is the North pole that stores Qì and supplies it for the functioning of the entire body. The Upper Dāntián (brain) is the South pole that directs and governs the quality of Qì manifestation.

When we compare these Two Poles with the Tàijí Yīn-Yáng symbol, we can easily see that the spirit (Shén, 神) residing in the Upper Dāntián is classified as Yáng, since it manifests the Qì into action. That is why the spirit is called "Yángshén" (陽神) in Chinese Qìgōng society. However, the area located in the Real Lower Dāntián is called "Sea Bottom" (Hǎidǐ, 海底) where it is able to store Qì to an abundant level. The Qì stored in the Real Lower Dāntián is thus called "Yīnshuǐ" (陰水), which means "Yīn Water" (Figure 4–1). It was believed that this Yīn water originates from the Original Essence (Yuánjīng, 元精) stored in the internal kidneys (Nèishèn, 內腎) and external kidneys (Wàishèn, 外腎). "External kidneys" are testicles or ovaries. In fact, it is now understood that the "Original Essence" is actually the hormones produced by the adrenals of the internal kidneys and by the gonads (the testicles or ovaries). Due to this reason, the water (Qì) produced in these glands is often called "kidney water" (Shènshuǐ, 腎水).

However, from another point of view, we can see that since the Real Lower Dāntián supplies the quantity of Qì, it can be considered Yáng, while the spirit, which governs the quality of Qì manifestation, can thus be considered Yīn. From this, you can see how Yīn and Yáng are defined according to different points of view. If we take a closer look, we can see this viewpoint clearly.

Again, if you observe the Tàijí Yīn-Yáng symbol closely, you can see that there is a hidden Yáng fountain (Yángquán, 陽泉) in the center of the Yīn water, and a concealed Yīn spirit (Yīnshén, 陰神) in the center of the Yáng spirit. In fact, in Qìgōng Embryonic Breathing training, you train these two pole centers of hidden Yáng and concealed Yīn. For example, if you are able to keep your mind at the center of the hidden Yáng within the Yīn water, the Qì at the Real Lower Dāntián will continue to be stored and preserved,

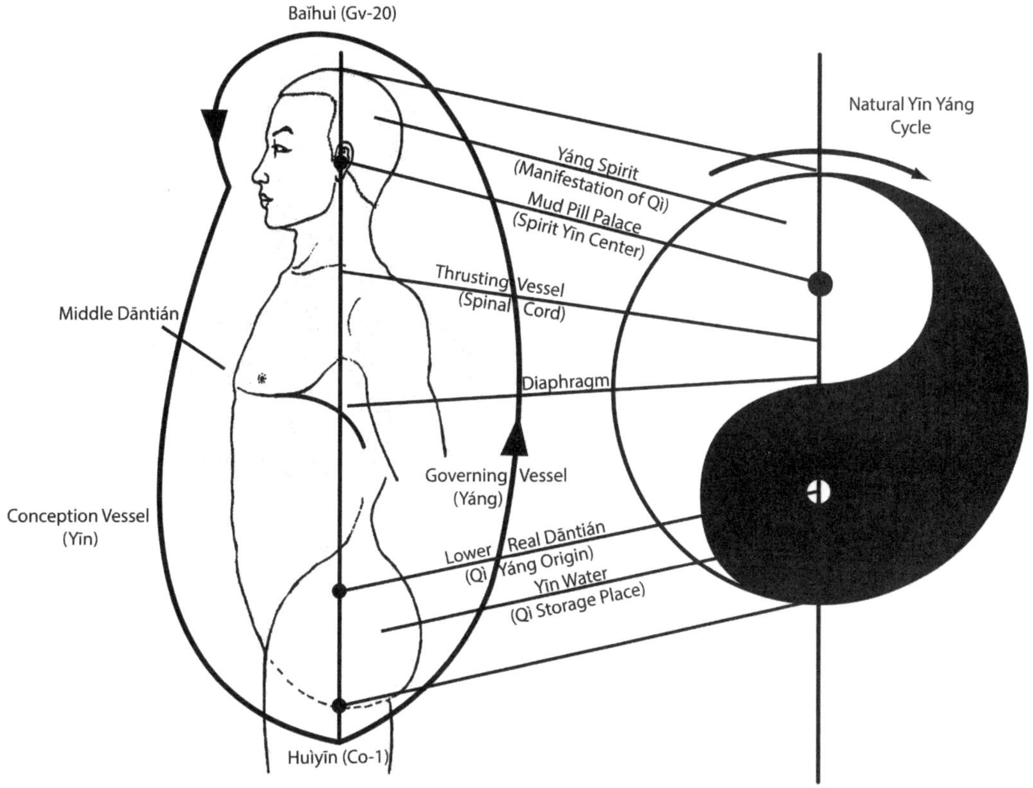

Figure 4-1. The Body's Yīn and Yáng, and the Two Polarity Centers

like a spring which is able to produce water continuously. Not only that, if you also know how to keep the spirit condensed at its center (concealed Yīn), then the quality of Qì manifestation will reach a higher level of efficiency.

These are two concealed Poles, one at the center of the head (Mud Pill Palace) and the other at the center of the gut. Though they are two, they function as one. If you are able to keep your mind at these two poles, the spirit and the Qì will stay in their residences. This process is called "Embracing Singularity" (Bàoyī, 抱一).

The Spirit is the Master of the Body (Shénwéi Zhǔzǎi, 神為主宰). The Spirit is related to your mind. This mind is what is called "Tàijí" (太極) (Grand Ultimate) in Small Human Heaven and Earth (Small Universe or Nature). When this mind acts properly, the spirit can be raised up to a high level and when this mind acts strangely, then the spirit will be disordered and the quality of Qì manifestation will be poor. Therefore, in order to have a condensed and focused spirit, you must first regulate your mind. To achieve this, you must not be attracted by human affairs, emotions and desires. You must see through to the reality that the material world is only temporary. In order to reach the goal of immortality or enlightenment, you must train to cultivate your spirit to a strong level so it can survive independently even when the physical body is dead. This is the concept of immortality (spiritual eternity).

In the Embryonic Breathing training, regulating your mind and spirit in the Upper Dāntián is more crucial than regulating your Qì. After all, it is your mind and spirit which govern your life and control the efficiency of Qì manifestation. When mind and spirit are strong and focused, the Qì can be stored to an abundant level. However, when the mind and spirit are scattered and confused, the spirit will become Yáng and naturally the Qì will also be manifested and wastefully consumed. In this case, the level of spiritual cultivation will be shallow.

However, regulating the mind and spirit is a very difficult and long process. Using your mind to deal with your mind is like trying to force yourself to fall asleep. The more you do so, the worse it will be. That is why nearly half of the available documents discuss the regulating of the mind and spirit. The key means of regulating the mind and spirit is through regulating the breathing.

Keep the Yì at the Dāntiáns (Yìshǒu Dāntián, 意守丹田). The first major key of Embryonic Breathing is to keep your Yì at the concealed Yīn located at the "Mud Pill Palace" (Níwángōng, 泥丸宮) in the Upper Dāntián, and also at the hidden Yáng in the center of the Real Lower Dāntián (Zhēn Xiàdāntián, 真下丹田). This training is called "the Yì is kept at the Dāntiáns" (Yìshǒu Dāntián, 意守丹田). When this happens, the spirit can stay at its residence (Shénshì, 神室) (Spiritual Residence or Upper Dāntián) and the Qì can be collected and stored at its center (Qìshě, 氣舍) (Qì's Dwelling or Real Lower Dāntián).

In order to have a condensed and focused spirit staying at the "Mud Pill Palace" (Yīnshén, 陰神), you must first regulate your mind. That means you must first calm down your mind and withdraw it from the attractions of surrounding affairs and emotional disturbances. This means regulating your Emotional Monkey Mind, by first regulating your breathing. Breathing is like a banana which is able to lead the monkey Xīn into the cage. When your breathing is calm, the physical body can be relaxed and the mental mind can be peaceful. Therefore, if you are able to breathe softly, gently, slenderly and deeply, the mind can be calmed down. Then the spirit can be focused and condensed at its residence. Once you have reached a profound stage, the spirit and the breathing will mutually depend on and harmonize with each other. This is the initial state of Embracing Singularity (Bàoyī, 抱一).

Mutual Dependence of Shén and Breathing (Shénxí Xiāngyī, 神息相依) (Mǔzǐ Xiāngyī, 母子相依). Once you have reached this stage, you have established a close connection between your Shén and Qì through breathing. This kind of breathing is also called "Cavity Breathing" (Xuéwèi Hūxī, 穴位呼吸) or "Dāntián Breathing" (Dāntián Hūxī, 丹田呼吸), which means breathing with the Shén and Qì staying at their cavities (residences).

Then, you will bring the Shén down from the Upper Dāntián to the Real Lower Dāntián to unite the Shén and Qì together. This is the state of "Mutual Dependence of Spirit and Breathing" (Shénxí Xiāngyī, 神息相依) or "Mutual Dependence of Son and Mother." "Son" represents "Shén" while "Mother" represents "Qì." When this happens, you have traced back to the origin of your life—the Wújí state. Therefore, I have named it "Wújí Breathing" (Wújí Hūxī, 無極呼吸) (breathing with no polarities) or "second brain breathing." In Wújí Breathing there is no discrimination of Yīn and Yáng either in Shén or Qì.

Hold the Breathing to Conceal the Shén and Qì (Bìxí Cángshén Yùnqì, 閉息藏神蘊氣). The key to bringing the Shén down to unite with the Qì is correct breathing. There are two schools of thought on how to do it correctly. One group believes that in order to contain the Shén and Qì at the Real Lower Dāntián, you must inhale deeply and then hold the breath as long as possible while keeping your mind (spirit) there. When you inhale to your maximum and then hold the breath, you are allowing the Shén and Qì to combine to their maximum. It is just like when you push a car. First you inhale deeply to absorb abundant oxygen for the biochemical reaction, then you exhale while pushing. After you exhale to the maximum, you hold the breath so the Qì can manifest in its most extreme and efficient way. Embryonic Breathing is just reversing the process. First, you exhale and relax your body and mind, then you inhale deeply, softly, and slenderly. When the inhalation has reached its maximum, then you hold your breath while keeping your mind at the Real Lower Dāntián. When this happens, the Shén will be condensed and the Qì will be gathered at the Real Lower Dāntián.

Another group of documents argue that "hold the breathing" does not mean the process which actually "stops the breathing." They explain that since the breathing is so slender, gentle, and soft, the breathing is as if it exists without existing. If you really hold your breath, your mental and physical bodies will be tensed. When this happens, the mind can be disturbed and the spirit and the Qì cannot be contained at the Real Lower Dāntián efficiently.

However, from my personal understanding, both sides have their good reasons and theories. The best way of breathing is inhaling slowly, slenderly, softly, and quietly as if the breathing does not exist. However, when you reach the final stage of inhalation, then you hold the breath. Begin with a few seconds only. Only after you have practiced for a long time and feel comfortable and natural holding it, can you then increase the length of time.

Unification of Shén and Qì (Shénqì Xiànghé, 神氣相合). There are two meanings to "Unification of Shén and Qì" (Shénqì Xiànghé, 神氣相合). One is that the mind stays at the Real Lower Dāntián so you are able to return yourself to the origin of life, as explained in the previous sub-section. That means the location where unification takes place is at the Real Lower Dāntián. This is the way of longevity. The other meaning is to conceive a Spiritual Embryo (Shéntāi, 神胎) at the Huángtíng (黃庭). Then this Spiritual Embryo is led upward to reopen "the Third Eye." Naturally, this second meaning is the first step towards reaching enlightenment.

In order to conceive a Spiritual Embryo, you must first learn how to lead the "Fire Qì" (Huǒqì, 火氣) or "Post-Heaven Qì" (Hòutiānqì, 後天氣) from the Middle Dāntián downward, and the "Water Qì" (Shuǐqì, 水氣) or "Pre-Heaven Qì" (Xiāntiānqì, 先天氣) upward, to meet each other at the Huángtíng cavity. This is the process of Kǎn-Lí (坎離) (water-fire). This process, also called "the intercourse of dragon and tiger" (Lónghǔ Jiāogòu, 龍虎交媾), will produce the "Water Mother" (Shuǐmǔ, 水母), which provides life for the Shén to reside and grow.

Therefore, you must also bring your Shén down to the Huángtíng. This Shén is considered the Son. Again this process is called "Mutual Dependence of Mother and Son" (Mǔzǐ Xiāngyī, 母子相依). When this happens, the Spiritual Embryo can be conceived. When this Spiritual Embryo has matured, then it is led upward to the Upper Dāntián for its birth (the reopening of the Third Eye). This is a necessary step for spiritual enlightenment.

To summarize this section, the important key theories and practicing methods are:

1. **To calm down the mind and physical body.** The first step of Embryonic Breathing is to keep the mind in a state of extreme calmness. In order to reach this goal, you withdraw from all of the surrounding emotional attractions, disturbances, and desires. When this happens, you are able to condense your spirit at the Mud Pill Palace at the center of the Upper Dāntián. Then the actions and excitement of the brain will gradually cease and the mind can be calmed, your physical body can be peaceful and relaxed, and you have found the way of Embracing Singularity (Bàoyī, 抱一).
   To further calm the mind and physical body, you should bring your mind down to the Real Lower Dāntián, to lead the body's Qì down to the lower section of the body. The brain cells will not be excited, and the mind can reach a calmer and more peaceful state. *Dào Dé Jīng* (道德經), Chapter 16, said: "Reach the extreme emptiness, and keep the profound calmness."[1] This implies the extreme calmness of the mind and the body. This is the first step in leading the Qì to the Real Lower Dāntián and storing it there.

2. **To condition the Real Lower Dāntián (bio-battery) and improve the capacity for Qì storage.** In order to increase the storage capacity of Qì to a level higher than that of normal people, the Real Lower Dāntián must be conditioned. How to condition the Real Lower Dāntián will be explained briefly in the last section of this chapter. Even though this method is not explained in ancient Embryonic Breathing documents, the method of conditioning

the Real Lower Dāntián has specifically been discussed in Muscle/Tendon Changing and Marrow/Brain Washing Classic. For a more thorough discussion, please refer to the book: *Qìgōng—The Secret of Youth*, published by YMAA Publication Center.

3. **To build up or store the Qì in the Real Lower Dāntián to an abundant level.** This is the process of charging the bio-battery. When Qì in the Real Lower Dāntián is charged to an abundant level, the practices of Muscle/Tendon Changing and Marrow/Brain Washing are possible. The key to storing the Qì to an abundant level is practicing the correct ways of breathing.
4. **To stimulate hormone (Original Essence) production in the Adrenals and Testicles (or Ovaries).** Hormones act as catalysts in the body's biochemical reaction. When the hormone level is properly regulated, the body's biochemical reaction will be smooth and healthy. Naturally, the Qì production will be smooth and abundant. It is well known today that maintaining healthy hormone levels is the key to longevity.
5. **To strengthen the physical body and health (Muscle/Tendon Changing).** When the Qì is abundantly stored in the Real Lower Dāntián, the Qì in the eight vessels (Bāmài, 八脈) will be highly charged as well. Then the Qì circulation in the Twelve Primary Qì Channels (Shíèrjīng, 十二經) can be regulated efficiently. This is the crucial key to maintaining and conditioning our physical bodies.
6. **For longevity and enlightenment (Marrow/Brain Washing).** When abundant Qì is led inward to the bone marrow, the production of blood cells from the marrow will be smooth and healthy. Plenty of healthy blood cells in the body is the key to slowing the aging process. This is because blood cells are the main carriers of oxygen and nutrition for the body's metabolism. In addition, when the abundant Qì is led upward through the spinal cord (Chōngmài, 衝脈) to nourish the brain, the Spirit of Vitality can be raised and the Third Eye (Tiānyǎn, 天眼) can be reopened. This is the goal of Buddhahood or enlightenment in Buddhist and Daoist society.

References

1. 《道德經・十六章》：〝致虛極，守靜篤。〞

Part III

Practice of Embryonic Breathing

CHAPTER 5

Practice of Embryonic Breathing

5.1 INTRODUCTION (JIÈSHÀO, 介紹)

From the previous chapters, we have recognized the importance of Embryonic Breathing in Nèidān (內丹) (Internal Elixir) Qìgōng practice. It does not matter what the goal of your practice is, whether health, longevity, or spiritual enlightenment—without Embryonic Breathing, your achievement will be shallow, if not impossible.

In this chapter, I would like, based on my past fifteen years of practice in Embryonic Breathing and continuous reading and pondering of hundreds of ancient documents, to introduce a practical and achievable Embryonic Breathing method for interested Qìgōng practitioners in today's society. You should understand that almost all of the available documents existing today were revealed to the public only since the 1980s. When you practice, you must use your logical mind and wise judgment to make decisions. Often the same practice can generate different effects and results for different people. Some of the practices may be appropriate for some and not for others. Therefore, you must study the theory behind the practice and adjust the methods recommended.

Before we enter the practice, I must emphasize one more thing, namely that the entire Embryonic Breathing practice occurs through self-inner-observation (Nèishì, 內視), or "self-inner-feeling." This feeling is the way that your mind communicates with your physical body, Qì, and Shén. This feeling can be shallow or profound, depending on how much you are able to calm down your mind and feel it. The level of feeling is unlimited, and normally follows the depth of your mind and awareness. Naturally, wrong feeling or mental perception can also lead you into fascination, illusion, and imagination (Rùmó, 入魔). These false and unrealistic feelings can lead you to a state of emotional disturbance, and further away from the correct practice of Qì cultivation (Zǒuhuǒ, 走火).

Therefore, when you practice, it is very important that you should not have an ego or even set up a plan for your progress. This will only generate a serious disturbance in your mind. It can also cause Qì stagnation. If you are not sure of the correct method, it is better to learn from an experienced teacher. Often, a couple of sentences of guidance will lead you to the correct path. However, honestly speaking, there are very few such experienced practitioners existing today.

When you read this chapter, be logical, patient, and understanding. Always go back to the ancient documents, study and ponder them. Often, you will find a nice, new, valuable clue that can unravel your confusion.

In the next section, I will summarize the important preparations, both physical and psychological. The actual practice will be discussed in Section 3.

5.2 Preparation for Embryonic Breathing (Tāixí Liànxí Zhī Zhǔnbèi, 胎息練習之準備)

The preparation for Embryonic Breathing can be divided into two parts, the physical and psychological. Usually, we can see that it is easy to understand the theory of the practice. However, it is not easy to carry out the practical side. Understanding can be quick, but the practice will take a great deal of patience and self-conquering. If you expect to see rapid results, it is more likely that you will quit after just a few weeks or months. Therefore, the psychological preparation is more important than the physical.

Physical Preparation

1. **Sitting Upright.** When you practice Embryonic Breathing, the best physical position is sitting upright (Figure 5–1). When you sit upright, it is easier for you to find your central energy line. Your mind will also be able to recognize the top and the bottom so that the locations of Upper Dāntián and Real Lower Dāntián can be registered by the mind easily. Naturally, there is no danger when you practice Embryonic Breathing, as long as you are not holding your breath. When you practice holding the breath, your conscious mind must be there to direct the practice, and be aware of what is happening; otherwise your physical body can tense up very easily.

   If you find that you cannot sit upright easily and the lower back tightens, it may be a good idea to find a support for your lower back (Figure 5–2). Often an arm-rest couch can provide you with a very relaxed position for your practice (Figure 5–3).

2. **Crossing Legs.** To prevent the Qì flowing downward to the legs, the best position for your legs is bending the hip joints with crossed legs. However, if you are a beginner, this can cause numbness of your legs and thus disturb your calm and concentrated mind for practice. Therefore, if you sit on a cushion, be sure it is of the proper height, depending on your personal needs. Try sitting on it for ten minutes and see whether you are still comfortable with it. You should be able to sit for thirty minutes without experiencing any discomfort.

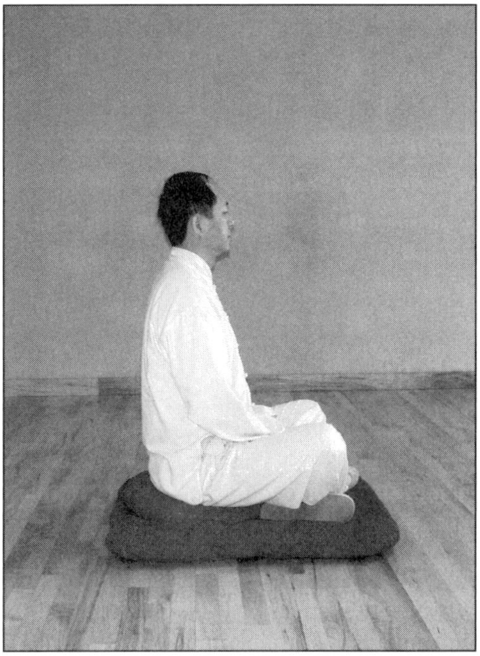

Figure 5-1. Sitting Meditation Posture

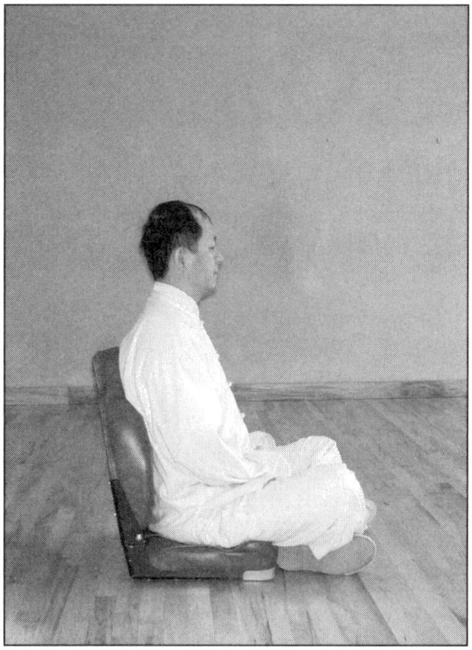

Figure 5-2. Sitting Meditation on a Fishing Chair

In addition, numbness of the legs can be caused by the floor you are sitting on. If the floor is hard, such as wood or concrete, then the pressure on your lower legs will be increased, causing numbness of the lower legs. Instead, sit on a piece of soft material (Figure 5-4). However, you should not use artificial material such as polyester, which tends to accumulate a lot of static charge in winter time. Natural materials such as cotton or silk are always the best, because our bodies have already grown used to them since the beginning of human history. Furthermore, you should keep your legs a short distance apart at the shin area. In this case, the downward pressure from the upper leg on the lower one can be avoided. This will make your sitting much more comfortable.

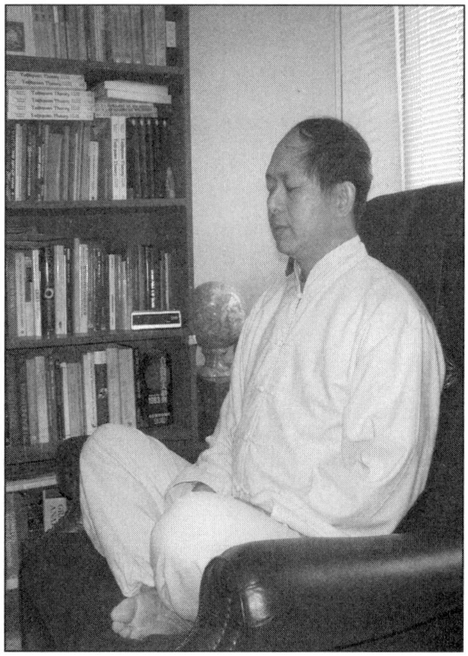

Figure 5-3. Sitting Meditation on a Couch

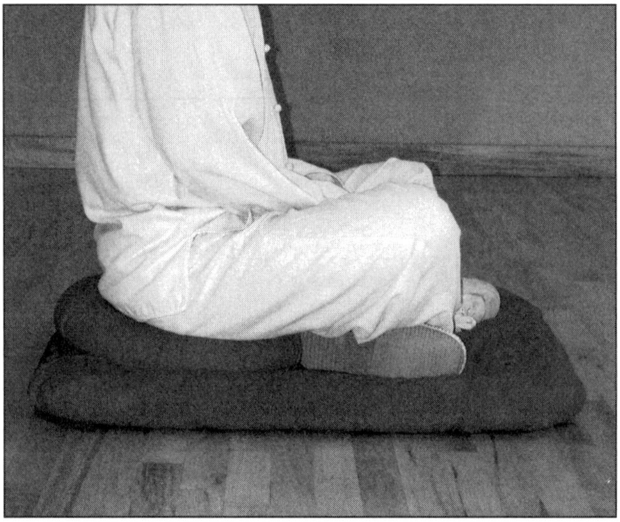

Figure 5-4. Mat on a Meditation Cushion

3. **Lying Down Position.** You may practice Embryonic Breathing lying down without danger. When you practice Embryonic Breathing, your mind is at the Upper and Real Lower Dāntián. You are not using your mind to lead the Qì to circulate in your body. In this case, you are not "driving" your Qì, rather you are simply charging your battery while parked. However, when you practice, you should not lie on your side. The face-up reclining position is the best. If you lie on your side, you will lose your feeling of balance. Not only that, lying sideways can cause uneven tension on both sides of the body.

   It is important to recognize that when you practice Embryonic Breathing in a lying down position, you will lose the clear feeling of the position of Upper Dāntián and Real Lower Dāntián, unless you have already become proficient in your practice. Not only that, it is easier for you to fall asleep if you practice Embryonic Breathing in this position. There is no danger, but if you fall asleep, your progress will also be shallow, and naturally you will lose the purpose of practice. Nevertheless, it will be a good way of falling asleep if that is what you wish to do. Using Embryonic Breathing to lead the Qì to the central energy line will make your sleeping more efficient and effective, because right before you fall asleep, your mind has already become calm and the Qì has already been led to its center.

4. **Practicing Environments.** When you practice, you should keep yourself in a quiet and comfortable room. Place a sign on the door, silence your telephone, keep the place dark, so your mind will not be disturbed. The air circulation and temperature are also important, as stagnant air and improper temperature or humidity can cause discomfort, which can distract your mind.

5. **Diet.** When your stomach is full or empty, do not practice. A couple of cookies or a glass of milk will make your stomach comfortable and cooperate with your mind. Concerning the diet for Embryonic Breathing, normally too much red meat will make your mind disturbed easily. Absorbing protein from fish, chicken, and soy beans is the best. If you practice Embryonic Breathing in the wintertime, you may eat more meat than in the summertime, when it is better if you eat more fruit and vegetables. This is because the Qì in your body is already Yáng in summertime. If you eat more red meat, your body will become too Yáng and the mind will be disturbed more easily. In wintertime, you may eat more fish and chicken so you have more protein for your immune system.
6. **Clothes.** The best way of practicing Embryonic Breathing is naked. In this case, there is no restrictive feeling of your physical body. Naturally, it is not easy to be naked when you meditate in the wintertime. In this case, you should wear loose clothes. When practicing Embryonic Breathing in the wintertime, since the mind is calm at the Dāntián and the body is relaxed, the Guardian Qì (Wèiqì, 衛氣) will be weaker, and you may catch cold easily.

Psychological Preparation. It is necessary to cultivate a mind that is peaceful and calm, able to recognize the fact and the truth of practice. Otherwise your mind will be disturbed, confused and scattered, and your accomplishment will be shallow. Therefore, before beginning the practice, you must have a clear understanding psychologically. Following are the common hindrances to success.

1. **Lack of Confidence.** Usually, for a beginner, the biggest drawback is lack of confidence. You are not sure you are able to accomplish your goal. You don't trust yourself that you can conquer your lazy mind and keep up the practice till the end. You don't know whether the theory and the practice methods are correct. The way of handling these problems is first answering such questions as: Why do you want to practice Embryonic Breathing? How much do you really want to practice? Do you know the theory and practice methods clearly? What do you expect to accomplish in the long run? If you don't have answers for these questions, then you need to reconsider your motives.
2. **Confused About Training.** Often, confusion arises, especially when you encounter some experiences which you don't understand or which are not explained in the book. In this case, you must know the theory clearly. You should know there are differences in each individual's Qì status, emotional mind, and lifestyle. Therefore, it is not easy to follow the book exactly. You need to adjust the methods and learn to adopt them in your life and

personality. Confusion can also be caused by lack of confidence or disturbances of your emotional mind.

3. **Disturbed Emotional Monkey Mind.** Emotional disturbances are one of the major hindrances to your practice. That is why there are so many documents discussing how to regulate your mind and spirit. If you cannot overcome serious emotional disturbances which always try to lead your mind away from concentration, then you will achieve nothingness. The emotional mind includes the seven passions and six desires (Qīqíng Liùyù, 七情六慾). The seven passions are happiness (Xǐ, 喜), anger (Nù, 怒), sorrow (Āi, 哀), joy (Lè, 樂), love (Ài, 愛), hate (Hèn, 恨), and lust (Yù, 慾). The desires are generated from the six roots which are the eyes, ears, nose, tongue, body, and mind (Xīn, 心). In addition, you must train yourself until you have a neutral mind that can be separated from the four emptinesses of earth, water, fire, and wind (Sìdà Jiēkōng, 四大皆空) (i.e., the material world).

   The first, unavoidable step in practicing Embryonic Breathing is to regulate your emotional mind. Naturally, this is not an easy task, especially in lay society. If your emotional mind cannot be regulated, then your Shén cannot be steady and stay at its residence at peace. In this case, the Qì will also be led away from its residence, the Real Lower Dāntián, and the accomplishments of the practice will be empty.

   When you practice, you should not force yourself. This will trigger the action of your emotional mind. At the beginning, you may get excited. However, once the honeymoon period is over, then it becomes more difficult. Only if you can enjoy sitting for a long time can your mind be calm. Therefore, psychologically, you must prepare yourself to enjoy the sitting.

   You should not set goals, as they include desire and this will trigger your emotional mind. Once you set goals, then you will have expectations and ego, and your emotional mind will be disturbed. Simply do it and enjoy it, focus on the present, and don't permit the possibility of failure to defeat you into giving up your efforts. Continue pondering and correct yourself onto the right path of practice. Follow the recommended practice procedures and stay with them. According to my personal teaching experience in Embryonic Breathing over more than ten years, I am confident that these procedures work, and will lead you gradually into the profound level of practice.

5.3. Practice of Embryonic Breathing (Tāixí Zhī Liànxí, 胎息之練習)

In this section, we will discuss the method of practicing Embryonic Breathing. First, your mind must be able to locate the Upper Dāntián and the Real Lower Dāntián. Next, you learn to condense the spirit to a higher level of focus, and to produce more abundant Qì. Then, we discuss how to lead the spirit and the Qì to their residences and keep them there. Finally, you unite the spirit and the Qì at the Real Lower Dāntián and store the Qì there to an abundant level.

We will briefly discuss the method of the Qì's Kǎn-Lí, and how to unite it with the Shén at the Huángtíng (黃庭) so the Spiritual Embryo can be conceived. The method of leading the Qì upward to nourish the brain and Shén will be discussed in the book *QìGōng—Grand Circulation for Spiritual Enlightenment.*

Timing of Practice. The best times for practicing, according to the documents, are dawn, noon, dusk, and midnight. However, this is not easy in today's lifestyle. I recommend the times of dawn and right before you go to sleep. If your schedule allows it and you normally take a nap, then you should use this time to practice Embryonic Breathing. This is because the Qì status in your body is the most Yáng during the early afternoon. If you practice Embryonic Breathing, you will be able to lead the surplus Qì inward for storage.

When your mind and body have reached a very calm, peaceful, and relaxed state, you may simply allow yourself to fall asleep. Remember that practicing Embryonic Breathing is not the same as other Nèidān meditation practices in which you are using your mind to lead the Qì. In Nèidān practice, you should not fall asleep since it will cause the Qì to enter the wrong path. However, when you practice Embryonic Breathing, you are not using your mind to lead the Qì, so falling sleep will not cause you any problem.

However, you should not be restricted to the timings suggested. According to some documents, once you have mastered the keys to Embryonic Breathing, you can practice anytime and anywhere.

Orientation of Practice. When you practice Embryonic Breathing, you should take advantage of the natural Qì, the most significant of which are the Qì of the sun, the moon, and the earth's magnetic field. Therefore, if possible, choose your meditation orientation accordingly (Table 4–1). If you wish to know more about this subject, please refer to the book: *The Root of Chinese Qìgōng*, published by YMAA Publication Center.

Timing	Purpose	Orientation	Natural Qì Source
Dawn	Nourishing	Face East	Sun
	Retreating*	Face West	Sun
Noon	To Calm Down	Any Direction	--
Dusk	Prevent Retreating	Face East	Sun
	Retreating	Face West	Sun
Night†	Nourishing	Face South	Earth's Magnetic Field
	Retreating	Face North	Earth's Magnetic Field

*Retreating means to remove some Qì away from your body so the body can be regulated into being more Yīn.

†If you wish to absorb the Qì from the moon, you should meditate facing the moon two to three days before it is full. After the full moon this is not recommended, since the moon can then drain your Qì away.

Table 4-1. Meditation Orientations and Timings

Recognizing the Yīn Center of the Upper Dāntián and the Yáng Center of the Real Lower Dāntián (Shàngdāntián Yīnhéxīn Yǔ Xiàdāntián Yánghéxīn Zhī Rènshí, 上丹田陰核心與下丹田陽核心之認識) (Xuéwèi Rèntóng, 穴位認同). The first step of Embryonic Breathing is to recognize the Yīn center of the Upper Dāntián (Yīnshén, 陰神) and the Yáng center of the Real Lower Dāntián (Yángquán, 陽泉). As explained before, the upper Yīn center is able to stabilize and control the status of Yángshén's manifestation (Yángshén, 陽神) while the lower Yáng center is the origin of the Yīn water's production (Yīnshuǐ, 陰水) (Figure 2–20). The recognition of these two centers must be accomplished through the self-inner-feeling, which is the only way to lead your Shén and Qì to these centers and keep them there.

The exact location of the Yīn center in the Upper Dāntián (Shàngdāntián, 上丹田) is at the central bottom of the Spiritual Valley (Shéngǔ, 神谷) (Figure 3–2) where the pineal and pituitary glands are located. This is the center of the Mud Pill Palace (Níwángōng, 泥丸宮) and of the spiritual residence (Shénshì, 神室) (Upper Dāntián). It is located at the central point of the line connecting the top part of the two ears, and also the central point of the line connecting the Yìntáng (M-HN-3) (印堂) and Qiángjiān (Gv-18) (強間), which is to say it is located where these two lines intersect. To recognize this point through feeling, you must first rid yourself of all emotional disturbances and also the external attractions of your mind. In this case, your mind will be clear and easily search for the location. If you search for it sincerely, it will take only a few days for you to recognize the point.

The exact location of the Yáng center in the Real Lower Dāntián (Zhēn Xiàdāntián, 真下丹田) is where the center of the large and small intestines is located, namely a couple of inches above the physical center of gravity. In fact, the entire digestive system constitutes the "Real Lower Dāntián." If you are able to find the center of this system, then you are able to keep the Qì there and store it to an abundant level. The Yáng center is located behind the Yīnjiāo (Co-7) (陰交) and in front of the cavity Shíqīzhuīxià (M-BW-25) (十七椎下) (below the 17th Vertebrae). In fact, it is at the center of these two cavities. Again, if you search for this point when you meditate, you will be able to find it in just a few days or weeks.

Condensing the Shén and Condensing the Qì to their Centers (Regulating the Mind and Spirit, Regulating the Qì) (Tiáoxīn, 調心) (Tiáoshén, 調神) (Tiáoqì, 調氣). After you have located the exact site of the Yīn center in the Upper Dāntián, then you will learn how to raise the spirit and keep it there. Then calm down your emotional mind (Xīn, 心) and cease outside distractions and material attractions. This will enable you to concentrate on raising your spirit and condensing it at the Yīn spiritual center. If you have difficulty reaching this goal, simply pay attention to your respiration. Regarding the inhalation, keep it soft, slender, and long. When you exhale, simply be natural and allow the carbon dioxide to be released by itself. In this case, your mind will be stabilized and then calm. Once you have achieved this, then use your mind to focus your spirit at the Yīn spiritual center. When this happens, the Yáng spirit (陽神) (manifestation of Qì by the spirit) can be controlled. Remember, on one hand you aim to raise your spirit to a high level, but on the other, you want to govern it so it can come under the control of the Yīn spirit.

To condense the Shén at this Yīn spiritual center, simply imagine your head as a ball, with the Mud Pill Palace (Níwángōng, 泥丸宮) at the center. Inhale deeply, using Reversed Abdominal Breathing (Nìhūxī, 逆呼吸), while gently holding up the Huìyīn (Co-1) or anus. The breathing must be soft and slender. While you are doing so, imagine that the ball is shrinking and condensing inward to the Mud Pill Palace. When you exhale, simply relax and allow the abdomen and Huìyīn area to return to their normal state. That means you should pay more attention to the inhalation. In this case, the Yì (Wisdom Mind) of inhalation is strong, which can therefore lead the Shén and Qì inward to condense at their centers.

Conditioning the Bio-battery (Real Lower Dāntián) (Zhēn Xiàdāntián Zhī Gǎiliáng, 真下丹田之改良). In order to store a large quantity of Qì in the Real Lower Dāntián, the first step is to condition it, so as to improve capability, storage potential (efficiency), and capacity. If you have a bio-battery which is only the same as other normal people, then how can you expect your Qì storage to be higher than others?

From the ancient *Muscle/Tendon Changing and Marrow/Brain Washing Classic* (*Yìjīnjīng, Xǐsuǐjīng*; 易筋經・洗髓經), it is recognized that the most efficient way of conditioning this bio-battery (False and Real Lower Dāntiáns) is through massage and stimulation. Massage gets rid of the fat hidden within so the circulation can be smoother, and stimulation will condition the sensitivity of the nerves in the area so they are able to handle a larger quantity of Qì stored there. The entire conditioning process is long and needs a great deal of training and patience. You must clearly understand the theory behind the conditioning. It is impossible to explain the entire conditioning process here. If you wish to know more about this training, please refer to the book: *Qìgōng—The Secret of Youth*, published by YMAA Publication Center.

Increase the Quantity of Qì (Qìliàng Zhī Jiāqiáng, 氣量之加強). There are various ways of producing extra Qì at the Lower Dāntián. For example, you may use herbs to increase the quantity of Qì in the body, or use massage methods to convert the fat at the Lower Dāntián area into Qì. You may also use the abdomen's up-and-down movements with the coordination of breathing.

When using herbs, you must find herbal stores that have all the ingredients required. However, it is not easy to find these herbs other than in Asia such as Táiwān, Hong Kong, and China. Even then, the cost of the herbs can be very high, and some special ingredients may not be available due to their seldom being used.

If you use massage methods, you will need a massage partner. In addition, both of you must know the correct massage techniques and how to regulate the power used at each step. If you use breathing techniques, you must know the "how" and "why," so your practice can be effective without causing problems. If you wish to know more about using herbal prescriptions and massage methods to increase the quantity of Qì, again please refer to the book: *Qìgōng—The Secret of Youth*.

Here, I would like to introduce the known methods of breathing that are able to increase the quantity of Qì in your body. There are two methods which have commonly been used by Buddhist and Daoist monks in the past. As long you know the theory and practice patiently, with these two methods you will be able to convert the fat stored at the abdominal area into extra Qì in your body. The theory of these two breathing methods has been introduced in previous chapters. They are Normal Abdominal Breathing (Zhèng Fùhūxī, 正腹呼吸) (Buddhist Breathing) and Reversed Abdominal Breathing (Fǎn, Nì Fùhūxī; 反・逆腹呼吸) (Daoist Breathing).

A. **Normal Abdominal Breathing (Buddhist Breathing)** (Zhèng Fùhūxī, 正腹呼吸) (Fójiā Hūxī, 佛家呼吸). In Normal Abdominal Breathing, when you inhale, the abdomen is gently pushed out, and when you exhale, the abdomen is withdrawn (Figures 5-5 and 5-6). In order to fill up the Qì to an abundant level in the lower abdominal area (Elixir Furnace or Elixir Field), when you inhale you should also gently push out your Huìyīn (Co-1) cavity (or anus), and when you exhale you hold it up gently. Remember, you should not tense this area during either inhalation or exhalation, unless you are doing some special training such as Hard Qìgōng. When you do so, you are converting the food essence (fat) into Qì through the abdominal movements.

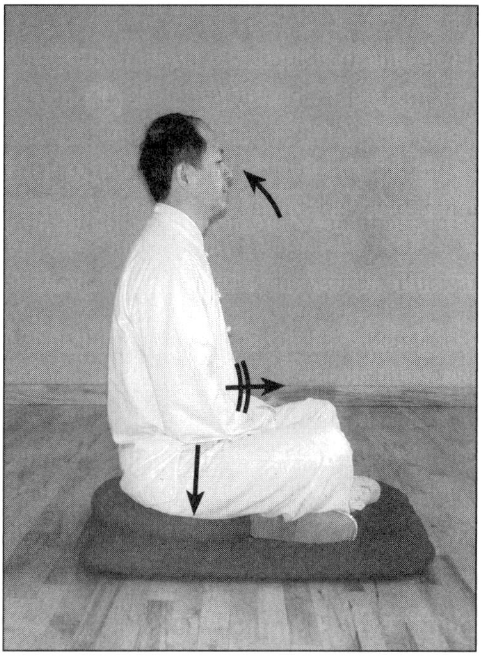

Figure 5-5. Normal Abdominal Breathing (Inhalation)

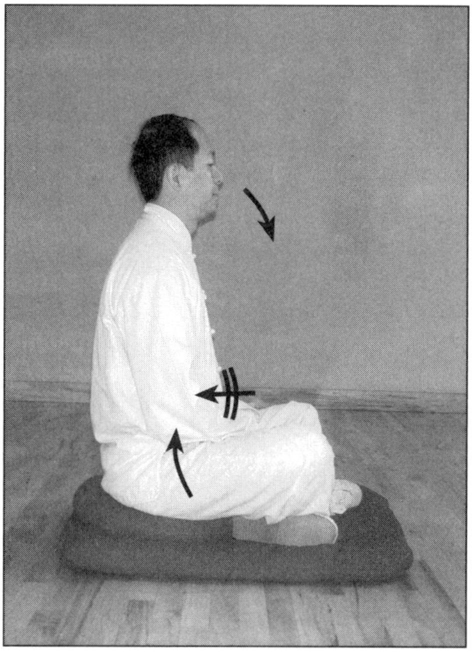

Figure 5-6. Normal Abdominal Breathing (Exhalation)

Not only that, through the movements of the abdomen and the Huìyīn cavity, the Original Essence (Yuánjīng, 元精) (Hormone) in the pancreas (islets of Langerhans) and gonads (sex glands) will also be produced.

After you have practiced for a few weeks, you will start to experience some warm feeling and even some trembling at the abdominal area. This signals the increase of the Qì in this area.

As a beginner, you should practice Normal Abdominal Breathing for at least six months until your mind is able to control the muscles around the abdominal area efficiently. Remember this kind of breathing is more relaxing and natural, and so will not cause any troublesome tension at the stomach area.

B. Reverse Abdominal Breathing (Daoist Breathing) (Fǎn Fùhūxī, 反腹呼吸) (Nì Fùhūxī, 逆腹呼吸) (Dàojiā Hūxī, 道家呼吸). After you have practiced Normal Abdominal Breathing for at least six months, then you may proceed to Reverse Abdominal Breathing. In Reverse Abdominal Breathing, when you inhale, the abdomen is gently pulled inward, and when you exhale, the abdomen is gently pushed outward (Figures 5-7 and 5-8). Again, the coordination of the Huìyīn (Co-1) cavity (or anus) is very important. The Huìyīn

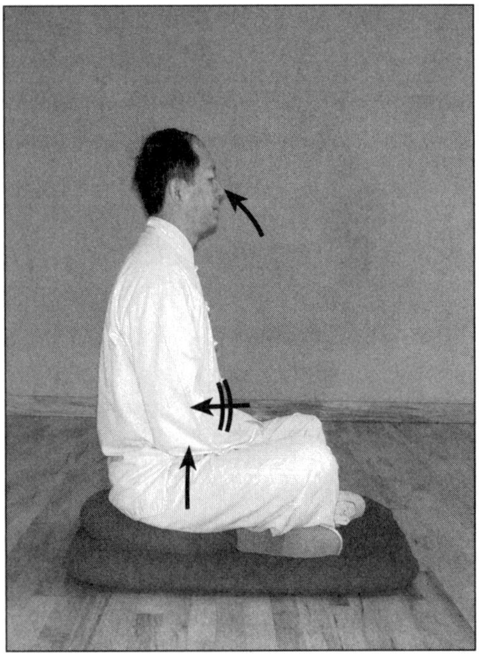

Figure 5-7. Reverse Abdominal Breathing (Inhalation)

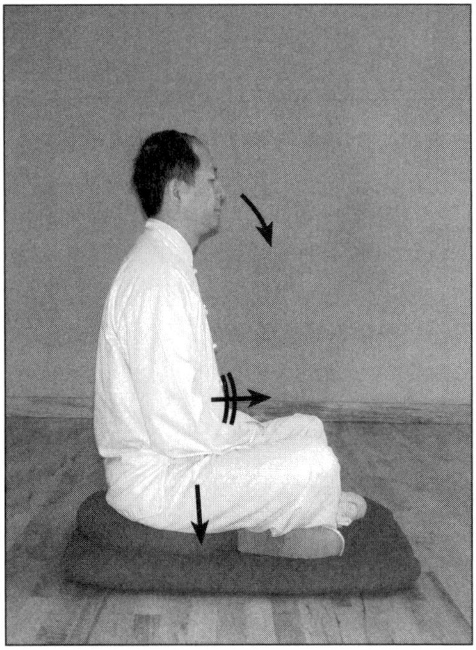

Figure 5-8. Reverse Abdominal Breathing (Exhalation)

cavity is a major gate that regulates the four Yīn vessels, and therefore controls the Qì status of the body. Again, you should not tense this area during either inhalation or exhalation unless you are doing some special training such as Hard Qìgōng. Traditionally, a master would not reveal this secret of Huìyīn control to any student until he was completely trusted by the master.

Often, a Qìgōng or martial arts beginner encounters the problem of tightness in the abdominal area. The reason for this is that when you inhale in Reverse Abdominal Breathing, the diaphragm is pulling downward while the abdominal area is withdrawing. This can generate tension in the stomach area. To reduce this problem, you must already have mastered the skill of Normal Abdominal Breathing and be able to control the abdominal muscles efficiently. In addition, you may start on a small scale with Reverse Abdominal Breathing, and only once you can control the abdominal muscles efficiently, can you then increase to a larger scale of abdominal movement. Naturally, this will take time.

Embryonic Breathing (Cavity Breathing) (Wújí Breathing) (Tāixí, 胎息) (Xuéwèixí, 穴位息) (Wújíxí, 無極息). The above two breathing techniques enable you to produce more Qì in your body. However, if you do not know how to store the extra Qì in the Real Lower Dāntián (bio-battery), this extra Qì will be led to the physical body and manifested (consumed). To store the Qì to an abundant level, you need the method of Embryonic Breathing.

In order to store the Qì in the human bio-battery, you must first recognize the center of the Real Lower Dāntián through feeling correctly and learning to keep your mind there. When your mind is in the Real Lower Dāntián, the Qì will not be led away from its residence. To conserve Qì by keeping the mind at the Real Lower Dāntián (Yìshǒu Dāntián, 意守丹田) is the crucial key of success.

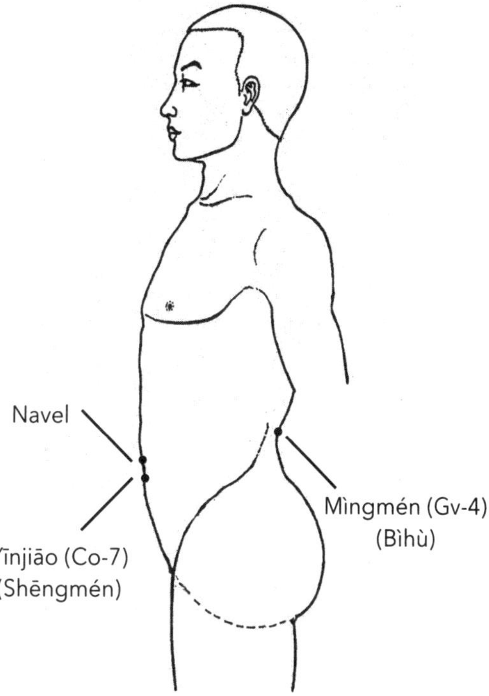

Figure 5-9. Shēgmēn (the Door of Life) and Bìhù (the Closed Door)

The way to keep the mind at the Real Lower Dāntián, so the Qì can be led there, is through the movement of the front abdominal area and the lower back area at the same time. The front abdominal area (Navel or Yīnjiāo cavity) is called "Shēngmén" (生門), which means "the door of life," while the rear lower back area is called "Bìhù" (閉戶) or "Mìhù" (密戶), meaning "the closed door," which implies the Mìngmén (Gv-4) (命門) cavity between L2 and L3 (Figure 5–9). Through this balanced front-and-back movement, you are able to locate the center (Yáng water) easily. Naturally, your mind will be at these two front and back places at the beginning. However, after you have practiced for a period of time and have reached the stage of "regulating without regulating," the mind will be at the center easily.

That means when you practice Embryonic Breathing, the first step is to find the above two doors and move them up and down at the same time. Naturally, extra Qì will be produced at both the front and the rear. While you are doing so, you must also coordinate with the up-down movements of the Huìyīn (Co-1) (會陰) or anus. Soon you will feel the Qì in the entire Girdle Vessel expanding and withdrawing at the same time (Figure 5–10).

The most amazing part of the practice is that, through these movements, the production hormones—insulin from the Islets of Langerhans in the pancreas, DHEA (dehydroepiandrosterone) in the adrenal glands, and testosterone (male) and estrogen and progesterone (female) in the sex glands—can be regulated and possibly increased. This is due to the stimulation of the glands through the exercises.

In addition, when you practice Embryonic Breathing, other than placing your mind at the Yáng center of the Real Lower Dāntián, you must also place your mind at the Yīn center of the Upper Dāntián. You should remember that the Upper Dāntián and the Real Lower Dāntián are the Two Poles of the central energy line. They correspond and synchronize with each other simultaneously. Though they are two places, they are the two faces of the same thing and cannot be separated. Remember, the Shén and the Qì are just like son and mother which cannot and should not be separated when you practice Embryonic Breathing.

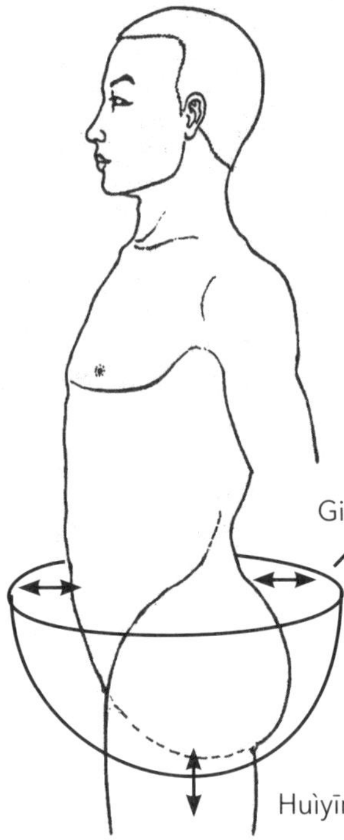

Figure 5-10. Embryonic Breathing

When this happens, due to the mind concentrating at the Yīn center of the Upper Dāntián, the production of melatonin (pineal gland) and growth hormone (pituitary gland) will also be regulated and increased. With these hormones, all of the biochemical reactions will become smooth and the metabolism of the body can be regulated and improved.

The final stage of Embryonic Breathing is to bring the Shén downward to the Real Lower Dāntián, so the Shén and Qì can be united at the Real Lower Dāntián. When this happens, the Qì can stay at its residence and be stored to a very high level. This is called "mutual harmonization or unification of Shén and Qì" (Shénqì Xiànghé, 神氣相合). In this case, the two Poles have unified and become a singularity—the Wújí state, the beginning of life. That is why I call this stage of Embryonic Breathing "Wújí Breathing" (Wújíxí, 無極息). Naturally, the way of leading the Shén down to the Real Lower Dāntián is through the concentrated mind with the coordination of breathing.

Two Ways of Leading the Qì and Shén to the Real Lower Dāntián. There are two possible ways of breathing that allow you to lead the Qì and Shén to the Real Lower Dāntián for effective unification. When the Qì is raised up to the brain, the Shén will be excited and the mind will become scattered. Consequently, the heartbeat will quicken and blood pressure will rise. This is because when the Shén is raised up, the manifestation of the Qì will be enhanced. However, if the Qì is led downward to the Real Lower Dāntián, then the Qì will stay at its residence and be conserved. When this happens, the mind can be calmed and relaxed. This will result in the cooling of the physical body and lowering of the blood pressure. When the Qì is led down, then the Shén can also be led down by the calm mind.

Buddhist Way: Inhale deeply while using the mind to lead the Qì downward through the Thrusting Vessel (central energy line) to the Real Lower Dāntián, and then, while keeping the mind there, exhale. Naturally, when you inhale, the abdomen is expanding while the Huìyīn cavity (or anus) is gently pushing downward. When you exhale, simply relax the abdominal area and Huìyīn (or anus) and allow them to return to the normal level naturally (Figure 5–11). When this happens, the Qì can be led down significantly and stay at its residence. The more you practice, the faster you are able to make it happen. This kind of breathing technique can be used to lower the blood pressure, ease the excited mind (mental body), and slow the heartbeat. This Buddhist way of breathing can be very effective to relax you both mentally and physically.

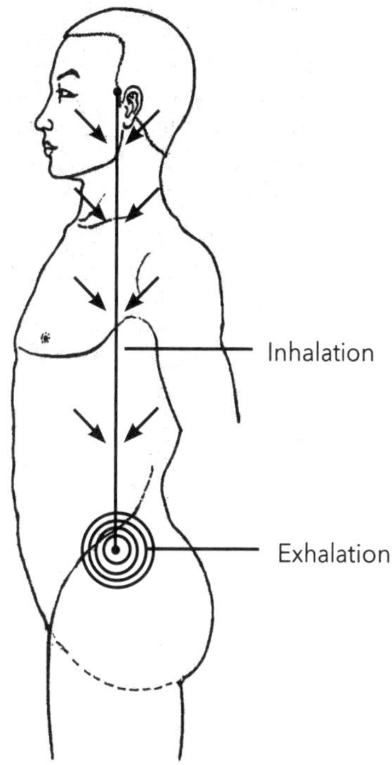

Figure 5-11. The Buddhist Way of Leading the Qì Down to the Real Lower Dāntián

Daoist Way: First, you inhale to condense the Qì inward to the center. Naturally, while you are doing so, you must also withdraw your abdominal area and hold up your Huìyīn cavity. In this case, you are shrinking the Guardian Qì (Wèiqì, 衛氣) and enhancing the Marrow Qì (Suǐqì, 髓氣). Once the Qì is led to the central energy line (Thrusting Vessel or spinal cord), exhale deeply, gently pushing out your abdomen and Huìyīn, and lead the Qì downward through the central energy line (Figure 5–12). In this way, Qì can also be stored at the Real Lower Dāntián. This Daoist way can be used to effectively cool down the excitement of the physical body.

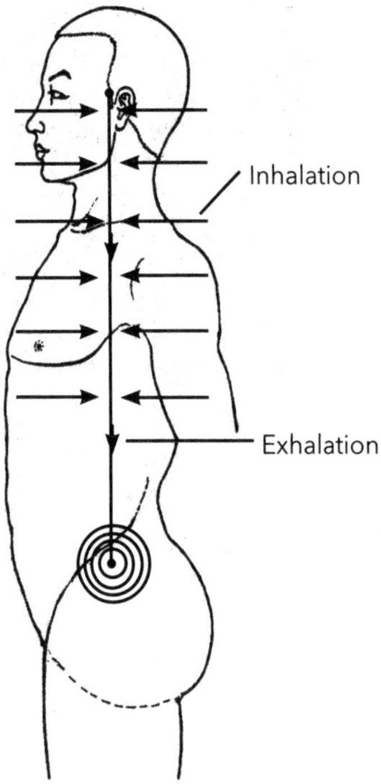

Figure 5-12. The Daoist Way of Leading the Qì Down to the Real Lower Dāntián

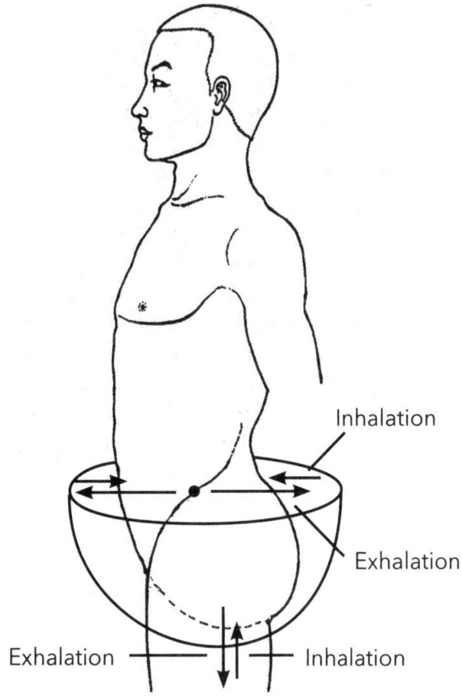

Figure 5-13. Girdle Vessel Breathing

Two Suggested Approaches:

1. Buddhist way first and then Daoist: This helps you to calm down the mind and Shén first and then use the calmed mind to lead the Qì inward.
2. Daoist way first and then Buddhist: This helps you to lead the Qì inward first to calm down the physical body and then calm down the mind.

Each of these approaches has its advantages and disadvantages. It also depends on each individual's preferences.

Once you can lead the Qì down and inward to store it at the Real Lower Dāntián, you must also be able to maintain your mind there. In this case, you are doing Embryonic Breathing. However, this Embryonic Breathing can be divided again into two practices. One is classified as Yáng and is called "Girdle Vessel Breathing" (Dàimàixí, 帶脈息) and the other one is classified as Yīn and is called "Marrow Breathing" (Suǐxí, 髓息). Since the Qì is led laterally, when you practice these two breathing techniques it is most effective if you use the Reverse Abdominal Breathing technique (Daoist breathing) instead of the Normal Abdominal Breathing Technique (Buddhist breathing).

Girdle Vessel Breathing (Dàimàixí, 帶脈息). In this form of breathing, you must concentrate your mind strongly on the exhalation. That means when you exhale, the breath is long, slender, and firmly leading the Qì outwards around the Girdle Vessel. Naturally, you are also gently pushing your abdomen out and Huìyīn (or anus) downward at the same time (Figure 5–13). The mind should continue to lead the Qì out a few feet or even a few yards horizontally. When this happens, the body is turning more Yáng and the entire body's Guardian Qì is also expanding. If you wish to enhance the expansion of Qì, once you have reached your maximum in your exhalation, simply hold your breath for a few seconds and allow the Qì to reach the place the mind wishes for. If you wish to strengthen this expansive Qì even more, while you are exhaling, make the sound "Hā" (哈), and when your exhalation has reached to its limit, hold your breath for a few seconds.

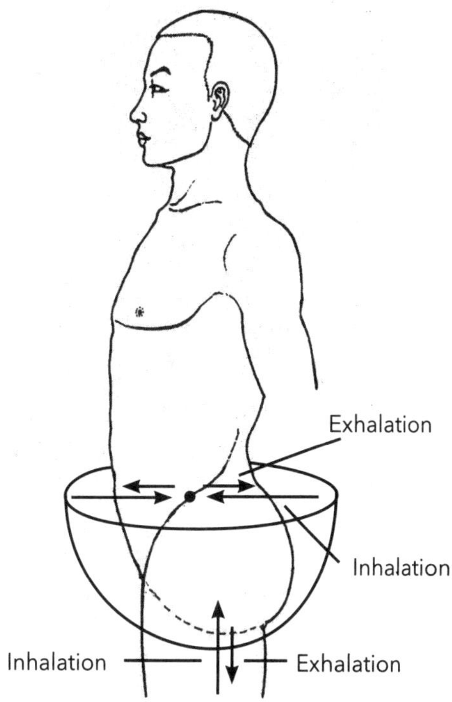

Figure 5-14. Marrow Breathing

When you inhale, simply relax and allow the abdomen and Huìyīn areas to return to their normal state.

The Qì manifestation in the Girdle Vessel is classified as Yáng, since it can make your body and mind Yáng. The Qì manifestation in the Thrusting Vessel is classified as Yīn since it is able to calm down your physical body and mind. Therefore, if you use Girdle Vessel Breathing, you can change the manifestation of your body's Qì from Yīn to Yáng. This means you can use this technique to strengthen your Guardian Qì and rid yourself of the feeling of cold or chill. This kind of practice is suitable for the wintertime, or when you are depressed. Naturally, you are consuming your Qì as well.

Marrow Breathing (Suǐxí, 髓息). In this breathing, you must concentrate your mind strongly on the inhalation. That means when you inhale, the breathing is long, slender, and firmly leading the Qì inward around the Girdle Vessel. Naturally, you are also drawing your abdomen in and Huìyīn (or anus) upward at the same time (Figure 5–14). The mind should continue to lead the Qì in until it has reached the Yīn center of the Real Lower Dāntián. Naturally, when this happens, the body is turning more Yīn and the entire body's Guardian Qì is shrinking. If you wish to lead the Qì in more effectively and keep it at the Real Lower Dāntián for storage, once you have reached your maximum in your inhalation, simply hold your breath for a few seconds and allow the Qì to reach to the Yáng center within the Yīn. When you exhale, simply relax and allow the abdomen and Huìyīn areas to return to their normal state.

When you do this, you are storing the Qì at the Real Lower Dāntián and also leading the Qì to the bone marrow for washing. Naturally, this will also make your body's Guardian Qì shrink, thus weakening your immune system against the cold. Therefore, you should not practice this in wintertime. Instead, you may start it in spring and enhance the practice in the summer. When the fall comes, you must change the practice to Girdle Vessel Breathing so you are able to strengthen your Guardian Qì.

Conceiving of Spiritual Embryo (i.e., Initiation of Enlightenment) (Shéntāi Zhī Yùnyù, 神胎之孕育). If you wish to conceive a Spiritual Embryo (Shéntāi, 神胎) and lead it up to the Upper Dāntián for its birth (i.e., enlightenment), then you must know the method, which I will describe here briefly. If you are interested in pursuing this goal, please read the book: *Qìgōng—Grand Circulation for Spiritual Enlightenment.*

The first step in conceiving the Spiritual Embryo is to lead the Fire Qì (Huǒqì, 火氣) (Post-Heaven Qì) downward from the Middle Dāntián (Zhōngdāntián, 中丹田) and the Water Qì (Shuǐqì, 水氣) (Pre-Heaven Qì) upward from the Real Lower Dāntián, and have them meet at the Huángtíng (黃庭), the inner space between the diaphragm and the Real Lower Dāntián (center of gravity). This process is commonly called "Kǎn-Lí" (坎離) in Qìgōng practice. When this happens, the Yīn and Yáng Qìs will interact with each other. In the presence of the Shén, life (the Spiritual Embryo) can be conceived. Therefore, you must also lead the Shén down to meet the Qì at the Huángtíng.

Further Spiritual Qìgōng Developments (Shén Zhī Jìnxiū, 神之進修). As mentioned before, according to Daoist society, there are four stages of spiritual cultivation, namely: 1. Refine the Essence and Convert it into Qì (Liànjīng Huàqì, 煉精化氣); 2. Refine the Qì and Convert it into Spirit (Liànqì Huàshén, 煉氣化神); 3. Refine the Spirit and Return It to Nothingness (Liànshén Fǎnxū, 煉神返虛); 4. Crushing the Nothingness (Fěnsuì Xūkōng, 粉碎虛空). Through Embryonic Breathing, you will be able to achieve the first stage of cultivation. This will provide you with an opportunity to conceive the Spiritual Embryo at the Real Lower Dāntián. Only then can you have a solid foundation for further spiritual cultivations. These include:

Breathing's Yin and Yang 呼吸陰陽圖

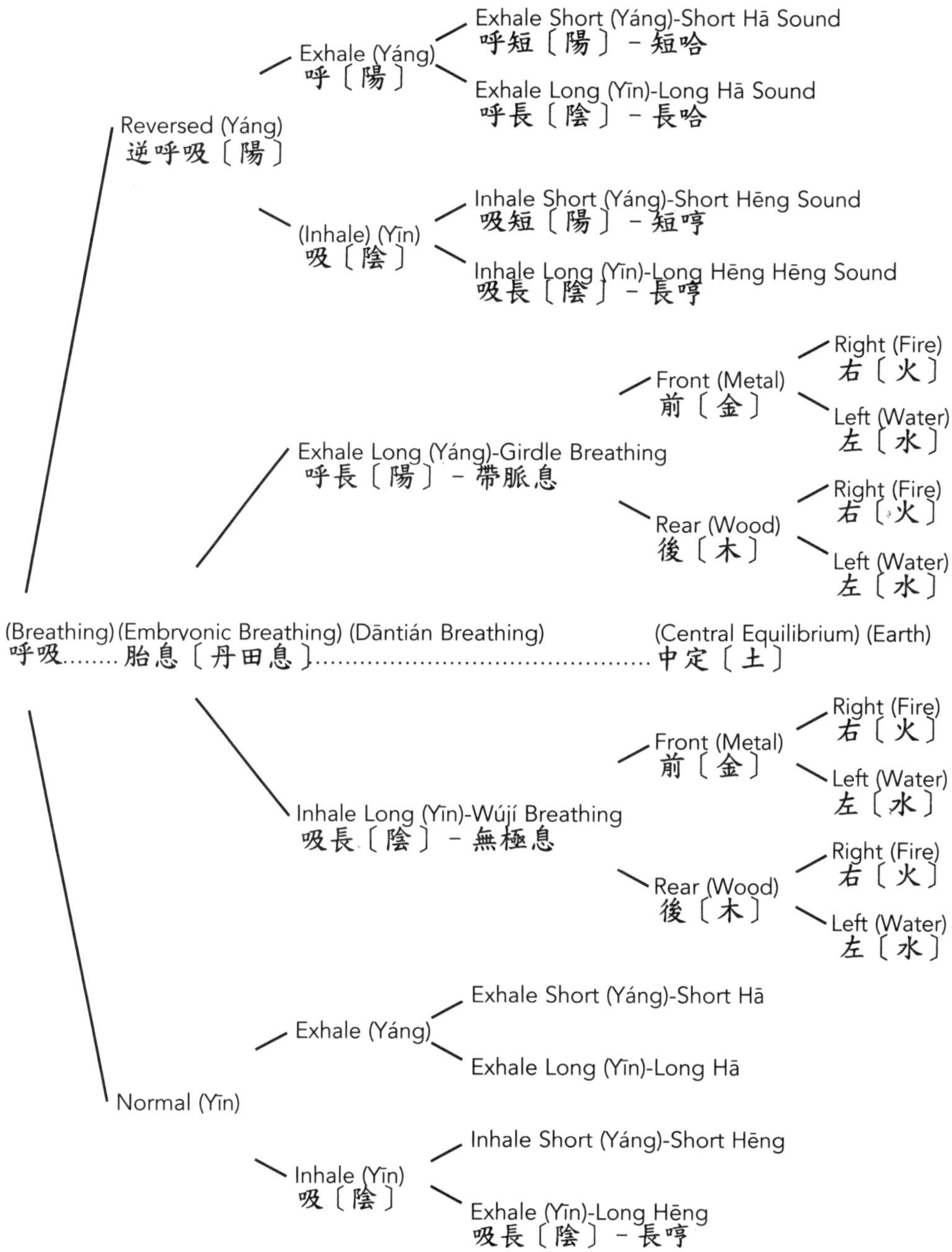

Figure 5-15. Breathing's Yīn and Yáng

1. **Small Circulation** (Xiǎozhōutiān, 小周天). Once you have learned Embryonic Breathing and are able to store the Qì to an abundant level, the next step is learning how to use the accumulated Qì to recondition your physical body and make it strong, healthy, and able to live long. This process is called "Small Cyclic Heaven" (Xiǎozhōutiān, 小周天) or simply "Small Circulation" Qìgōng meditation. That means you will learn how to lead the Qì to the Conception and Governing Vessels (Rènmài, Dūmài; 任脈・督脈) to increase the Qì's circulation to a more abundant level. These two vessels regulate and govern the Qì circulation in the twelve primary Qì channels, which can condition the physical body, in the process of "Muscle/Tendon Changing" (Yìjīn, 易筋) Qìgōng. Remember, only if you have a healthy and long physical life, can you have enough time for your spiritual cultivation. We will discuss the training of "Small Circulation" meditation in the book: *Qìgōng Meditation—Small Circulation*.
2. **Grand Circulation** (Dàzhōutiān, 大周天). "Grand Cyclic Heaven" or simply "Grand Circulation" (Dàzhōutiān, 大周天) meditation includes: Self-Inner Body Grand Circulation, Dual Qì Exchange Grand Circulation with a partner, and also Qì Exchange Grand Circulation with nature. Self-Inner Body Grand Circulation includes how to lead the Qì to circulate in the twelve channels or to any part of the body, and how to lead the Qì upward through the Thrusting Vessel for "brain washing" (Xǐsuǐ, 洗髓) for spiritual enlightenment. The last process is the process of "refining the Qì and converting it into spirit" (Liànqì Huàshén, 煉氣化神). In order to achieve this goal, you must first lead the Qì upward through the Thrusting Vessel. This process is called "refining the Qì to sublimate it" (Liànqì Shēnghuá, 煉氣昇華). We will discuss it in the book: *Qìgōng—Grand Circulation for Spiritual Enlightenment*.
3. **Spiritual Enlightenment** (Shéntōng, 神通). In Buddhist and Daoist societies, the final goal of spiritual cultivation is the "unification of heaven and human" (Tiānrén Héyī, 天人合一). At this stage there is no differentiation between the natural spirit and human spirits. In this case, the human spirit will have its eternal life and will not have to reenter the natural cycle of reincarnation (Bùzài Lúnhuí, 不再輪迴).

   In order to reach this goal, you must first conceive a holy Spiritual Embryo in the Huángtíng (黃庭). When this embryo is matured, then you lead it up to the Upper Dāntián to give birth to this Spiritual Embryo. In order to do so, the "heaven eye" (Tiānyǎn, 天眼) (the Third Eye) must be reopened, which allows the spiritual baby to be born. When this happens, since your spiritual energy will be re-attached to the natural spirit, you will suddenly understand all natural events, resume the capability of telepathy, and also see the possibilities of the future. This is the process of "spiritual enlightenment." In order to reach this goal, you must first "refine the spirit and return it to nothingness" (Liànshén Fǎnxū, 煉神返虛). This means you must get rid of human thinking, emotional bondage, and desires. You must be as truthful as nature. Only then can you expect the reopening of the Third Eye.

However, in order to have an independent external spiritual life, you must train the spiritual baby and make it stronger. This includes the processes of "three years of nursing" (Sānnián Bǔrǔ, 三年哺乳) and "nine years of facing the wall" (Jiǔnián Miànbì, 九年面壁). These two processes also mean the process of "crushing the nothingness" (Fěnsuì Xūkōng, 粉碎虛空). Once the new spiritual life is strong and can be independent, then the physical will not mean anything any more. This is the final process of "unification of heaven and human."

5.4 Recovery from the Meditative State (Jìngzuòhòu Zhī Huīfù, 靜坐後之恢復)

When you meditate, once your conscious mind decides to wake up and return to normal activity, you must know how to handle it properly. If you do not know how to recover from your meditative state properly, you may experience headache (mental imbalance) or some physical tightness, especially in the spine. Correct recovery methods can prevent or remove any Qì stagnation that occurs during meditation. Therefore, how to recover from the meditative state remains one of the most important parts of meditation practice.

The methods of recovering from the meditative state are both mental and physical. The trick of recovery is to reverse the normal regulating procedures for meditation. This means first regulating your mind, next your breathing, and finally your body. Next, the general methods of recovery that have been passed down and gained through my personal experience will be introduced.

Regulate the Mind, Qì, and Breathing. The first step of recovery from your meditation is to continue keeping your mind calm. Slowly awaken from your semi-sleeping or semi-hypnotic state. It seems that you have just woken up from a deep sleep, yet your conscious mind is still in control.

Second, if you know Skin-Marrow Breathing very well, you may practice it for a few minutes. Try to exhale longer than you inhale. This will lead the Qì to the skin surface and arouse the physical body from the sleeping state.

Third, move your mind to the Upper Dāntián (or the third eye) and relocate your spiritual center. Sit there for a couple of minutes. When you do this mentally, you will have woken yourself up completely and comfortably.

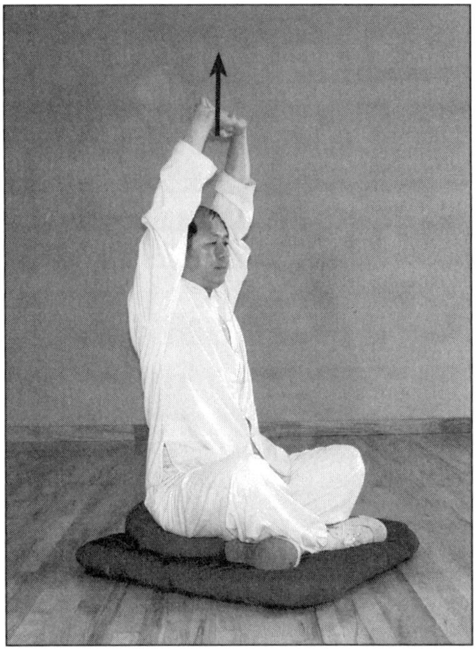

Figure 5-16. Upward Torso Stretching

Remember, when you recover from your meditative state mentally, you should not resist and speed up. You should take it easy, be natural and comfortable. From this, you will obtain a great level of mental satisfaction in peace and harmony.

Regulate the Body. After you have brought your mind to the real world, you should next regulate your body and to help it recover from the semi-sleeping state. In addition, through correct movement, you should also learn how to disperse the stagnant Qì that may be caused from a long sitting position or an improper sitting posture. Next, some effective recovering movements and stretching will be introduced.

1. **Upward Torso Stretching.** The first step of the recovery of your body is stretching your torso. Simply interlock your hands and then push upward (Figure 5-16). This action is very similar to waking up and lifting your arms to stretch yourself. From this upward pushing, you are able to untie any possible locking of the torso or spine caused by a long time sitting.
   After your hands have reached the highest position, stay there, inhale deeply and then exhale. Finally, inhale again and lower your arms. Repeat twice more.

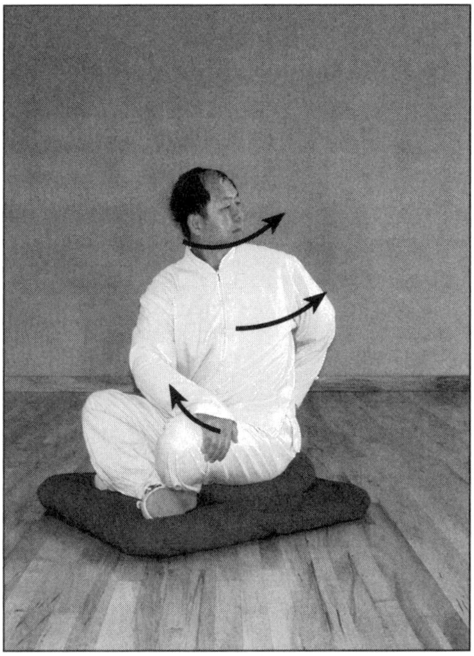

Figure 5-17. Sideways Torso Twisting

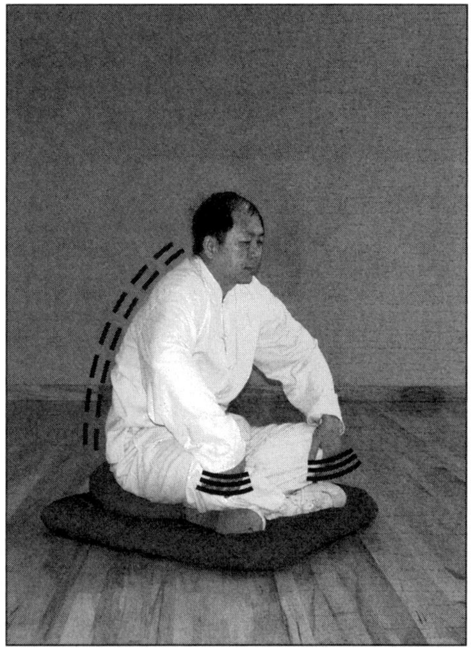

Figure 5-18. Spine Waving

2. **Sideways Torso Twisting.** After you have completed the upward stretching, you should next twist your torso to stretch it sideways. When you do this, simply turn your body to your left first and use your right hand to pull your left thigh while pushing your left shoulder backward (Figure 5–17). Stay in this position, inhale and then exhale. Next, twist to the other side.
3. **Spine Waving.** After you have completed the upward and sideways stretching of the torso, loosen your vertebrae, section by section, from the sacrum upward to the neck. To do this, place both your hands on the knees and use the pulling of the hands to generate the waving spine motion (Figure 5–18). When you begin to pull, the lower torso is thrusting forward, and you should inhale deeply at this time. When the waving motion has reached the upper spine, you should exhale. You should move the spine comfortably and naturally. This waving spine movement is the same spine action as a sigh. That means when you are depressed and feel a great emotion is stuck in your body, you generally inhale deeply and generate a waving motion from the lower back. When the motion reaches the upper torso, you exhale and make the "Hen" sound. This is the most natural torso movement that allows you to relax the torso and release any possible emotional energy. Therefore, it is used for the torso relaxation movement.

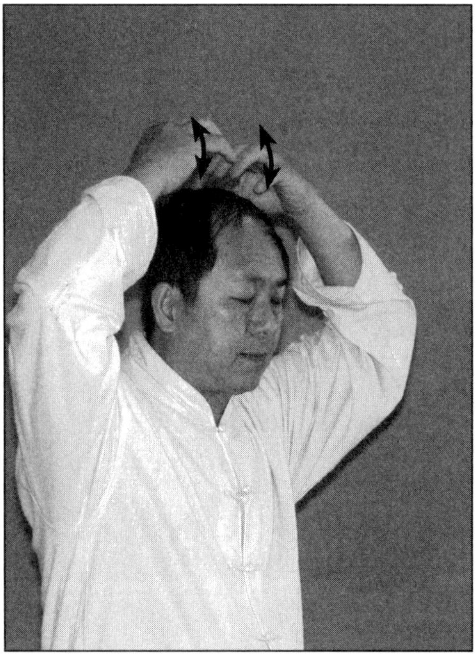

Figure 5-19. Tap the Head

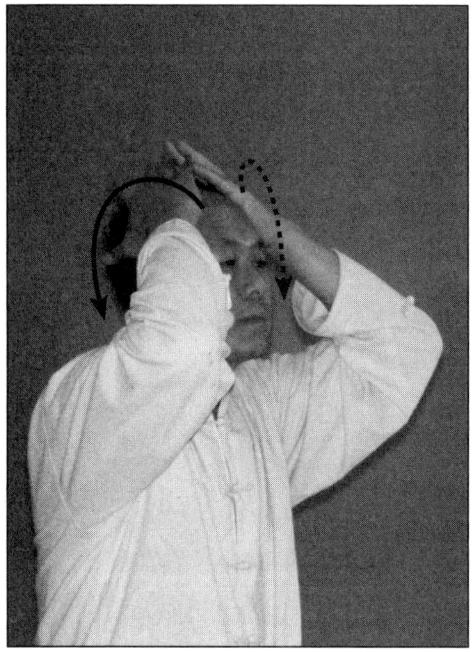

Figure 5-20. Brush the Hair

4. **Tap the Head.** Next, use the fingertips to tap your head from the front backward and from the center to the sides for a few minutes (Figure 5–19). This tapping action will lead the accumulated Qì inside the head to the skin surface. After tapping, then use both your hands to brush your head lightly from the front backward (Figure 5–20).
5. **If Necessary, Walk for a Couple of Minutes.** After you have finished the above recovery massaging and exercises, if you wish, you may walk or simply lie down to rest for a few minutes.

CHAPTER 6

Conclusion

Before finishing this book, I would like to summarize a few important points:

1. The earliest record of Embryonic Breathing is from *Dào Dé Jīng* (*Classic on the Virtue of the Dào*) (道德經) written by Lǎozi (老子) (604–531 BCE). As a matter of fact, this is the origin of the entire Embryonic Breathing. This origin offers a clear concept of the training and the essence of Dào in scholar Daoism (Dàoxué, 道學). This concept was studied and practiced and became one of the most important and essential practices of Nèidān Qìgōng (內丹氣功) (Internal Elixir) practice.
2. From the number of documents about Embryonic Breathing existing today, we can see how important and essential this practice is to Internal Elixir Qìgōng. Most of the documents were hidden in Buddhist and Daoist monasteries in the past, and it was not until the late 20th century that almost all of the documents were revealed to the public.
3. Though the theory behind these documents is not hard to understand, it is extremely hard to practice, especially the part concerning cultivation of "human temperament," meaning the cultivation of human nature which allows us to find the root and the meaning of human origin. This is especially difficult in today's societies.
4. This book has provided you with a scientific viewpoint both in theory and practice. Many people believe that it is impossible to learn from a book, which is sometimes true, depending upon the individual. In order for you to get to the right path of practice, it is extremely important to study and understand the theory. When you understand the theory, it is like having a map and being able to read it. In this case, you will not need a teacher to direct you step-by-step. The teacher will only show you the direction and offer you his personal experience.
5. You must read the documents translated and commented in Chapter 3 repeatedly. Remember, each document is just a road sign to direct you to the right path of training. Nevertheless, you must always place a question mark in each one of them. Always question whether it makes logical sense. How much can

> you trust this article? You should know that each document or book you read, each statement or a saying of a person, is only that person's personal opinion. They are for your reference, not to believe blindly. Which, naturally, includes this book. Therefore, you must learn to be wise and make a logical judgement. Then ponder and practice it cautiously. In no time, you will see the practice clearly.

After you practice Embryonic Breathing for a period of time, you will discover that it seems there is another world (spiritual world) which other regular people cannot reach. This world has not yet been understood by today's science. If you are able to get involved in this practice, you will become a pioneer of the study and practice of spiritual science. Compared to the state of today's material science, spiritual science still lags far behind. This is why we have encountered the most serious crises and challenges today. On one hand we have developed a material science which is able to destroy the entire world, while on the other, we still don't know how to control human desires and temperament.

Western spiritual science and understanding, in my personal opinion, lags far beyond the development of the East. This is simply because of the involvement of Western religion in politics. Glory, dignity, and wealth have become the major concerns in Western religious society. For this reason, those people who had natural inborn spiritual feelings and capabilities were accused of being witches and burned to death.

In China, the situation was very different. Spiritual people would usually hide themselves in the mountains for spiritual cultivation. Many of them would write down their experiences, and these writings have been passed down to us. Commonly, when those spiritually talented people were found, Chinese said they had the affinity of the Buddha (Fóyuán, 佛緣) or of the Dào (Dàoyuán, 道緣). These people were usually sent to the monasteries for further training.

I sincerely believe that in order to promote human spiritual science further, the first priority is to translate the existing ancient documents written by experienced spiritual practitioners. However, there are very many documents now available to society. I realize that even though I have spent the last forty years collecting, studying, and interpreting them, all my effort has only contributed possibly 0.1% to the entire study. To expedite the spiritual study, we will need a huge, well-funded non-profit organization to translate these documents, thus allowing the general public to study and practice them.

Acknowledgments

Thanks to Tim Comrie for his photography and typesetting. Thanks to Erik Elsemans, Ciaran Harris, and Susan Bullowa for proofing the manuscript and contributing many valuable suggestions and discussions. Special thanks to Tony Richard Chee for the cover design on the first edition, to Keith Brown for the first editing, and James O'Leary for final editing. Also, special thanks to Dr. Thomas G. Gutheil for his foreword.

Additional thanks to Johnny Houx for proofreading this second edition, to Doran Hunter for copyediting, and Axie Breen for the cover design and illustration enhancements..

APPENDIX A

Translation and Glossary of Chinese Terms

Āi 哀 Sorrow.

Ài 愛 Love, kindness.

Ānlú 安爐 "To install a furnace," implying the establishment of abundant Qì at the Real Lower Dāntián in this book. In order to do so, you must know the method of Embryonic Breathing.

Ànmó 按摩 Literally: press rub. Together they mean massage.

Āntiān Lèmìng 安天樂命 "Peace with heaven and delight in your destiny."

Bāduànjǐn 八段錦 Eight Pieces of Brocade. A Wàidān Qìgōng (外丹氣功) practice which is said to have been created by Marshal Yuè, Fēi (岳飛) during the Southern Sòng Dynasty (1127–1280 CE) (南宋).

Bāfāng 八方 "Eight directions," implying the space or air around us.

Bāguà 八卦 Literally, "Eight Divinations." Also called the Eight Trigrams. In Chinese philosophy, the eight basic variations; shown in the *Yìjīng* (易經) (*Book of Changes*) as groups of single and broken lines.

Bāguàzhǎng 八卦掌 Eight Trigrams Palm. One of the internal martial styles, believed to have been created by Dǒng, Hǎi-Chuān (董海川) between 1866 and 1880 CE

Báihè 白鶴 White Crane. A well-known southern Chinese martial style which originated in the Shàolín Temple (少林寺).

Bǎihuì (Gv-20) 百會 Literally, "hundred meeting." An important acupuncture cavity located on the top of the head. The Bǎihuì cavity belongs to the Governing Vessel (Dūmài, 督脈).

Bǎirì Zhújī 百日築基 One Hundred Days to Build the Foundation. In Yìjīnjīng (易筋經) and Xǐsuǐjīng (洗髓經), the training of the first hundred days is the most important because you lay the foundation for further progress.

Bāmài 八脈 Referred to as the Eight Extraordinary Vessels. These eight vessels are considered to be Qì reservoirs, which regulate the Qì status in the primary Qì channels.

Bào 抱 Can be translated as embrace, hold together, stick together, enfold, harbor, or cherish.

Bāoxī (2852–2737 BCE) 包羲 An ancient ruler of China.

Bàoyī 抱一 Embracing (i.e., maintaining) a state of singularity (singleness). It means to keep the spirit (or mind) and Qì at the central energy line and later unify the spirit and Qì together at the Real Lower Dāntián.

Biǎnquè 扁鵲 A well-known physician who wrote the book *Nánjīng* (難經) (*Classic on Disorders*) during the Chinese Qín and Hàn Dynasties (255 BCE–220 CE, 秦・漢).

Bìhù 閉戶 Also called "Mìhù" (密戶) and means "the closed door," implying the Mìngmén (Gv-4) (命門) cavity between L2 and L3.

Bóyáng 伯陽 A nickname of Lǎozi (老子). Lǎozi was also called Lǐěr (李耳) or Lǎodān (老聃).

Bùtiáo Értiáo 不調而調 "Regulating without regulating." This implies that when regulating is no longer necessary, all of the regulating processes will naturally cease. This is the stage of Wúwéi (無為), or "doing nothing."

Bùzài Lúnhuí 不再輪迴 "Will not re-enter the natural cycle of reincarnation." According to Buddhist philosophy, once you have reached a stage of spiritual enlightenment, your spirit will not have to reincarnate. This spirit will have eternal life.

Cǎiyào 採藥 "Pick the herb." A term used in Daoist Qìgōng practice that means to receive the generated Qì.

Chán 禪 1. Practices which are related or associated with Buddhism, including the cultivation, the refinement, and pursuing the study of Buddhahood. 2. Buddhist term for "meditation," meaning to regulate the Xīn until it is calm and steady. 3. A Chinese school of Mahayana Buddhism (known as "Zen" in Japan) that asserts enlightenment can be attained through meditation, self-contemplation, and intuition.

Cháng 常 "The natural constant routines or patterns."

Chángquán 長拳 "Long range fist" or "long sequence." Chángquán includes all northern Chinese long-range martial styles. Tàijíquán is also called Chángquán simply because its sequence is long.

Chànǚ 姹女 The shy lady (i.e., mother), implying Qì.

Chén 塵 "Dust," which implies the dirty mind generated from the seven emotions and six desires.

Chéng 乘 Means the Buddhist teaching, a conveyance to bring the truth to men and help them.

Chéngfó 成佛 Achieving Buddhahood is called "Chéngfó."

Chēng, Gīn-Gsào (1911–1976) 曾金灶 Dr. Yáng, Jwing-Ming's White Crane master.

Chénshì 塵世 A word for lay society meaning a "dust world" which is filled with emotional disturbances.

Chéntǔ 塵土 Dust. In Buddhism, the emotions and desires found in lay society are considered "emotional mud" or "dust."

Chì (Qì) 氣 The general definition of Qì is: universal energy, including heat, light, electromagnetic energy, and any other type of energy. A narrower definition of Qì refers to the energy (i.e., bioelectricity) circulating in human or animal bodies.

Chì Kūng (Qìgōng) 氣功 The Gōngfū (功夫) of Qì, which means the study of Qì.

Chílǎo Fǎnjī Yùndòng 遲老返機運動 Slowing of aging and returning the function exercises. It means those Qìgōng practices which are able to slow down the aging process and return the practitioner to a healthy state.

Chín (Qín) 擒 "To catch" or "to seize."

Chín Ná (Qínná) 擒拿 Literally, "seize control." A type of Chinese Gōngfū which emphasizes grabbing techniques to control the opponent's joints in conjunction with attacking certain acupuncture cavities. One of the main fighting categories in Chinese martial arts. These four categories are: kicking (Tī, 踢), striking (Dǎ, 打), wrestling (Shuāi, 摔), and controlling (Ná, 擒拿).

Chōngmài 衝脈 Thrusting Vessel. One of the Eight Extraordinary Vessels.

Chúgǒu 芻狗 Chúgǒu were sacrificial dogs which were made from straw and used for ceremonies of worship in ancient China.

Chūnqiū 春秋 Spring and Autumn Period. One of the Chinese warring periods (722–484 BCE) (Zhànguó, 戰國).

Confucius (Kǒngzǐ) (551–479 BCE) 孔子 A Chinese scholar, during the Spring and Autumn Period (722–484 BCE) (Chūnqiū, 春秋), whose philosophy has significantly influenced Chinese culture.

Cùn 寸 Chinese measurement of length. One cun of Chinese length approximately equals one-third of a decimeter.

Cúnshén 存神 "To retain the Shén" at its residence.

Dàchéng 大乘 Great conveyance. A high level of Buddhist study.

Dàdān 大丹 Great Elixir. Means the Qì is led upward to the brain for enlightenment training in meditation.

Dàdào 大道 Great Dào. Means "great nature."

Dàdìng 大定 Great steadiness. Implies a very high level of steadiness both in mind and physical body.

Dàdǐnglú 大鼎爐 Large tripod and furnace. The final stage of conceiving a Spiritual Embryo at the Huángtíng (黃庭) cavity is to unite the Shén in the head with the Qì at the Huángtíng. Head is a tripod while Huángtíng is a furnace.

Dàfǎn 大返 Great returning, meaning to "return the human temperament to the natural state."

Dàimài 帶脈 Girdle (or Belt) Vessel. One of the Eight Extraordinary Vessels.

Dàimàixí 帶脈息 Girdle Vessel Breathing. Also known as Skin Breathing (Fūxí, 膚息) or Body Breathing) (Tǐxí, 體息).

Dámó 達磨 The Indian Buddhist monk who is credited with creating the Yìjīnjīng (易筋經) and Xǐsuǐjīng (洗髓經) while at the Shàolín monastery (少林寺) during the Liáng Dynasty (梁朝) (502–557 CE). His last name was Chadili (剎地利), and he was also known as Bodhidharma. He was once the prince of a small tribe in southern India.

Dān 丹 "Elixir."

Dāndǐng Dàogōng 丹鼎道功 The Elixir Cauldron Way of Qìgōng. Daoist Qìgōng training.

Dānlú 丹爐 Elixir Furnace. Abdominal area (False Lower Dāntián) which is able to produce elixir.

Dāntián 丹田 Literally: Elixir Field. Locations in the body which are able to store and generate Qì (elixir) in the body. The Upper, Middle, and Lower Dāntiáns are located respectively between the eyebrows (brain), at the lower section of the sternum (Jiūwěi, Co-15, 鳩尾), and a few inches below the navel.

Dāntián Hūxī 丹田呼吸 Dāntián Breathing.

Dào 道 The "way," by implication the "natural way."

Dào Dé Jīng 道德經 *Classic on the Virtue of the Dào*. Written by Lǎozi (老子) during the Zhōu Dynasty (1122–255 BCE) (周朝).

Dàojiā (Dàojiào) 道家〔道教〕 The Dào family. Daoism. Created by Lǎozi (老子) during the Zhōu Dynasty (1122–255 BCE) (周朝). In the Hàn Dynasty (c. 58 CE) (漢朝), it was mixed with Buddhism to become the Daoist religion (Dàojiào) (道教).

Dàojiā Hūxī 道家呼吸 Daoist Breathing.

Dàojiào 道教 Dào religion created by Zhāng, Dào-Líng (張道陵) who combined the traditional Daoist principles with Buddhism during the Chinese Eastern Hàn Dynasty (25–220 CE) (東漢).

Dàowài Cǎiyào 道外採藥 To pick up the herb outside of the Dào (道). A Daoist Qìgōng training.

Dàoxué 道學 Scholar Daoism. Its philosophical foundation is "Dào Dé Jīng" written by Lǎozi. Dàoxué is different from Dàojiào (道教) (i.e., Dào religion) which was created by Zhāng, Dào-Líng (張道陵) who combined the traditional Daoist principles with Buddhism during the Chinese Eastern Hàn Dynasty (25–220 CE) (東漢).

Dǎoyǐn 導引 Direct-lead. Another name of "Qìgōng."

Dàoyuán 道緣 "The affinity of the Dào," implying that a person has a pre-birth relationship associated with the Dào.

Dāqiáo 搭橋 To build a bridge. Refers to the Qìgōng practice of touching the roof of the mouth with the tip of the tongue to form a bridge or link between the Governing and Conception Vessels (Rèn-Dūmài, 任・督脈).

Dàzhōutiān 大周天 Literally, "Grand Cyclic Heaven." Usually translated "Grand Circulation" and called "Macrocosmic Meditation" in Indian Yoga. After a Nèidān Qìgōng practitioner completes Small Circulation (Xiǎozhōutiān, 小周天), he will circulate his Qì through the entire body or exchange Qì with nature.

Dǎzuò 打坐 Meditation is called "Dǎzuò" in Daoism which means "engaging sitting."

Dé 德 The manifestation of the Dào or the activities (actions) of nature.

Dì 地 The Earth. Earth (Dì, 地), Heaven (Tiān, 天) and Man (Rén, 人) are the "Three Natural Powers" (Sāncái, 三才).

Dì 蒂 The stalk of a fruit or flower, connecting to the root of life.

Dì Wǔxīn Hūxī 第五心呼吸 "Fifth Gate Breathing" is also called "Bǎihuì Breathing" (百會呼吸), or "Upper Dāntián Breathing" (Shàngdāntián Hūxī, 上丹田呼吸).

Diǎnmài 點脈 Mai means "the blood vessel" (Xuěmài, 血脈) or "the Qì channel" (Qìmài, 氣脈). Diǎnmài means "to press the blood vessel or Qì channel."

Diànqì 電氣 Dian means "electricity" and so Diànqì means "electrical energy" (electricity). In China, a word is often placed before "Qì" to identify the different kinds of energy.

Diǎnxuè 點穴 Diǎn means "to point and exert pressure" and Xuè means "cavities." Qínná (Chín Ná) (擒拿) techniques that specialize in attacking acupuncture cavities to immobilize or kill an opponent.

Diǎnxuè Massages 點穴按摩 One of Chinese massage techniques in which the acupuncture cavities are stimulated through pressing. Diǎnxuè massage is also called acupressure and is the root of Japanese Shiatsu.

Dìlǐshī 地理師 Dìlǐ (地理) means "geomancy" and Shī (師) means "teacher." Therefore Dìlǐshī is a teacher or master who analyzes geographic locations according to the formulas in the *Yìjīng* (易經) (*Book of Changes*) and the energy distributions in the Earth. Also called Fēngshuǐshī (風水師).

Dìng 定 "To stabilize" or "to firm." The goal is to reach the steadiness, the firmness of the body, the mind, and the spirit.

Dìngshén 定神 To stabilize the spirit. To keep the spirit at one place (usually the Shàngdāntián located at the Third Eye). One of the exercises for regulating the Shén (神) (spirit) in Qìgōng.

Dòngfáng 洞房 The space between the two eyebrows, two inches inward is called "Dòngfáng."

Dōnghàn 東漢 East Hàn. A Chinese dynasty during the period from 25–220 CE

Dōngmiánxí 冬眠息 Hibernation breathing.

Dǒuniú 斗牛 "Big Dipper," which implies the process of condensing the Shén at the Upper Dāntián.

Dūmài 督脈 Usually translated "Governing Vessel." One of the Eight Extraordinary Vessels.

Éméi 峨嵋 Name of a mountain in Sìchuān Province (四川), China.

Fǎn 返 Return. Means to return your breathing to its natural way.

Fǎn Fùhūxī 反腹呼吸 Reverse abdominal breathing. One of the Qìgōng breathing methods. Also called "Fǎnhūxī" (反呼吸) (reverse breathing) or "Daoist breathing."

Fǎnhūxī (Nìhūxī) 反呼吸 (逆呼吸) Reverse breathing. Also commonly called "Daoist Breathing."

Fǎnjīng Bǔnǎo 返精補腦 A special Daoist Qìgōng terminology which means "to return the Jīng to nourish the brain."

Fǎntóng 返童 Back to childhood. A training in Nèidān Qìgōng (內丹氣功) through which the practitioner tries to regain control of the muscles of the lower abdomen.

Fǎntóng Hūxī 返童呼吸 Back to childhood breathing. A breathing training in Nèidān Qìgōng (內丹氣功) through which the practitioner tries to regain control of the muscles in the lower abdomen. Also called "abdominal breathing" (Fùhūxī, 腹呼吸)

Fēishēng 飛升 Spiritual ascending. Means the separation of the spiritual body and the physical body.

Fēn 分 Chinese measurement of length. One Fēn approximately equals one-third of a centimeter.

Fēng 風 Wind.

Fēngshuǐ 風水 Literally, "wind-water."

Fēngshuǐshī 風水師 Literally, "wind water teacher." Teacher or master of geomancy. Geomancy is the art or science of analyzing the natural energy relationships in a location, especially the interrelationships between "wind" and "water," hence the name. Also called Dìlǐshī (地理師).

Fěnsuì Xūkōng 粉碎虛空 To crush the nothingness. One of the Daoist training processes for enlightenment wherein the illusion which connects the physical world and the spiritual plane is destroyed.

Fénxiāng 焚香 Burning incense.

Fójiā (Fójiào) 佛家 (佛教) Literally, Buddhism family. Jiào means religion. Therefore, the Buddhist Religion.

Fójiā Hūxī 佛家呼吸 Buddhist breathing. Implies "normal abdominal breathing."

Fóyuán 佛緣 Affinity for Buddhahood.

Fúshēng 浮生 Literally, "floating life." The life is just like a floating duckweed without a root.

Fùshì Hūxī 腹式呼吸 Literally, "abdominal way of breathing." As you breathe, you use the muscles in the lower abdominal area to control the diaphragm. It is also called "back to childhood breathing."

Fūsuǐxí 膚髓息 Skin and marrow breathing.

Fùxí 腹息 Abdominal breathing.

Fūxí 膚息 Skin breathing. One of the Nèidān Qìgōng (內丹氣功) breathing practices.

Gāowán Yùndòng 睪丸運動 Testicle exercises. Qìgōng exercises.

Gēnjī 根基 Foundations.

Gōng (Kūng) 功 Energy or hard work.

Gǒng 汞 Mercury. Mercury and lead are terms commonly used in Daoist society. Lead and mercury were used in Daoist alchemy to adjust the Yīn and Yáng of the elixir.

Gōngfū (Kūng Fū) 功夫 Literally: energy-time. Any study, learning, or practice which requires a lot of patience, energy, and time to complete. Since practicing Chinese martial arts requires a great deal of time and energy, Chinese martial arts are commonly called Gōngfū.

Gù 固 "To solidify and to firm."

Guān 觀 "To look," "to observe," or "to pay attention." "Look" here means to feel and to sense.

Guānxīn 觀心 Observing the Xīn. Implies to pay attention to the activities of the emotional mind.

Guānyuán 關元 Key Origin. Different name of the Lower Dāntián, where the Pre-Birth Qì (Original Qì) is converted from the Original Essence (Yuánjīng, 元精).

Guānzhǐ 觀止 Means the observation is stopped and is no longer necessary. Once you have regulated your emotional mind, then no more regulating is necessary. Therefore, the observation of the Xīn will naturally stop.

Guǐ 癸 Implies "kidneys" and means the production of the Original Essence (i.e., hormone).

Guǐ 鬼 Ghost. When you die, if your spirit is strong, your soul's energy will not decompose and return to nature. This soul energy is a ghost.

Guǐqì 鬼氣 The Qì residue of a dead person. It is believed by the Chinese Buddhists and Daoists that this Qì residue is a so-called ghost.

Guīxí 龜息 Turtle breathing. In Chinese Qìgōng society, it is believed that a turtle is able to live for a long time because it knows how to breathe slow and deep. Through this breathing, the Qì can be led to the surface of the skin and to the marrow efficiently.

Gùjīng 固精 To solidify the Essence. A Qìgōng exercise for keeping and firming the Essence.

Guóshù (Kuóshù) 國術 Literally: national techniques. It is an abbreviation of "Zhōngguó Wǔshù" (中國武術) which means "Chinese Martial Techniques." Another name for Chinese martial arts. First used by President Chiang, Kai-Shek (蔣介石) in 1928 at the founding of the Nánjīng Central Guóshù Institute (南京中央國術館).

Gǔqífēng 古奇峰 Name of a mountain located in Xīnzhú, Táiwān (臺灣・新竹), where Dr. Yáng, Jwing-Ming learned White Crane Gīngfū from Master Chēng, Gīn-Gsào (曾金灶) (1911–1976).

Gǔshén 谷神 Valley Spirit.

Gùshén 固神 Gu means to firm and solidify. An exercise for regulating the Shén (神) in which you firm and strengthen the spirit at its residence.

Hǎidǐ 海底 Means "Sea Bottom." This is a name given by martial artists to the Huìyīn cavity (Co–1) (會陰) in Chinese medicine. Perineum.

Hàn (206 BCE–220 CE) 漢 A dynasty in Chinese history.

Hán, Chìng-Táng (1900–1976) 韓慶堂 A well-known Chinese martial artist, especially in Táiwān. Master Hán is also Dr. Yáng Jwìng-Mǐng's Long Fist grandmaster.

Hé 和 Harmony or peace.

Hèn 恨 Hate.

Hēng 哼 A Yīn Qìgōng sound that is the opposite of the Yáng Hā (哈) sound. This sound is commonly used to lead the Qì inward and to store it in the bone marrow. This sound can also be used for an attack when the manifestation of only partial power is desired. Hēng is one of the two sounds commonly used in Tàijíquán.

Hòutiānqì 後天氣 "Post-Birth Qì" or "Post-Heaven Qì." This Qì is converted from the Essence of food and air and is classified as "fire Qì" since it can make your body too Yáng.

Hǔ 虎 Tiger.

Huánjīng Bǔnǎo 還精補腦 Literally, to return the Essence to nourish the brain. A Daoist Qìgōng training process wherein Qì which has been converted from Essence is lead to the brain to nourish it.

Huángpó 黃婆 "Old yellow lady." Means the "match-maker" who brings the Yīn (female) and Yáng (male) together.

Huángtáng 黃堂 Different name of The Middle Dāntián.

Huángtíng 黃庭 Literally, "yellow yard." It implies the area called "Jade Ring" (Yùhuán, 玉環) in Daoist society. The area is located at the solar plexus. In Daoist Qìgōng, Huángtíng is the place where Fire Qì and Water Qì are mixed to generate a spiritual embryo (Shéntāi, 神胎). Huángtíng has also implied The Middle Dāntián.

Huátuó 華佗 A well-known physician during the Chinese Jìn Dynasty (晉) in the 3rd century CE

Huì 慧 "Intelligence" or "wisdom" through pondering, analyzing, and comprehension so you are able to handle millions of events without being confused.

Huìyīn (Co-1) 會陰 Literally, "meet Yīn." An acupuncture cavity belonging to the Conception Vessel located at the perineum area.

Hún 魂 The soul. Commonly used with the word Líng (靈), which means spirit. Daoists believe that a human being's Hún (魂) and Pò (魄) originate with his Original Qì (Yuánqì, 元氣), and separate from the physical body at death.

Huǒqì 火氣 Fire Qì (Post-Heaven Qì). Qì from the Middle Dāntián, which tends to make the body positive or Yáng.

Huóqì 活氣 Living Qì or vital Qì. When something is alive it has "vital Qì."

Huózǐshí 活子時 Alive Zǐ timing. Special timings adequate for meditation.

Jiǎ Xiàdāntián 假下丹田 False Lower Dāntián. Daoists believe that the Lower Dāntián located on the front side of the abdomen is not the real Dāntián. The Real Lower Dāntián corresponds to the physical center of gravity. The False Lower Dāntián is called Qìhǎi (Co-6) (氣海) (Qì ocean) in Chinese medicine.

Jiànggōng 絳宮 Crimson Palace. The space under the heart. A different name of the Middle Dāntián. Often it is used as an alternative name of the "heart" (Xīn, 心). The Middle Dāntián provides you with Post-Birth Qì converted from food and air.

Jiè 界 "World, boundaries, circles, and societies."

Jiétāi 結胎 Conceive the embryo.

Jiětuō 解脫 Self-liberation from spiritual bondage.

Jīn 金 Metal. One of the Five Elements (Wǔxíng, 五行) and implies lungs.

Jīn, Shào-Fēng 金紹峰 Dr. Yáng, Jwìng-Mǐng's White Crane grand-master.

Jīndān 金丹 Golden Elixir. Implies precious Qì.

Jīndān Dàdào 金丹大道 Golden Elixir Large Way. Major Daoist Qìgōng training in which the elixir is produced in the body through training, and later used to extend life.

Jīndiàn 金殿 Also called "Jīnshì" (金室) and means "Golden Palace" and implies "lungs." It also often implies "the brain."

Jīng 經 Channels. Sometimes translated as "meridians." Refers to the twelve organ-related "rivers" which circulate Qì throughout the body.

Jìng 靜 Calm and silent.

Jīng 精 Essence. The most refined part of anything. What is left after something has been refined and purified. In Chinese medicine, Jīng can mean semen, but it generally refers to the basic substance of the body which the Qì and Spirit enliven.

Jīngliàn 精煉 To refine or purify a liquid to a high quality.

Jīngliáng 精良 "Excellent quality" (literally "pure and good").

Jīngmíng 精明 "Keen and clever."

Jīngōng 金公 "Golden Male," which implies "Original Essence" (Yuánjīng, 元精).

Jīngqì 精氣 Essence Qì or semen Qì. The Qì which has been converted from Original Essence (Yuánjīng, 元精).

Jīnguān 金關 "Golden Gate," which implies "Upper Dāntián."

Jīngshén 精神 Essence-Spirit. Often translated as the "Spirit of Vitality." Raised spirit (raised by the Qì which is converted from Essence), which is restrained by the Yì (意).

Jīngshì 精室 "Semen residence." Implies the testicles.

Jīngxì 精細 Delicate and painstaking (literally, "pure and fine").

Jīngzǐ 精子 Literally, "essence son." The most refined part of human essence. The sperm.

Jìngzuò 靜坐 Meditation is commonly called "Jìngzuò" which means "sit quietly."

Jīnniǎo 金鳥 "Golden Bird." Implies "Original Spirit" (Yuánshén, 元神).

Jīnpǐn 金品 "Golden Material." Implies "Spiritual Embryo."

Jīnquè 金闕 Golden Palace. The space under the heart. A different name of the Middle Dāntián.

Jīnshì 金室 "Golden Residence." Also called Jīndiàn (金殿) and implies "the brain" (Upper Dāntián) or "the lungs."

Jīnyè 金液 "Golden Liquid," which implies the generation of precious saliva during Enlightenment Grand Cyclic Heaven meditation.

Jīnzhōngzhào 金鐘罩 Literally, "Golden Bell Cover." A higher level of Iron Shirt training.

Jiǔnián Miànbì 九年面壁 Nine years of facing the wall. The last stage of the Xǐsuǐjīng (洗髓經) training for enlightenment or Buddhahood.

Jīxíng 積行 Accumulate good deeds. Implies doing good things for others.

Juéhǎi 覺海 "Awaken Ocean." The conscious mind.

Jùjīng Huìshén 聚精會神 "Gathering your Jīng to meet your Shén." That means concentration.

Jūnqiàn 君倩 A Daoist and Chinese doctor during the Chinese Jìn Dynasty (265–420 CE) (晉). Jūnqiàn is credited as the creator of the Five Animal Sports (Wǔqínxì, 五禽戲) Qìgōng practice.

Kāiqiào 開竅 Opening the tricky gate. In Qìgōng, opening the gate of the Upper Dāntián.

Kāitiānyǎn 開天眼 Literally, "opening the heaven eye," and implies reopening the Third Eye.

Kǎn 坎 One of the Eight Trigrams, meaning "water."

Kǎn-Lí 坎離 Kǎn represents "water" and Lí represents "fire." Kǎn-Lí means to use water and fire to adjust the body's Yīn and Yáng.

Kǎn-Lí Jìngzuò 坎離靜坐 Kǎn-Lí Meditation. It implies the Wind Path of meditation circulation.

Kāo, Táo 高濤 Dr. Yáng, Jwìng-Mǐng's first Tàijíquán master.

Kōngmén 空門 Literally "empty door." Means the door leading you to the "Four Emptinesses" (Sìdà Jiēkōng, 四大皆空).

Kōngqì 空氣 The air is called "Kōngqì" which means "the Qì in space."

Kōngdòng 崆峒 Name of a mountain. There are three Kongdong mountains, located at Hénán (河南), Jiāngxī (江西), and Gānsù (甘肅) provinces.

Kǒngzǐ (Confucius) (551–479 BCE) 孔子 A Chinese scholar, during the Spring and Autumn Period (722–484 BCE) (Chūnqiū, 春秋), whose philosophy has significantly influenced Chinese culture.

Kòuchǐ 扣齒 Biting the teeth.

Kūn 坤 One of the Eight Trigrams (Bāguà, 八卦). Corresponds to Earth.

Kūntǔ 坤土 "Kūn" (坤) represents the earth (Tǔ) in the Eight Trigrams, that is why it is called "Kūntǔ" (坤土).

Kūng (Gōng) 功 Means energy or hard work.

Kūng Fū (Gōngfū) 功夫 Literally "energy-time." Any study, learning, or practice which requires a lot of patience, energy, and time to complete. Since practicing Chinese martial arts requires a great deal of time and energy, Chinese martial arts are commonly called Gōngfū.

Kūnlún 崑崙 One of the highest mountains in the west of China including Xīnjiāng (新疆), Xīzàng (西藏), and Qīnghǎi (青海) provinces.

Lǎma 喇嘛 Tibetan priests are called Lǎmas.

Lǎodān 老聃 Nickname of Lǎozi (老子). Lǎozi was also called Lǐěr (李耳) or Bóyáng (伯陽).

Láogōng (P-8) 勞宮 "Labor Palace." Cavity name. On the Pericardium Primary Qì Channel in the center of the palm.

Lǎojūn 老君 Means Lǎozi. Lǎojūn is the name given by Daoist followers.

Lǎozi (604–531 BCE) 老子 The creator of Daoism, also called Lǐěr (李耳) or Lǎodān (老聃), by his nickname, Bóyáng (伯陽).

Lè 樂 Joy or happiness.

Léi 雷 Thunder.

Lí 離 One of the Eight Trigrams (Bāguà, 八卦). Corresponds to Fire.

Lǐ, Mào-Chīng 李茂清 Dr. Yáng, Jwìng-Mǐng's Long Fist master.

Lǐ, Shí-Zhēn (1518–1593 CE) 李時珍 A well-known Chinese physician and Qìgōng master who wrote a book about the eight Qì vessels, *Qíjīng Bāmài Kǎo* (奇經八脈考) (*The Study of Strange Meridians and Eight Vessels*) in the 16th century.

Lǐěr 李耳 Nickname of Lǎozi (老子), also called Lǎodān (老聃), or Bóyáng (伯陽).

Liàn 煉 "To refine" or "to purify" the Shén and Qì so the Original Qì (Yuánqì, 元氣) can be returned to its origin.

Liàn 練 To refine, to train, or to discipline.

Liànjǐ 煉己 "Train the self." Means self-discipline.

Liànjīng Huàqì 煉精化氣 To refine the Essence and convert it into Qì. One of the Qìgōng training processes through which you convert Essence into Qì.

Liànqì 煉氣 Liàn means "to train, to strengthen and to refine." A Daoist training process through which your Qì grows stronger and more abundant.

Liànqì Huàshén 煉氣化神 To refine the Qì to nourish the spirit. Part of the Qìgōng training process in which you learn how to lead Qì to the head to nourish the brain and Shén (神) (spirit).

Liànqì Shēnghuá 煉氣昇華 To train the Qì and sublimate. A Xǐsuǐjīng (洗髓經) training process by which the Qì is led to the Huángtíng (黃庭) or the brain.

Liànshén 煉神 To train the spirit. To refine, strengthen, and focus the Shén.

Liànshén Fǎnxū 煉神返虛 To train the spirit to return to nothingness (i.e., freedom from emotional bondage). An advanced stage of enlightenment and Buddhahood training in which the practitioner learns how to lead his spirit to separate from his physical body.

Liànshén Liǎoxìng 煉神了性 To refine the spirit and end human nature. The final stage of enlightenment training where you learn to keep your emotions neutral and try to be undisturbed by human nature.

Liáng (502–557 CE) 梁 A dynasty in Chinese history.

Liǎo 了 Implies "the end" or "the completion" of the cultivation.

Liǎowù 了悟 "The end of comprehension." Implies enlightenment.

Líng 靈 1. The spirit of being, which acts upon others. Líng only exists in highly spiritual animals such as humans and apes. It represents an emotional comprehension and understanding. When you are alive, it implies your intelligence and wisdom. When you die, it implies the spirit of the ghost. Líng also means divine or supernatural. Líng is often used together with Shén (Língshén, 靈神) to mean "supernatural spirit." It is believed that Qì is the source which nourishes the Líng and is called "Língqì" (靈氣), meaning "supernatural energy, power, or force." 2. Supernatural Shén is called "Líng." "Líng" describes someone who is sharp, clever, nimble, and able to quickly empathize with people and things. Líng can also be a supernatural psychic capability which allows you to communicate with nature or other spiritual beings. Often, Líng also means "Supernatural Inspiration" which allows you to comprehend and understand the changes or variations of nature.

Língfēng 靈風 "Spiritual Wind." Implies the flow of spiritual energy which passes through your body.

Línggǔ 靈谷 Divine Valley. Different name of the Lower Dāntián.

Língguān 靈關 Spiritual Gate. Implies "Spiritual Valley" (Shéngǔ, 神谷), between the two hemispheres of the brain, the residence of the spirit.

Língguāng 靈光 Supernatural divine light.

Línggǔi 靈鬼 Means "spiritual ghost."

Línghún 靈魂 Spiritual soul.

Língshān 靈山 "Spiritual Mountain." A Buddhist term which is equivalent to the "Spiritual Valley" (Shéngǔ, 神谷) referred to in Daoist society.

Língshén 靈神 "Supernatural spirit" or "divine."

Língtāi 靈胎 Spiritual embryo.

Língtái 靈臺 Means "Spiritual Platform or Station" and implies "Spiritual Valley" (Shéngǔ, 神谷).

Língzhī 靈芝 Ganoderma lucidum, a special herbal fungus supposed to possess supernatural powers ("Reishi" in Japan and the West). Língzhī can also mean a similar species of hard, dark brown fungus, Fomes Japonica. In Qìgōng society, sometimes Língzhī means the elixir which enables you to have a long life.

Liùgēn 六根 Six Roots. Means the eyes, ears, nose, tongue, body, and Yì (mind) which can generate emotions and desires.

Liùhé Bāfǎ 六合八法 Literally: six combinations eight methods. One of the Chinese internal martial arts; its techniques are combined from Tàijíquán (太極拳), Xíngyìquán (形意拳), and Bāguàzhǎng (八卦掌). This style of Chinese internal martial arts was reportedly created by Chén, Bó (陳博) during the Sòng Dynasty (960–1280 CE) (宋朝).

Liùmén 六門 "Six Doors." Implies the two eyes, the two ears, the nose, and mouth; the six sense organs.

Liùqì 六氣 Means "Six Qìs," including the body's Qì (air), blood, saliva, liquid, essence, and meridians (vessels). Sometimes "Liùqì" implies the six different climates including wind, heat, damp, fire, dry, and cold.

Liùqíng 六情 A special Buddhist term which means "six compassions" derived or generated from the eyes, ears, nose, tongue, body, and mind.

Liùyù 六慾 Six Desires. The six desires are the temptations generated from the six roots which are the eyes, ears, nose, tongue, body, and mind (Xīn, 心).

Liùzéi 六賊 Six Thieves. Means: eyes, ears, nose, tongue, body, and emotional mind which could disturb your feeling and increase your six desires (Liùyù, 六慾).

Lóng 龍 Dragon.

Lónghǔ Jiāogòu 龍虎交媾 The intercourse of dragon and tiger. Implies the interaction of Yīn and Yáng.

Luò 絡 The small Qì channels which branch out from the primary Qì channels and are connected to the skin and to the bone marrow.

Mǎ 馬 Horse.

Mài 脈 Means "vessel" or "Qì channel." The eight vessels involved with transporting, storing, and regulating Qì.

Mǎo 卯 One of the twelve Terrestrial Branches (Shíèr Dìzhī, 十二地支) (i.e., 5–7 a.m.).

Mencius (Mèngzǐ) (372–289 BCE) 孟子 A well-known scholar who followed the philosophy of Confucius during the Chinese Warring States Period (403–222 BCE) (Zhànguó, 戰國).

Mìhù 密戶 Also called "Bìhù" (閉戶). Means "Concealed Door" which implies the Mìngmén (Gv-4) (命門) cavity located between L2 and L3 vertebrae.

Miànbì 面壁 Face the wall.

Mìng 命 The physical body is called "Mìng," which means "life."

Míng 冥 Represents the Yīn Space (Yīnjiān, 陰間) (spiritual world) which is opposite to the Yáng Space (Yángjiān, 陽間) of the material world.

Míng Dynasty (1368–1644 CE) 明朝 A Chinese dynasty.

Mìngdì 命蒂 Life Stalk, the stalk connecting to the root of life.

Mìnggēn 命根 Life Root.

Míngxīn 冥心 Míngxīn means to keep the mind in the Yīn world. "Yīn world" (Yīnjiān, 陰間) is the spiritual world where we go after death.

Míngxīn Jiànxìng 明心見性 Understand your Xīn so you can see your human temperament.

Mìngmén (Gv-4) 命門 "Life door." An acupuncture cavity belonging to the Governing Vessel located on the lower back (between L2 and L3). Sometimes, it means the two kidneys in Qìgōng society. In Chinese martial arts, Mìngmén means the area between the shoulder blades. Mìngmén also implies the Lower Dāntián.

Míngtáng 明堂 The space between the two eyebrows, one inch inward is called "Míngtáng."

Mìzōng 密宗（秘宗） "Secret style." Tibetan Qìgōng is commonly called Mìzōng simply because it is not known by outside people.

Mù 木 Wood. One of the five basic elements (Wǔxíng, 五行) and implies liver.

Mùmǔ 木母 Means "Wood Mother" and implies "liver" (Shén).

Mǔzǐ Xiāngyī 母子相依 "Mutual Dependence of Son and Mother." "Son" represents "Shén" while "Mother" represents "Qì."

Nà 納 Means "to receive" and implies inhalation.

Nèi 內 Internal.

Nèidān 內丹 Internal Elixir. A form of Qìgōng in which Qì (the elixir) is built up in the body and spread out to the limbs.

Nèidān Qìgōng 內丹氣功 Internal Elixir Qìgōng practice.

Nèiguān 內觀 "Internal Observation." Implies pay attention to the inner body.

Nèiqì 內氣 Lower Level Qì, also called "Inner Qì" (Xiàcéngqì, 下層氣).

Nèishèn 內腎 Literally, internal Kidneys. In Chinese medicine and Qìgōng, the real Kidneys; while Wàishèn (外腎) (external Kidneys) refers to the testicles or ovaries.

Nèishì Gōngfū 內視功夫 Nèishì means "to look internally," so Nèishì Gōngfū refers to the art of looking inside yourself to read the state of your health and the condition of your Qì.

Nì Fùhūxī 逆腹呼吸 Reverse Abdominal Breathing. Also called "Fǎn Fùhūxī" (反腹呼吸).

Níwángōng 泥丸宮 Mud pill palace. The place where the Mud Pills reside. Qìgōng terminology for the brain. Mud pills imply pineal and pituitary glands.

Níng 凝 Means "to concentrate, to condense, to refine, to focus, and to strengthen."

Níngshén 凝神 To condense or focus on the spirit. In Qìgōng training, after you are able to keep your spirit in one place, you learn how to condense it into a tiny spot and make it stronger.

Nù 怒 Anger.

Péng, Zǔ 彭祖 A legendary Qìgōng practitioner during the period of emperor Yáo (堯) (2356–2255 BCE) who was said to have lived for 800 years.

Píng 平 Peace and harmony.

Píngcháng Hūxī 平常呼吸 Normal regular breathing.

Pò 魄 Vigorous life force. The Pò is considered to be the inferior or animal soul. It is the animal or sentient life which is an innate part of the body which, at death, returns to the earth with the rest of the body. When someone is in high spirits and gets vigorously involved in some activity it is said he has Pòlì (魄力), which means he has "vigorous strength or power."

Pòlì 魄力 When a person has strong, vital energy to accomplish something, it is called "Pòlì," and means "the strength of vigor."

Qì (Chì) 氣 The general definition of Qì is: universal energy, including heat, light, and electromagnetic energy. A narrower definition of Qì refers to the energy circulating in human or animal bodies. A current popular model is that the Qì circulating in the human body is bioelectric in nature.

Qì Ànmó 氣按摩 Qì massage. One of the high levels of massage techniques in which a massage doctor will use his or her Qì to remove the Qì stagnation in a patient's body. Qì massage is also called "Wàiqì Liáofǎ" (外氣療法) which means "healing with the external Qì."

Qǐhuǒ 起火 To start the fire. In Qìgōng practice, when you start to build up Qì at the Lower Dāntián (Xiàdāntián, 下丹田).

Qíjīng Bāmài 奇經八脈 Literally, "strange (odd) channels eight vessels." Usually referred to as the Eight Extraordinary Vessels or simply as the vessels. Called odd or strange because they are not well understood and some of them do not exist in pairs.

Qìpò 七魄 Means "Seven Vital Forces" which are related to the seven emotions (Qīqíng, 七情).

Qīqíng 七情 The seven emotions, which include happiness (Xǐ, 喜), anger (Nù, 怒), sorrow (Āi, 哀), joy (Lè, 樂), love (Ài, 愛), hate (Hèn, 恨), and lust (Yù, 慾).

Qīqíng Liùyù 七情六慾 The seven passions and six desires. The seven passions are happiness (Xǐ, 喜), anger (Nù, 怒), sorrow (Āi, 哀), joy (Lè, 樂), love (Ài, 愛), hate (Hèn, 恨), and desire (Yù, 慾). The six desires are the six sensory pleasures derived from the eyes, ears, nose, tongue, body, and mind.

Qìshě 氣舍 "Qì's Dwelling." Implies the Real Lower Dāntián.

Qìshì 氣勢 Shi means the way something looks or feels. Therefore, the feeling of Qì as it expresses itself. For example, the spiritual state or morale of an army is called "energy state."

Qīyuán 七元 "Seven Origins." Implies the original function of the seven orifices of eyes, nose, mouth, and ears, which are related to the five internal organs, liver, lungs, heart, spleen, and kidneys. Qīyuán also means the original Qì level of the five internal organs.

Qìxuě 氣血 Literally, "Qì blood." According to Chinese medicine, Qì and blood cannot be separated in our body and so the two words are commonly used together.

Qiān 鉛 "Lead." Lead and mercury are terms commonly used in Daoist society. Lead and mercury were used in Daoist alchemy to adjust the Yīn and Yáng of the elixir.

Qiángjiān (Gv-18) 強間 An acupuncture cavity, belonging to the Governing Vessel.

Qiào 竅 Implies the changes or variations of nature.

Qìgōng (Chì Kūng) 氣功 Gōng (功) means Gōngfū (功夫) (lit. energy-time). Therefore, Qìgōng means the study, research, and/or practices related to Qì.

Qìhǎi (Co-6) 氣海 Means Qì ocean. An acupuncture cavity belonging to the Conception Vessel (Rènmài, 任脈) which is about one to two inches under the navel.

Qín and Hàn Dynasties (255 BCE—220 CE) 秦、漢 Two dynasties in Chinese history.

Qīng Dynasty (1644–1912 CE) 清朝 A dynasty in Chinese history.

Qīngchéng 青城 A mountain located in Sìchuān Province (四川省).

Qīngxiūpài 清修派 Peaceful Cultivation Division. A branch of Daoist Qìgōng.

Qínná (Chín Ná) 擒拿 Grasp and Control. An aspect of Chinese martial arts training, Qínná specializes in controlling the enemy through "misplacing the joint" (Cuògǔ, 錯骨), "dividing the muscle" (Fēnjīn, 分筋), "sealing the breath" (Bìqì, 閉氣), and "cavity press" (Diǎnxuè, 點穴).

Qiūyuè 秋月 "The moon in the Fall." Means the full moon, which implies the shining result of forming the Spiritual Embryo.

Qūjiāng 曲江 Means "Curved Rivers," and implies "intestines" (Real Lower Dāntián).

Rèqì 熱氣 "Re" means "warmth" or "heat." Generally, Rèqì is used to represent heat Qì.

Rén 仁 Humanity, kindness or benevolence. When Dào and Dé are applied in human society, it is benevolence (Rén, 仁) and righteousness (Yì, 義).

Rén 人 Man or mankind. One of the Three Powers (Sāncái, 三才). The Three Powers are Heaven (Tiān, 天), Earth (Dì, 地), and Man (Rén, 人).

Rènmài 任脈 Conception Vessel. One of the Eight Extraordinary Vessels in Chinese medicine and Qìgōng.

Rénqì 人氣 Human Qì.

Rénshì 人事 Literally, human relations. Human events, activities and relationships.

Rénxiān 人仙 Means "human immortality."

Ruǎnquán 軟拳 Soft style. Tàijíquán is a typical soft martial style.

Rùdào 入道 "Enter the Dào." Means getting involved in Daoism study.

Rùdìng 入定 Entering the state of steadiness both mentally and physically.

Rújiā 儒家 Literally, "Confucian family." Scholars following Confucian thoughts; Confucianists.

Rùmó 入魔 "Entering the devil." Wrong feeling or mental perception can lead you into fascination, illusion, and imagination.

Ruòcún 若存 Means "as if it were existing."

Sān 三 Three.

Sānbǎo 三寶 Three treasures. Essence (Jīng) (精), energy (Qì) (氣) and spirit (Shén) (神). Also called Sānyuán (三元) (three origins).

Sānběn 三本 The Three Foundations.

Sāncái 三才 The "Three Powers": Heaven (Tiān, 天), Earth (Dì, 地), and Man (Rén, 人).

Sānchóng 三蟲 Three Worms, also called "Sānshī" (三尸) (Three Copses). These are: the worm of desire which likes treasure and precious things; the worm which likes the tastes, easily loses temper, despise those who are good and kind; and the worm that likes sex and makes one confused.

Sàngōng 散功 Literally, "energy dispersion." A state of premature degeneration of the muscles where the Qì cannot effectively energize them. It can be caused by earlier overtraining.

Sānguān 三關 Three Gates. Three obstacles in Small Circulation meditation practice. These three gates are: Wěilǘ (尾閭) (i.e., tailbone), Jiājí (夾脊) (i.e., Squeeze Spine between shoulder blades), and Yùzhěn (玉枕) (i.e., jade pillow).

Sānguān 三觀 Three observations, including: 1. Observing Emptiness—to observe the emptiness of all natural laws and events; 2. Observing Falseness—to observe the falseness of all natural laws; 3. Observing Between.

Sānhuā Jùdǐng 三花聚頂 Three flowers reach the top. One of the final goals of Qìgōng whereby the three treasures (Essence, Qì, and Shén) (精・氣・神) are led to the top of the body to nourish the brain and spirit center (Upper Dāntián) (Shàngdāntián, 上丹田).

Sānjiào 三教 Means three schools. The three schools are Buddhism, Daoism, and Confucianism.

Sānjiè 三界 Three worlds and implies the laymen matrix. These three worlds are: 1. The world of desires (for sex and food); 2. The world of colors (material world); 3. The world of no color (generated from extreme calmness through the meditation).

Sānnián Bǔrǔ 三年哺乳 Three years of nursing.

Sānqì Guīyuán 三氣歸元 The "three Qì's" (essence, Qì, and spirit) all return to their origins.

Sānshī 三尸 Three Corpses, also called "Sānchóng" (三蟲) (Three Worms). Three Corpses are the three desires which could lead you to your death. They are the temptations of money, taste (food), and sex.

Sānyuán 三元 Three origins. Also called "Sānbǎo" (三寶) (three treasures). Human Essence (Jīng, 精), energy (Qì, 氣) and spirit (Shén, 神).

Shàngcéngqì 上層氣 Means "Upper Level Qì." Also called "Wàiqì" (外氣) (External Qì).

Shàngdāntián 上丹田 Upper Dāntián. Located at The Third Eye, it is the residence of the Shén (神) (spirit). Often, Shàngdāntián means "brain."

Shàngdǎo 上島 Different name of the Upper Dāntián.

Shàng Tiānguān 上天關 Different name of the Upper Dāntián.

Shàng Tǔfǔ 上土釜 Different name of the Upper Dāntián.

Shānzhōng 膻中 The central area between the nipples. Some Qìgōng practitioners consider Shānzhōng is the location of the Middle Dāntián.

Shàolín 少林 "Young woods." Name of the Shàolín Temple, a Buddhist temple in Hénán Province (河南), famous for its martial arts.

Sèyùn 色蘊 Color concealment.

Shén 神 Spirit. The consciousness within which the mind and thought function. According to Chinese Qìgōng, the Shén resides at the Upper Dāntián (Shàngdāntián, 上丹田) (the Third Eye).

Shénbù Shǒushè 神不守舍 Means "the spirit is not kept at its residence."

Shéngǔ 神谷 Spirit valley. Formed by the two hemispheres of the brain, with the Upper Dāntián (Shàngdāntián, 上丹田) at the exit.

Shénguī 神龜 Means "Spiritual Turtle."

Shénhún 神魂 Refers to the spirit of a dying person since his spirit is between "Shén" and "Hún."

Shénlú 神廬 Means "the spiritual residence," namely the head.

Shénlú 神爐 Spiritual Furnace. Different name of the Lower Dāntián.

Shénmíng 神明 Spiritually divine or spiritually enlightened beings.

Shénníng 神寧 Means the spirit is calm and peaceful.

Shénqì Xiànghé 神氣相合 "Mutual harmonization or unification of Shén and Qì." The final stage of regulating the Shén.

Shénshì 神室 Spirit residence. An alternative name of the "heart" (Xīn, 心). Shénshì also represents the Upper Dāntián.

Shènshuǐ 腎水 "Kidney water," water (Qì) produced by essence from the Internal and External Kidneys."

Shéntāi 神胎 Spiritual embryo. It is also called "Língtāi" (靈胎).

Shéntōng 神通 Spiritual Enlightenment.

Shénxí 神息 Spirit breathing. The stage of Qìgōng training where the spirit is coordinated with the breathing.

Shénxí Xiāngyī 神息相依 "Mutual Dependence of Spirit and Breathing." A stage in Qìgōng practice.

Shénxīan 神仙 Since "Xīan" originated with the Shén, the "Xīan" is sometimes called "Shénxīan," which means "immortal spirit."

Shēnxīn Pínghéng 身心平衡 Body and heart (mind) balanced. This means a balance between the physical body and the mental body.

Shénzhì 神志 The mind generates the will, which keeps the Shén firm. The Chinese commonly use Shén (spirit) and Zhì (will) together as "Shénzhì" because they are so related.

Shénzhì Bùqīng 神志不清 Means "the spirit and the will (generated from Yì) are not clear." That is, the mind is confused and not steady.

Shēngmén 生門 "Life Door." Implies navel, since it provides the life before your birth.

Shèngtāi 聖胎 Holy embryo. Another name for the spiritual embryo (Shéntāi, 神胎).

Shīchóng 尸蟲 Means "corpse worms" and implies "three emotional worms" which are able to agitate your emotions and lead you to the path of death. These three worms are: 1. Desires at the Upper Dāntián; 2. Seven emotional attachments at the Middle Dāntián; and 3. Desires for alcohol and sex.

Shíèr Dìzhī 十二地支 The Twelve Terrestrial Branches or Horary Characters, which include: Zǐ (子) (11 p.m.–1 a.m.)—Rat, Chǒu (丑) (1–3 a.m.)—Ox, Yīn (寅) (3–5 a.m.)—Tiger, Mǎo (卯) (5–7 a.m.)—Hare, Chén (辰) (7–9 a.m.)—Dragon, Yǐ (巳) (9-11 a.m.)—Snake, Wǔ (午) (11 a.m.–1 p.m.)—Horse, Wèi (未) (1–3 p.m.)—Sheep, Shēn (申) (3–5 p.m.)—Monkey, Yǒu (酉) (5–7 p.m.)—Cock, Shù (戌) (7–9 p.m.)—Dog, and Hài (亥) (9–11 p.m.)—Boar.

Shíèrjīng 十二經 The Twelve Primary Qì Channels in Chinese medicine.

Shíèr Jīngluò 十二經絡 The Twelve Primary Qì Channels and Their Branches.

Shíèrshí 十二時 "Twelve Timings." Means Shíèr Dìzhī (十二地支) (The Twelve Terrestrial Branches) which are the traditional Chinese divisions for a day.

Shítiāngān 十天干 The Ten Celestial Stems. Chinese use The Ten Celestial Stems together with Twelve Terrestrial Branches (Shíèr Dìzhī, 十二地支) to form a cycle of sixty. From this, they distinguish the different natural cycles of the year. The Ten Celestial Stems include: Jiǎ (甲), Yǐ (乙), Bǐng (丙), Dīng (丁), Wù (戊), Jǐ (己), Gēng (庚), Xīn (辛), Rén (壬), and Guǐ (癸).

Shíyuè Huáitāi 十月懷胎 Ten months of pregnancy. A stage in Daoist Qìgōng when the spiritual embryo is nourished.

Shíyùn 識蘊 Discriminating concealment.

Shìzūn 世尊 A respectful name for Buddha (Fó, 佛) (Sakyamuni).

Shíqīzhuīxià (M-BW-25) 十七椎下 Name of an acupuncture cavity located below the 17th vertebrae.

Shǒu 守 Means "to keep and to protect."

Shǒu Juéyīn Xīnbāoluòjīng 手厥陰心包絡經 Arm Absolute Yīn Pericardium Primary Qì Channel. One of the twelve primary Qì channels.

Shǒu Shǎoyáng Sānjiāojīng 手少陽三焦經 Arm Lesser Yáng Triple Burner Primary Qì Channel. One of the twelve primary Qì channels.

Shǒu Shǎoyīn Xīnjīng 手少陰心經 Arm Lesser Yīn Heart Primary Qì Channel. One of the twelve primary Qì channels.

Shǒu Tàiyáng Xiǎochángjīng 手太陽小腸經 Arm Greater Yáng Small Intestine Primary Qì Channel. One of the twelve primary Qì channels.

Shǒu Tàiyīn Fèijīng 手太陰肺經 Arm Greater Yīn Lung Primary Qì Channel. One of the twelve primary Qì channels.

Shǒu Yángmíng Dàchángjīng 手陽明大腸經 Arm Yáng Brightness Large Intestine Primary Qì Channel. One of the twelve primary Qì channels.

Shǒushén 守神 To keep the mind at the spirit. A Qìgōng meditation training.

Shǒuyìn 手印 "Hands' stamp." Stamp here means to press against.

Shòuyùn 受蘊 Perception concealment.

Shuāngxiū 雙修 Double cultivation. A Qìgōng training method in which Qì is exchanged with a partner in order to balance the Qì in both people. It also means the dual cultivation of both the physical body and the human temperament.

Shuǐmǔ 水母 "Water Mother," which provides life for the Shén to reside and grow.

Shuǐqì 水氣 Water Qì. Qì created from Original Essence, which is able to calm your body.

Sìdà Jiēkōng 四大皆空 "Four large are empty." A stage of Buddhist training where all of the four elements (earth, water, fire, and air) are absent from the mind so that one is completely indifferent to worldly temptations.

Sǐqì 死氣 Dead Qì. The Qì remaining in a dead body. Sometimes called "ghost Qì" (Guǐqì, 鬼氣).

Sìshí 四時 Means nature's four seasons.

Sìwēiyí 四威儀 Means "four solemn living manners," which include walking, residing, sitting, and lying.

Sìxiàng 四象 Means "Four Phases" which are derived from Two Poles (Liǎngyí, 兩儀).

Sìzhèng 四正 Nature, or the universe, (i.e., heaven and earth) is called "Sìzhèng," which means four directions, east, west, south, and north.

Sòng and Yuán Dynasties (960–1367 CE) 宋、元 Two dynasties in Chinese history.

Suànmìngshī 算命師 Literally, "calculate life teacher." A fortune teller who is able to calculate your future and destiny.

Suǐqì 髓氣 Marrow Qì.

Suǐxí 髓息 Suǐ means the marrow or brain. Therefore, Suǐxí means the Qìgōng breathing technique which is able to lead the Qì to the bone marrow and brain.

Tài Chí Chuán (Tàijíquán) 太極拳 Great ultimate fist. An internal Chinese martial art.

Tàihé 太和 "Grand Harmonization." Implies the stage of extreme harmonization and peace.

Tàijí 太極 Means "grand ultimate." According to Chinese philosophy, Tàijí is an invisible force which is able to make Wújí (無極) (i.e., no extremity) derive into Yīn and Yáng poles and also vice versa.

Tàijíquán (Tài Chí Chuán) 太極拳 A Chinese internal martial style which is based on the theory of Tàijí (太極) (grand ultimate).

Táipěi 台北 The capital city of Táiwān located in the north of Táiwān.

Tàishàng 太上 Means "Grand Uppermost" and is an abbreviation of "Tàishàng Lǎojūn" (太上老君) which means "Grand Uppermost Old Gentleman." Religious title of Lǎozi (老子).

Tàishàng Lǎojūn 太上老君 Old Lord of the Ultimate. Religious title of Lǎozi (老子), used by religious Daoists.

Tàisù 太素 State of Grand Simplicity. Implies emptiness of mind.

Tāixí 胎息 Embryo breathing. A Qìgōng breathing technique which can be used to store the Qì in the Real Dāntián (Zhēn Dāntián, 真丹田).

Tàixū 太虛 Means "Grand Emptiness," which implies the great nature of the universe (Dào, 道).

Táiwān 台灣 An island to the southeast of mainland China. Formerly known as "Formosa."

Táiwān University 台灣大學 A well-known university located in Táipěi, Táiwān.

Tàizǔquán 太祖拳 A southern style of Chinese external martial arts.

Tamkang (Dànjiāng) 淡江 Name of a University in Táiwān.

Tiān 天 "Heaven" or "sky." One of the Three Powers (Sāncái, 三才). In ancient China, people believed that Heaven was the most powerful natural energy in this universe.

Tián 田 Means "Field."

Tiānchíshuǐ 天池水 "Heavenly water." Means "saliva."

Tiāngēn 天根 "Heaven's root." Different name of the Lower Dāntián.

Tiāngǔ 天谷 "Heaven Valley." The space between the two hemispheres of the brain is called "Heaven Valley."

Tiānlínggài 天靈蓋 Literally, "heaven spiritual cover." Implies the crown. It is called Bǎihuì (Gv-20) (百會) in acupuncture.

Tiānmén 天門 "Heaven Gate," and means "the Third Eye." Also called "Yìntáng" (印堂).

Tiānmù 天目 "Heaven Eye." Means the Third Eye referred to by some Western religious societies. There are several variations of this belief. The Chinese believe that prior to our evolution into humans, our race possessed an additional sense organ in our forehead. This "third eye" also provided a means of spiritual communication between one another and the natural world. As we evolved and developed means to protect ourselves from the environment, and as societies became more complex and human vices were developed, this third eye slowly closed and disappeared.

Tiānqì 天氣 Heaven Qì. It is now commonly used to mean the weather, since weather is governed by Heaven Qì.

Tiānrén Héyī 天人合一 Literally, "Heaven and man unified as one." A high level of Qìgōng practice in which a Qìgōng practitioner, through meditation, is able to communicate his Qì with the heaven's Qì.

Tiānshān 天山 Literally, "Sky Mountain." The name of a mountain located in Xīnjiāng Province (新疆), China.

Tiānshí 天時 Heavenly timing. The repeated natural cycles generated by the heavens such as seasons, months, days and hours.

Tiānxiān 天仙 "Heaven Immortality," which means the eternal nature of spirit.

Tiānxiānfó 天仙佛 Heavenly immortal Buddhahood.

Tiānyǎn 天眼 Literally, "the heaven eye." It is equivalent to the Third Eye or Yìntáng (M-NH-3) (印堂) cavity in acupuncture.

Tiáo 調 A gradual regulating process resulting in that which is regulated achieving harmony with others.

Tiáoqì 調氣 To regulate the Qì.

Tiáoshén 調神 To regulate the spirit.

Tiáoshēn 調身 To regulate the body.

Tiáoxí 調息 To regulate the breathing.

Tiáoxīn 調心 To regulate the emotional mind.

Tiěbùshān 鐵布衫 Iron shirt. Gōngfū training which toughens the body externally and internally.

Tiěshāzhǎng 鐵砂掌 Literally, "iron sand palm." A special martial arts conditioning for the palms.

Tǐxí 體息 "Body Breathing." Also called "Fūxí" (膚息), which means "skin breathing." This is a Qìgōng breathing technique which allows you to use your mind to lead the Qì to the skin surface to strengthen the Guardian Qì.

Tù 吐 Means "to utter," and implies exhalation.

Tǔ 土 Earth. One of the Five Elements (Wǔxíng, 五行).

Tǔfǔ 土府 Different name of The Middle Dāntián.

Tǔ-Nà 吐納 Qìgōng was also commonly called "Tǔ-Nà." Tǔ-Nà means to "utter and admit" which implies uttering and admitting the air through the nose (i.e., respiration).

Tuīná 推拿 Means "to push and grab." A category of Chinese massages for healing and injury treatment.

Tuōtāi Huàngǔ 脫胎換骨 To disembody and become a human immortal.

Tuóyuè 橐籥 Bellows. A tube which is used to blow up the fire in a furnace.

Wài 外 External or outside.

Wàidān 外丹 External elixir. External Qìgōng exercises in which a practitioner will build up the Qì in his limbs and then lead it into the center of the body for nourishment.

Wàidān Chì Kūng (Wàidān Qìgōng) 外丹氣功 External Elixir Qìgōng. In Wàidān Qìgōng, a practitioner will generate Qì in the limbs and then allow the Qì to flow inward to nourish the internal organs.

Wàijiā 外家 External family. Those martial schools which practice the external styles of Chinese martial arts.

Wàiqì 外氣 External Qì, also called "Upper Level Qì" (Shàngcéngqì, 上層氣).

Wàiqì Liáofǎ 外氣療法 Literally, "external Qì healing." One of the high levels of Qì massage in which a doctor will use his or her Qì to remove Qì stagnation in the patient.

Wàishèn 外腎 "External Kidneys." Chinese define the kidneys as internal kidneys and also external kidneys. Internal kidneys (Nèishèn, 內腎) are the same kidneys defined by Western medicine. However, the external kidneys means testicles or ovaries.

Wèiqì 衛氣 Protective Qì or Guardian Qì. The Qì at the surface of the body which generates a shield to protect the body from negative external influences such as colds.

Wénhuǒ 文火 Scholar fire. One of the soft types of breathing used in Chinese Qìgōng practice.

Wògù 握固 Means "to hold and firm."

Wù 悟 Comprehending the meaning of life and the truth of nature is called "Wù." (enlightenment).

Wǔ 午 Noon. One of the twelve Terrestrial Branches (Shíèr Dìzhī, 十二地支) (i.e., 11 a.m.–1 p.m.).

Wù-Jǐ 戊己 Two of The Ten Celestial Stems (Shítiāngān, 十天干). Wù-Jǐ implies the natural timings.

Wǔdāng Mountain 武當山 Located in Húběi Province (湖北省) in China.

Wújí 無極 No Extremity. This is the state of undifferentiated emptiness before a beginning.

Wújí Hūxī 無極呼吸 Wújí Breathing, also called Cavity Breathing (Xuéwèixí, 穴位息).

Wújíxí 無極息 Wújí Breathing, also called Cavity Breathing (Xuéwèixí, 穴位息).

Wǔhuǒ 武火 Martial fire. One of the hard and fast types of breathing used in Chinese Qìgōng practice. Martial breathing is commonly used in external martial arts.

Wǔqínxì 五禽戲 Five Animal Sports. A set of medical Qìgōng practice created by Jūnqiàn (君倩) during the Chinese Jìn Dynasty (265–420 CE) (晉). Name of medical Qìgōng set which imitates the movements of the tiger, deer, bear, ape, and bird. There is another saying that this Qìgōng set was created by Dr. Huátuó (華佗).

Wǔshù 武術 Literally, "martial techniques." A common name for the Chinese martial arts. Many other terms are used, including: Wǔyì (武藝) (martial arts), Wǔgōng (武功) (martial Gōngfū), Guóshù (國術) (national techniques), and Gōngfū (功夫) (energy-time). Because Wushu has been modified in mainland China over the past forty years into gymnastic martial performance, many traditional Chinese martial artist have given up this name in order to avoid confusing modern Wǔshù with traditional Wǔshù. Recently, mainland China has attempted to bring modern Wǔshù back toward its traditional training and practice.

Wǔtiáo 五調 Five regulating methods in Qìgōng practice which include: regulating the body, regulating the breathing, regulating the mind, regulating the Qì, and regulating the spirit.

Wúwéi 無為 Means "doing nothing," and implies "regulating without regulating."

Wúxīn 無心 The mind is not paying attention to something. Means "no intention."

Wǔxīn Hūxī 五心呼吸 One of the Nèidān Qìgōng (內丹氣功) practices in which a practitioner uses his mind in coordination with breathing to lead the Qì to the center of the palms, feet and head.

Wǔxíng 五行 Five Elements: Metal (Jīn, 金) (Lungs, Fall); Wood (Mù, 木) (Liver, Spring); Water (Shǔi, 水) (Kidneys, Winter); Fire (Huǒ, 火) (Heart, Summer); and Earth (Tǔ, 土) (Spleen, Four Seasons).

Wǔyá 五牙 Means the "living Qì of the Five Elements" (Wǔxíng, 五行): metal, wood, water, fire, and earth.

Wǔyùn 五蘊 "Five concealments," which implies "five internal organs: heart, lungs, liver, kidneys, and spleen." There is another interpretation of Wǔyùn. Wǔyùn includes: 1. Color concealment (Sèyùn, 色蘊); 2. Perception concealment (Shòuyùn, 受蘊); 3. Thinking concealment (Xiǎngyùn, 想蘊); 4. Acting concealment (Xíngyùn, 行蘊); 5. Discriminating concealment (Shíyùn, 識蘊). All of these concealments are able to generate desires and emotional unbalance.

Wǔyùn 五運 Means "the transportation of Five Elements" (Wǔxíng, 五行).

Wǔzéi 五賊 Five thieves. The "five emotions" which are related to the five internal organs: anger-wood (liver), happiness-fire (heart), pensiveness-earth (spleen), sadness-metal (lungs), and fear-water (kidneys).

Wùzhēn 悟真 To comprehend the truth. Implies reaching spiritual enlightenment.

Xí 息 Implies embryonic respiration.

Xǐ 喜 Joy, delight and happiness.

Xíhuǒ 熄火 Cease the fire.

Xiàcéngqì 下層氣 The bioelectricity stored at the Real Lower Dāntián is called "Xiàcéngqì" which means "Lower Level Qì" or "Nèiqì" (內氣) (Inner Qì).

Xian 仙 An immortal. A person who has attained enlightenment or Buddhahood, whose spirit can separate from and return to his physical body at will.

Xiāndào Jìngzuò 仙道靜坐 Enlightenment Meditation. Meditation to reach the Buddhahood or enlightenment.

Xiāndào Wùzhēn Jìngzuò 仙道悟真靜坐 Divine Enlightenment Meditation.

Xiānrén 仙人 Means those persons who have reached spiritual immortality (i.e., enlightenment).

Xiǎngyùn 想蘊 Thinking concealment.

Xiāntāi 仙胎 Immortal Embryo.

Xiāntiānqì 先天氣 Pre-Birth Qì or Pre-Heaven Qì. Also called Dāntián Qì (丹田氣). The Qì which is converted from Original Essence and is stored in the Lower Dāntián. Considered to be "water Qì," it is able to calm the body.

Xiāntiān Zhī Zhēn 先天之真 Pre-Heaven truth. The truthful mind before birth.

Xiào 孝 Filial Piety.

Xiǎodǐnglú 小鼎爐 Small Tripod and Furnace. Huángtíng (黃庭) is a tripod while the Real Lower Dāntián is a furnace.

Xiǎotōng 小通 Means "little smoothness" and means the smooth circulation of the Qì.

Xiǎozhōutiān 小周天 "Small Cyclic Heaven" or "Small Circulation Meditation." This is also commonly known as "Microcosmic Meditation" in Yoga or "Turning the Wheel of Natural Law" (Zhuǎnfǎlún, 轉法輪) by Buddhist society. A Nèidān Qìgōng (內丹氣功) training in which Qì is generated at the Dāntián (丹田), and then moved in a circle through the Conception and Governing Vessels (Rèn, Dūmài, 督脈).

Xiǎozhōutiān Jìngzuò 小周天靜坐 "Small Cyclic Heaven Meditation" or "Small Circulation Meditation."

Xīn 心 Means "heart." Xīn means the mind generated from emotional disturbance.

Xìn 信 Trust.

Xìng 性 Human nature or temperament.

Xíng 形 "Shape," and means physical body.

Xínggōng 行功 "To carry out the Gōng," and implies to train.

Xìngmìng Shuāngxiū 性命雙修 "Human nature life double cultivation." Originally Buddhist, though now predominantly Daoist approach to Qìgōng, emphasizing the cultivation of both spirituality (human nature) and the physical body.

Xíngyìquán (Xíngyì) 形意拳 Literally: Shape-Mind Fist. An internal style of Gōngfū in which the mind or thinking determines the shape or movement of the body. Creation of the style attributed to Marshal Yuè, Fēi (岳飛) during the Chinese Southern Sòng Dynasty (1127–1280 CE) (南宋).

Xíngyùn 行蘊 Acting concealment.

Xīnshén Bùníng 心神不寧 Means "the (emotional) mind and spirit are not peaceful." That means the mind is scattered.

Xīnxí Xiāngyī 心息相依 Heart (mind) and breathing (are) mutually dependent.

Xīnyuán Yìmǎ 心猿意馬 Literally, "heart monkey Yì horse." Xīn (heart) is used to represent the emotional mind which is acting as a monkey, unsteady and disturbing. Yì is the mind which is generated from calm and clear thinking and judgment (i.e., Wisdom Mind). The Yì is like a horse, calm and powerful.

Xīnzhāi 心齋 Means "purified Xīn" and implies a simply calm and sincere mind.

Xīnzhúxiàn 新竹縣 Birthplace of Dr. Yáng, Jwing-Ming in Táiwān.

Xiōngbù Hūxī 胸部呼吸 Chest breathing.

Xǐsuǐgōng 洗髓功 Gōngfū of marrow and brain washing Qìgōng practice.

Xǐsuǐjīng 洗髓經 "*Washing Marrow/Brain Classic,*" usually translated as "*Marrow/Brain Washing Classic.*" A Qìgōng training which specializes in leading Qì to the marrow to cleanse it or to the brain to nourish the spirit for enlightenment. It is believed that Xǐsuǐjīng training is the key to longevity and achieving spiritual enlightenment.

Xiū 修 Means "to regulate, to cultivate, to repair," or "to maintain in good condition."

Xiūqì 修氣 Cultivate the Qì. Cultivate implies to protect, maintain and refine. A Buddhist Qìgōng training.

Xū 虛 Means "emptiness" (nihility).

Xuán 玄 Means "marvellous" or "incredible" and when this word is used in Daoist documents, it means "mysterious."

Xuándé 玄德 Profound natural virtue.

Xuánguān 玄關 Tricky gates. The many key places in Qìgōng training.

Xuánpìn 玄牝 Means "the marvellous and mysterious Dào, the mother of creation of millions of objects."

Xuányuán 玄元 Means "the mysterious origin" and implies Dāntiáns (丹田).

Xuéwèi Hūxī 穴位呼吸 Cavity breathing. Means the Lower Dāntián breathing or Wújí breathing (Wújíxí, 無極息).

Xuéwèixí 穴位息 Cavity breathing. Implies Wújí breathing (Wújíxí, 無極息) or Embryonic Breathing (Tāixí, 胎息).

Xūmí 須彌 Xūmí is the Daoist term for the human spiritual being in the fullness of human virtue.

Xúndàozhě 尋道者 Meaning "Dào searcher," those who are studying the truth of the Dào.

Xùnfēng 巽風 Means "great wind."

Xūwú 虛無 Means "nothing."

Yán 言 Means "speaking" or "negotiating."

Yàn 咽 Means "to swallow the saliva."

Yǎnguānbí 眼觀鼻 Means "to use the eyes to look at the nose tip," which implies to pay attention to the breathing.

Yǎng 養 Means "to nourish, to increase, to raise," and "to cultivate."

Yáng 陽 One of the two poles (Liǎngyí, 兩儀). The other is Yīn. In Chinese philosophy, the active, positive, masculine pole is classified as Yáng. In Chinese medicine, Yáng means excessive, too sufficient, overactive, or overheated. The Yáng (or outer) organs are the Gall Bladder, Small Intestine, Large Intestine, Stomach, Bladder, and Triple Burner.

Yáng, Jwing-Mǐng 楊俊敏 Author of this book.

Yáng Style Tàijíquán 楊氏太極拳 A style of Tàijíquán created by Yáng, Lù-Chán (楊露禪) (1799–1872 CE).

Yángjiān 陽間 "Yáng World," the material world in which we live.

Yángjīng 陽精 Yáng Essence.

Yángquán 陽泉 Yáng Fountain. The Yáng center of the Real Lower Dāntián.

Yǎngshén 養神 Yáng means "to raise, nourish, and maintain." Shén means spirit. Yángshén is the main Buddhist approach to regulating the Shén.

Yángshén 陽神 When spirit (Shén, 神) is used to manifest the Qì into action, it is powerful. Therefore, though Shén itself is considered Yīn, it is called "Yángshén."

Yángqiāomài 陽蹺脈 Yáng Heel Vessel. One of the eight Qì vessels.

Yángwéimài 陽維脈 Yáng Linking Vessel. One of the Eight Extraordinary Vessels.

Yǎngyīng 養嬰 Nursing the baby.

Yànxí 晏息 Meditation or profound breathing.

Yào 藥 "Herb." Implies elixir.

Yǎomíng 杳冥 Means "Profound Abyss," which represents the Yīn spiritual world (Yīnjiān, 陰間).

Yī 一 Means "singularity."

Yì 義 Justice, righteousness.

Yì 意 Mind. (Pronounced "ee") Specifically, the mind which is generated by clear thinking and judgment, and which is able to make you calm, peaceful, and wise.

Yìjīng 易經 *Book of Changes*. A book of divination written during the Zhōu Dynasty (1122–255 BCE) (周).

Yìjīnjīng 易筋經 Literally: *Changing Muscle/Tendon Classic*, usually called the *Muscle/Tendon Changing Classic*. Credited to Dámó (達磨) around 550 CE This work discusses Wàidān Qìgōng (外丹氣功) training for strengthening the physical body.

Yīn 陰 In Chinese philosophy, the passive, negative, feminine pole. In Chinese medicine, Yīn means deficient. The Yīn (internal) organs are the Heart, Lungs, Liver, Kidneys, Spleen, and Pericardium.

Yīnjiān 陰間 "Yīn world." The spirit world after death is considered a Yīn world.

Yīnjiāo (Co-7) 陰交 Yīn junction. A junction of two vessels, Conception Vessel (Rènmài, 任脈) and Thrusting Vessel (Chōngmài, 衝脈). Yīnjiāo belongs to the Conception Vessel.

Yīnqiāomài 陰蹺脈 Yīn Heel Vessel. One of the Eight Extraordinary Vessels.

Yīnshén 陰神 "Yīn Spirit." The Yīn center of the Upper Dāntián.

Yīnshuǐ 陰水 Yīn Water. Implies that the Qì stored at the Lower Dāntián is calm and pure.

Yìntáng (M-HN-3) 印堂 Seal Hall. An acupuncture cavity belonging to miscellaneous cavities. Yìntáng is located at The Third Eye area. Also called "Tiānmén" (天門) (Heaven Gate) which implies "The Third Eye."

Yīnwéimài 陰維脈 Yīn Linking Vessel. One of the Eight Extraordinary Vessels.

Yīnyáng Xiétiáo 陰陽諧調 The harmony and balance of Yīn and Yáng.

Yìshǒu Dāntián 意守丹田 Keep your Yì on your Lower Dāntián (Xiàdāntián, 下丹田). In Qìgōng training, you keep your mind at the Lower Dāntián in order to build up Qì. When you are circulating your Qì, you always lead your Qì back to your Lower Dāntián before you stop.

Yǒngbǎo 永寶 "Forever treasure" and means the treasure that you are able to keep forever.

Yǒngquán (K-1) 湧泉 Gushing Spring. Name of an acupuncture cavity belonging to the Kidney Primary Qì Channel.

Yǒu 酉 One of the twelve Terrestrial Branches (i.e., 5–7 p.m.) (Shi Er Zhi, 十二支).

Yǒuxīn 有心 To have a heart. Means to have an intention.

Yǔ 雨 Rain.

Yù 慾 Desire or lust.

Yuán 猿 An ape.

Yuándào 元道 Original Dào.

Yuánhǎi 元海 Original Ocean.

Yuánjīng 元精 Original Essence. The fundamental, original substance inherited from your parents, it is converted into Original Qì (Yuánqì, 元氣).

Yuánqì 元氣 Original Qì. Created from the Original Essence (Yuánjīng, 元精) inherited from your parents.

Yuánshén 元神 Original Spirit. The spirit you already had when you were born.

Yùchí 玉池 Jade Pond. Implies the place underneath the tongue which is able to generate an abundance of saliva during meditation.

Yuè, Fēi 岳飛 A Chinese hero in the Southern Sòng Dynasty(1127–1280 CE) (南宋). Said to have created Bāduànjǐn (八段錦), Xíngyìquán (形意拳), and Yuè's Yīngzhǎo (岳家鷹爪).

Yùguǎn 玉館 Means "Jade Hall." An alternative name of the "heart" (Xīn, 心).

Yùhú 玉壺 Means "Jade Kettle." An alternative name of the "heart" (Xīn, 心).

Yùhuán 玉環 Jade ring.

Yùhuánxué 玉環穴 Jade ring cavity. It means the space inside the solar plexus area (Huángtíng).

Yújiā 瑜珈 Indian Yoga.

Yùmén 玉門 "Jade Gate" and means "the Third Eye."

Yún 雲 Cloud.

Yùtáng 玉堂 Means "Jade Hall" and implies "the palate of the mouth."

Yùtù 玉兔 Means "Jade Rabbit" and implies "Original Essence" (Yuánjīng, 元精).

Zāijiēpài 栽接派 Plant and Graft Division. A division of Daoist Qìgōng training.

Zen (Chán) (禪) The Japanese name of Chán.

Zhàng 丈 A Chinese unit of length which is a little bit longer than 10 feet (3m).

Zhāng, Dào-Líng 張道陵 A Daoist who combined scholarly Daoism with Buddhist philosophies and created Religious Daoism (Dàojiào, 道教) during the Chinese Eastern Hàn Dynasty (25–220 CE) (東漢).

Zhànguó 戰國 Warring States Period. A period in Chinese history (403–222 BCE).

Zhēn 真 Truth.

Zhēn Dāntián 真丹田 The Real Dāntián, which is located at the physical center of gravity.

Zhēn Xiàdāntián 真下丹田 Real Lower Dāntián, which is the main Qì reservoir or bioelectric battery in our body.

Zhēnqì 真氣 Means "Real Qì."

Zhēnrén 真人 Means "real person" or "truthful person." A Daoist aims to be truthful and is therefore called "truthful man."

Zhēnrú 真如 Means "Real Buddhahood."

Zhēnxí 真息 The real breathing or true breathing. That means the breathing has been regulated to a deep and profound level. It implies Embryonic Breathing.

Zhēnyī 真一 Means "Real One," "Real Singularity," or "Real Singleness." "One" or "singularity" implies the main energy pole of a human constructed by spiritual center and the Qì center.

Zhēnyuán 真元 Means "Real Origins" and implies the "Original Essence, Qì, and Shén" (Yuánjīng, Yuánqì, and Yuánshén, 元精、元氣、元神).

Zhèng Fùhūxī 正腹呼吸 Formal Abdominal Breathing. More commonly called Buddhist Breathing.

Zhèngqì 正氣 Righteous Qì. When a person is righteous, it is said that he has righteous Qì which evil Qì cannot overcome.

Zhǐ 止 Stop.

Zhǐguān 止觀 Literally means "to stop the observation" and implies that the observation of the Xīn's activities is stopped.

Zhǐguānfǎ 止觀法 Stop Looking Method. One of the methods used to regulate the mind.

Zhōng 忠 Loyalty.

Zhōngdāntián 中丹田 The Middle Dāntián which is believed to be located on the Shānzhōng (膻中) area which is the center between the nipples.

Zhǒngxí 踵息 Sole breathing.

Zhōu 周 Means "to be complete," "to be perfect," or "to be round."

Zhōu Dynasty (1122–255 BCE) 周朝 A dynasty in Chinese history.

Zhuǎnfǎlún 轉法輪 "Turning the Wheel of Natural Law." A Buddhist term meaning "Small Circulation.

Zhuāngzhōu 莊周 Zhuāngzi, Warring States Period (403–222 BCE). A Daoist scholar. He wrote a book called *Zhuāngzi* (莊子).

Zhuāngzi 莊子 A book written by the Daoist scholar Zhuāngzhōu (莊周) during the Chinese Warring States Period (403–222 BCE) (戰國).

Zǐ 子 Midnight. One of the twelve Terrestrial Branches (Shíèr Dìzhī, 十二地支) (i.e., 11 p.m.–1 a.m.).

Zìguān 自觀 Self-Internal-Vision. Means to observe the self-inner-mental activities.

Zìjué 自覺 Self-awareness.

Zǐshí 子時 Midnight, 11 p.m.—1 a.m.

Zìshì 自識 Self-recognition.

Zìtuō 自脫 Freedom of emotional or spiritual bondage.

Zìwù 自悟 Self-awakening.

Zìxǐng 自醒 Self-awakening.

Zǐ-Wǔ 子午 Means "midnight and noon."

Zǒuhuǒ 走火 Entering the fire path. False and unrealistic feelings can lead you to a state of emotional disturbance, and farther away from the correct practice of Qì cultivation.

Zǒuhuǒ Rùmó 走火入魔 Walk into the fire and enter into the devil. In Qìgōng training, if you have led your Qì into the wrong path it is called "walking into the fire," and if your mind has been led into a confused state, it is called "entering into the devil."

Zú Juéyīn Gānjīng 足厥陰肝經 Leg Absolute Yīn Liver Primary Qì Channel. One of the twelve primary Qì channels.

Zú Shǎoyáng Dǎnjīng 足少陽膽經 Leg Lesser Yáng Gall Bladder Primary Qì Channel. One of the twelve primary Qì channels.

Zú Shǎoyīn Shènjīng 足少陰腎經 Leg Lesser Yīn Kidney Primary Qì Channel. One of the twelve primary Qì channels.

Zú Tàiyáng Pángguāngjīng 足太陽膀胱經 Leg Greater Yáng Bladder Primary Qì Channel. One of the twelve primary Qì channels.

Zú Tàiyīn Píjīng 太陰脾經 Leg Greater Yīn Spleen Primary Qì Channel. One of the twelve primary Qì channels.

Zú Yángmíng Wèijīng 足陽明胃經 Leg Yáng Brightness Stomach Primary Qì Channel. One of the twelve primary Qì channels.

Zuòchán 坐禪 Meditation in Buddhist society is called "Zuòchán" which means "sit for Chán."

Index

abdomen 120
acupressure 10–11
acupuncture 10–11, 20, 23–24
air 118–119
alcohol 178
ancient documents 112, 155, 156, 313
Anthology of Daoist Village 236–237
Arm Absolute Yīn Pericardium Channel 38
Arm Greater Yáng Small Intestine Channel 36–38
Arm Greater Yīn Lung Channel 36–38
Arm Lesser Yáng Triple Burner Channel 36–38
Arm Lesser Yīn Heart Channel 36–38
Arm Yáng Brightness Large Intestine Channel 35–38
back to childhood breathing 124–125
Bāguàzhǎng 24–25
Bǎihuì (Gv-20) 61
Bao Pu Zi 292
Bìhù (the Closed Door) 335
Big Tripod Furnace 227–228
bio-battery 116, 140, 281, 318, 331, 335
bioelectricity 113–114, 222–223, 229–230
bladder 184
blood 45–46, 239–240
blood cells 42, 131
blood pressure 337
blood vessels 46
bone marrow 41–42, 131–132
brain 60, 170–171, 268–269
Brain Washing Enlightenment Meditation 15
brain wave patterns 144
breathing
  about 26–29, 66, 67, 132–133, 305, 316
  and Shén 30
  Dāntián 316
  embryonic 73
  five gates 74
  marrow 339
  normal 68
  normal abdominal 68, 71, 332
  reverse abdominal 69, 71, 333
  skin—marrow 73
  spiritual 77
Buddhahood 18–19, 52, 62, 149–150, 204–205, 282
Buddhism 23, 39, 40, 50, 96–97, 204–205, 232–233, 258–259
Buddhism, Tibetan 40–41
calming the mind 318
Canoderma lucidum 202
Cao Xian Gu 304
carbon dioxide 127–128
cell replacement 127–128, 130
center of self-being 146–147
Central Lǎojūn 264
Chen, Xi-Yi 265
Chōngmài 33
Chong Xu Zi 185–186
Classic of Huángtíng's External Scene 226–227
climate 9–10
clothes 327
Concealed Secret of Fong's Family 169
conception 123–125
Conception Vessel 33, 134–135, 200
Confucius 21, 247
corpse worms 178
Crushing the Nihility 340
Crushing the Nothingness 62, 188
cun 219–220
Dámó 23, 30–31, 40–41, 86
Dámó Chán 298
Dàimài 31
Dāntián 34–35, 49–50, 82, 94–95, 95–96, 116–117, 120–121, 221, 222–223, 224
Dāntián (Elixir Field) 13, 18
Dāntián Breathing 316
Dāntián, general 316
Dāntián, Lower 120–121, 122–123, 123–125, 140, 306
Dāntián, Real Lower 162, 163, 168, 304, 307, 314, 316, 330
Dāntián, Upper 121–123, 163, 314, 316, 330
dancing 13–15
Dào 107–108, 136–138, 209–210
Dào Dé Jīng (*Classic on the Virtue of the Dào*)

21, 107–108, 157, 158, 160, 173–174, 229, 241–242
Daoism 21, 39, 50, 96–97, 148–149, 176–177, 232–233
daytime 136–138
desire 178, 218, 304
Detailed Outline of Galenical 268–269
diaphragm 132–133, 133–134, 222–223
diet 327
Dūmài 31
earth's magnetic field 118–119
Eastern Medical Advices of Maintaining Health 221–224
Eight Pieces of Brocade 19–20, 177–178
Eight Trigrams (Bāguà) 9–10, 306
Eight Vessels (Ba Ma) 11–12, 31
electroencephalogram (EEG) 144–145
electromagnetic field 8–9
electromotive forces (EMF) 66, 113–114, 116, 118, 126–127
Embracing Simplicity 221–222
Embracing Singularity 192, 193–194, 194–195, 195–196, 197–198, 200, 205
embryo 59–60, 186–187, 213, 218–219
Embryonic Breathing, definition 94
Embryonic Breathing, practice 201
EMF (Electromotive Force) 66, 113–114, 116, 118, 126–127
emotion 218
emotional desires 216
emotional disturbance 210–211
emotional disturbances 328
emotional mask 173–174
emotional mind 3, 50–51
energy supply (body) 46
enlightenment 18–19, 52, 62, 149–150, 187–188, 199, 201, 319
exercise 119
extending life 177–178
External Elixir 6
External Elixir Wàidān 63
fasciae 134–136, 222–223
Fēngshuǐ 10
Fire Path 89–90
Five Animal Sports 11–12, 19–20
Five Elements 198, 244
Five Regulatings 63
food 118–119
Four Gates Breathing Circulation 92–93
Four Phases 303
geomancy 10
Girdle Vessel 134–138, 335, 336, 339
Glossary Talking of Zhu Zi 110
Golden Elixir 220–221
Governing Vessel 31, 34–35, 136, 200
Grand Circulation 342
Grand Circulation and Enlightenment Meditation 329
Grand Circulation Meditation 15
Grand Cyclic Heaven 228–229
Grand Cyclic Heaven Meditation 88–89
Guardian Qì 48
Gui Gu Zi 302
Guo Zhēnrén 282
Hai Chan Zhēnrén 213
halo 62
He Xian Gu 300
health 18–19, 146–147, 228–229, 319
Heaven Gate 159
herbal remedies 332
Holy Embryo 53–54, 59, 165, 305
hormones 56, 131–132, 200, 319, 336
Hou Zhēnrén 263
Huan Zhen 306
Huángtíng 55, 142–143, 172, 226, 227
Huìyīn 137–138, 139–140
Huìyīn (Co-1) 230, 332, 335
human 3
immortality 190
Internal Elixir 6, 236–237
Internal Elixir Nèidān 63
internal martial styles 24–25
internal vision 215
Interpretation of Embryonic Breathing Classic 169
intestines 125–126
Jīng 44–45
Jīng (essence) 43–44, 44–45
Joints Grand Circulation Meditation 92
Kan 25–26
Kan adjustment 29–30
Kǎn and Lí 6, 87–88
Kan Cang Zi 261

Kǎn-Lí 111
kidneys 314
Lang Ran Zi 214
Lǎojūn 297
Lǎozi 21
lead 42
Leading the Qì 337
Leg Absolute Yīn Liver Channel 38
Leg Greater Yáng Bladder Channel 36–38
Leg Greater Yīn Spleen Channel 36–38
Leg Lesser Yáng Gall Bladder Channel 36–38
Leg Lesser Yīn Kidney Channel 36–38
Leg Yáng Brightness Stomach Channel 35–38
Li 25–26
Li adjustment 29–30
Li Shan Lao Mu 215
Li Zhēnrén 235, 291
Ling Jian Zi 167
Língzhī 202
Lingtai 199–200
Liùhé Bāfǎ 24–25
Liùqì 303
Liu Zhēnrén 211, 299
longevity 201, 216, 319
Lu, Yan 164
Mao, Ri-Xin 286
martial society 149
massage 332
medical society 45–46
meditation
  benefits of 5
  hindrances to 327
  general 19, 21–22, 88–89, 145–146
  orientations 330
  posture 324
  psychological preparation 327
  recovery from 343
mercury 42
metabolism 182–184
Microcosmic Meditation 18
mind 27–28
Mìngmén (Gv-4) 55, 226, 335
Mr. Huan Zhen 286
Mud Pill Palace 99, 170–171, 207–208, 278
Muscle/Tendon Changing 41–42, 85–86, 87–88, 228–229
Muscle/Tendon Changing and Marrow/Brain Washing Qìgōng 331
Muscle/Tendon Changing Classic 40–41
natural spirit 4–5
Nèidān 6, 15–16, 58–59
Nèidān (Internal Elixir) 24–25, 323
Nèishì Gōngfū 215, 301
night time 135–138
Ohm's Law 127
Original Essence 172–173, 187–188, 314
Original Jīng 45
Original Qì 47, 159, 213–214, 239, 302
Original Shén 51–52
ovaries 314
Péng, Zǔ 11–12
perineum 137–138, 235–236
philosophers 3–4
physical body 46, 301
pineal gland 336
pituitary gland 336
Po 158
Post-Birth Qì 47
potential difference (EMF) 61
practice 329
practicing environment 326
pre-birth essence 119
pre-birth Qì 47
pregnancy 59, 167, 186–187, 213
primary Qì channels 31, 35–38
PurifYíngqì and Converting it into Spirit 188
Qì,
  about 5
  and breathing 67
  Center (Wújí Center) 95
  channels 11–12, 31, 58, 135–138
  definition 6–7, 8, 113
  Earth 7, 10
  external 133–134
  flow of 12, 20, 135–138, 200, 324
  function of 46, 117–118
  Heaven 7, 9–10
  Human 10
  poles 314
  research 114
  and Shén 30–31
  stagnation 66, 323

storage 17–18, 54–55, 318, 319, 335
Vessels 31
Qìgōng
about 10–11, 11–12
Buddhist 81
Daoist 41, 81, 201, 223–224
definition 116
from a scientific point of view 113
in martial arts society 13
martial 23
medical 19, 34
practice 12–13, 13–14, 14–15, 18–19, 81
religious 22–23, 34–35, 38–39, 52–53, 176–177
Qìhǎi (Co-6) 184
raising the Shén 83
Records of Recent Pondering 109–110
Refine the Essence 53–54
Refine the Essence and Convert it into Qì 340
Refine the Qì and Convert it into Spirit 340
Refine the Spirit and Return It to Nihility 340
Refining Spirit and Returning it to Nothingness 188
Regulating the Body 344
Regulating the Breathing 65, 201, 234–235, 343
Regulating the Mind 21–22, 300, 343
Regulating the Qì 81, 343
Regulating the Spirit 83
religious society 82, 87–88, 146–147, 222, 268
Rènmài 33
Required Anthology of Reaching the Dao's Entrance 290–291
scholar fire 236–237
scholar society 21–22, 148–149
science, modern Western 114–115
seasonal changes 20–21
seasons 9–10
Self Grand Circulation Meditation 91
Self Primary Qì Channel Circulation Meditation 92
self-awareness 147
semen 56–57, 57–58, 184
Seventh Bamboo Slips of the Bamboo Bookcase 223–224
sexual activity 57–58, 175, 178
Shàolín monks 23
Shén
about 28–29, 48–49, 49–50, 139–140, 331
and breathing 30, 317
and Qì 30–31
in Qìgōng 84
raising the 83
refining 60
Shēngmén (the Door of Life) 335
Sìxiàng 303
sickness 12–13, 307
Skin/Marrow Breathing Circulation 92–93
Small Circulation 18, 342
Small Circulation Meditation 15
Small Cyclic Heaven 228–229
Small Cyclic Heaven Meditation 88–89
Small Tripod Furnace 227–228
spine 345
spiritual baby 62
spiritual cultivation 100, 236–237, 251, 342
Spiritual Embryo 53–54, 59–60, 97, 201, 318, 340
spiritual enlightenment 342
spiritual freedom 147–148
Spiritual Turtle 220
Spiritual Valley 170–171, 278
stagnation 117–118, 166
stretching 344
Tàishàng 168
Tàishǐgōng 281
Tàijí 110
Tàijíquán 24–25
Taishi Family 209
terminology 157
testicle Essence 56–57
testicles 314
Thesis of Retaining the Shén and Firming the Qì 206–207
Thesis on the Origins and Symptoms of Various Diseases 290–291
thinking 119
Third Eye 61, 149–150, 159, 167, 222
Third Eyes 136–138
Three Corpses 237–238, 304
Three Powers (Sāncái) 6–7
Three Treasures 194
Thrusting Vessel 33, 34–35, 47–48, 134–138, 200
Tiānmén (Heaven Gate) 159

translation of ancient documents 156–157, 313
Transliteration of Wisdom Garden 247
two pole centers 139–140, 161, 189, 314, 315
unification of Shén and Qì 317
vegetarian diet 129–130, 300
vertebrae 345
Wàidān 6, 15–16, 58–59
Wàidān (External Elixir) 24
Wang Lu Shi Yu 55
Wang, Fang-Ping 295
Wang, Wen-Lu 180
Water Path 90
weather 9–10
Wind Path 90–91
Wisdom Mind 50–51, 64
Wu, Chong Zi 185–186
Wu, Shou-Yang 185–186
Wújí Breathing 140–142
Xǐsuǐjīng 87–88
Xǐsuǐjīng Qìgōng 56–57
Xǐsuǐ Qìgōng 56–57
Xiao Yao Zi 216
Xin 78
Xīn (emotional mind) 164, 166, 331
Xing Kong Zi 210
Xíngyìquán 24–25
Xú Shén Gōng 283
Xu, Qi-Yan 237
Xuán Hu Zhēnrén 262
Yan Ling 238
Yan Meng Zi 217
Yang 20, 98–99
Yang center 330
Yang channels 35–38
Yang Girdle Vessel 34–35
Yang Heel Vessel 31–33, 136–138
Yang Linking Vessel 31–33, 136–138
Yang Vessels 134
Yángqiāomài 31–33
Yángwéimài 31–33
Yellow Emperor 303
Yellow Yard Classic 187
Yi 78, 316
Yìjīnjīng 41–42, 86–87, 87–88, 331
Yìjīnjīng training 55–56
Yìjīng 232–233
Yìjīng (*Book of Changes*) 9–10, 107–108, 148–149
Yīn 20, 100
Yīn and Yáng 25–26
Yīn and Yáng, interaction of 140–141
Yīn center 330
Yīn channels 35–38
Yīn Heel Vessel 33, 136–138
Yīn Linking Vessel 33, 136–138
Yīn Vessels 134
Yīn-Yáng 6, 111
Yīnqiāomài 33
Yīnwéimài 33
Yu Zhēnrén 259
Yuan Huang 293
Yuan Xian Zhēnrén 260
Yuan, Tian-Gang 305
Zhang Tiānshí 302
Zhang, Guo-Lao 218
Zhang, Jing-He 169
Zhi You Zi 254
Zhuāngzi 11–12, 232–233, 255

About the Author

Yáng, Jwìng-Mǐng, PhD (楊俊敏博士)

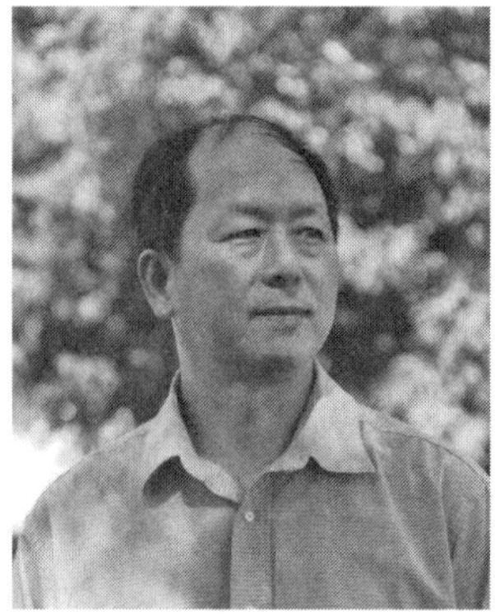

Dr. Yáng, Jwìng-Mǐng was born on August 11, 1946, in Xīnzhúxiàn (新竹縣), Táiwān (台灣), Republic of China (中華民國). He started his Wǔshù (武術) (Gōngfū or Kūng Fū, 功夫) trainingat the age of fifteen under Shàolín White Crane (Shàolín Báihè, 少林白鶴) Master Chēng, Gīn-Gsào (曾金灶). Master Chēng originally learned Tàizǔquán (太祖拳) from his grandfather when he was a child. When Master Chēng was fifteen years old, he started learning White Crane from Master Jīn, Shào-Fēng (金紹峰) and followed him for twenty-three years until Master Jīn's death.

In thirteen years of study (1961–1974) under Master Chēng, Dr. Yáng became an expert in the White Crane style of Chinese martial arts, which includes both the use of bare hands and various weapons, such as saber, staff, spear, trident, two short rods, and many others. With the same master he also studied White Crane Qìgōng (氣功), Qín Ná or Chín Ná (擒拿), Tuīná (推拿), and Diǎnxué massage (點穴按摩) and herbal treatment.

At sixteen, Dr. Yáng began the study of Yáng Style Tàijíquán (楊氏太極拳) under Master Kāo, Táo (高濤). He later continued his study of Tàijíquán under Master Lǐ, Mào-Chīng (李茂清). Master Lǐ learned his Tàijíquán from the well-known Master Hán, Chìng-Táng (韓慶堂). From this further practice, Dr. Yáng was able to master the Tàijí bare-hand sequence, pushing hands, the two-man fighting sequence, Tàijí sword, Tàijí saber, and Tàijí Qìgōng.

When Dr. Yáng was eighteen years old, he entered Tamkang College (淡江學院) in Taipei Xiàn to study physics. In college, he began the study of traditional Shàolín Long Fist (Chángquán or Cháng Chuán, 少林長拳) with Master Lǐ, Mào-Chīng at the Tamkang College Guóshù Club (淡江國術社), 1964–1968, and eventually became an assistant instructor under Master Lǐ. In 1971, he completed his MS degree in physics at the National Táiwān University (台灣大學) and then served in the Chinese Air Force of the Republic of China from 1971 to 1972. In the service, Dr. Yáng taught physics at the Junior Academy of the Chinese Air Force (空軍幼校) while also teaching Wǔshù (武術). After being honorably discharged in 1972, he returned to Tamkang College to teach physics and resumed study under Master Lǐ, Mào-Chīng. From Master Lǐ, Dr. Yáng learned Northern Style Wǔshù, which includes both bare hand and kicking techniques, and numerous weapons.In 1974, Dr. Yáng came to the United States to study mechanical engineering at Purdue University. At the request of a few students, Dr. Yáng began to teach Gōngfū, which resulted in the establishment of the Purdue University Chinese

Kūng Fū Research Club in the spring of 1975. While at Purdue, Dr. Yáng also taught college-credit courses in Tàijíquán. In May of 1978, he was awarded a PhD in mechanical engineering by Purdue.

In 1980, Dr. Yáng moved to Houston to work for Texas Instruments. While in Houston, he founded Yáng's Shàolín Kūng Fū Academy, which was eventually taken over by his disciple, Mr. Jeffery Bolt, after Dr. Yáng moved to Boston in 1982. Dr. Yáng founded Yáng's Martial Arts Academy in Boston on October 1, 1982.

In January of 1984, he gave up his engineering career to devote more time to research, writing, and teaching. In March of 1986, he purchased property in the Jamaica Plain area of Boston to be used as the headquarters of the new organization, Yáng's Martial Arts Association (YMAA). The organization expanded to become a division of Yáng's Oriental Arts Association, Inc. (YOAA).

In 2008, Dr. Yáng began the nonprofit YMAA California Retreat Center. This training facility in rural California is where selected students enroll in a five to ten-year residency to learn Chinese martial arts.

Dr. Yáng has been involved in traditional Chinese Wǔshù since 1961, studying Shàolín White Crane (Báihè), Shàolín Long Fist (Chángquán), and Tàijíquán under several different masters. He has taught for more than forty-six years: seven years in Táiwān, five years at Purdue University, two years in Houston, twenty-six years in Boston, and more than eight years at the YMAA California Retreat Center. He has taught seminars all around the world, sharing his knowledge of Chinese martial arts and Qìgōng in Argentina, Austria, Barbados, Botswana, Belgium, Bermuda, Brazil, Canada, China, Chile, England, Egypt, France, Germany, Holland, Hungary, Iceland, Ireland, Italy, Latvia, Mexico, New Zealand, Poland, Portugal, Saudi Arabia, Spain, South Africa, Switzerland, and Venezuela.

Since 1986, YMAA has become an international organization, which currently includes more than fifty schools located in Argentina, Belgium, Canada, Chile, France, Hungary, Iran, Ireland, Italy, New Zealand, Poland, Portugal, South Africa, Sweden, the United Kingdom, Venezuela, and the United States.

Many of Dr. Yáng's books and videos have been translated into many languages, including French, Italian, Spanish, Polish, Czech, Bulgarian, Russian, German, and Hungarian.

Books by Dr. Yáng, Jwìng-Mǐng

Analysis of Shàolín Chín Ná, 2nd ed. YMAA Publication Center, 1987, 2004

Ancient Chinese Weapons: A Martial Artist's Guide, 2nd ed. YMAA Publication Center, 1985, 1999

Arthritis Relief: Chinese Qìgōng for Healing & Prevention, 2nd ed. YMAA Publication Center, 1991, 2005

Back Pain Relief: Chinese Qìgōng for Healing and Prevention, 2nd ed. YMAA Publication Center, 1997, 2004

Bāguàzhǎng: Theory and Applications, 2nd ed. YMAA Publication Center, 1994, 2008

Comprehensive Applications of Shàolín Chín Ná: The Practical Defense of Chinese Seizing Arts. YMAA Publication Center, 1995

Essence of Shàolín White Crane: Martial Power and Qìgōng. YMAA Publication Center, 1996

How to Defend Yourself. YMAA Publication Center, 1992

Introduction to Ancient Chinese Weapons. Unique Publications, Inc., 1985

Meridian Qìgōng, YMAA Publication Center, 2016

Northern Shàolín Sword, 2nd ed. YMAA Publication Center, 1985, 2000

Qìgōng for Health and Martial Arts, 2nd ed. YMAA Publication Center, 1995,1998

Qìgōng Massage: Fundamental Techniques for Health and Relaxation, 2nd ed. YMAA Publication Center, 1992, 2005

Qìgōng Meditation: Embryonic Breathing. YMAA Publication Center, 2003

Qìgōng Meditation: Small Circulation, YMAA Publication Center, 2006

Qìgōng, the Secret of Youth: Dá Mó's Muscle/Tendon Changing and Marrow/Brain Washing Qìgōng, 2nd ed. YMAA Publication Center, 1989, 2000

Root of Chinese Qìgōng: Secrets of Qìgōng Training, 2nd ed. YMAA Publication Center, 1989, 1997

Shàolín Chín Ná. Unique Publications, Inc., 1980

Shàolín Long Fist Kūng Fū. Unique Publications, Inc., 1981

Simple Qìgōng Exercises for Health: The Eight Pieces of Brocade, 3rd ed. YMAA Publication Center, 1988, 1997, 2013

Tài Chí Ball Qìgōng: For Health and Martial Arts. YMAA Publication Center, 2010

Tài Chí Chuán Classical Yáng Style: The Complete Long Form and Qìgōng, 2nd ed. YMAA Publication Center, 1999, 2010

Tài Chí Chuán Martial Applications, 2nd ed. YMAA Publication Center, 1986, 1996

Tài Chí Chuán Martial Power, 3rd ed. YMAA Publication Center, 1986, 1996, 2015

Tài Chí Chuán: Classical Yáng Style, 2nd ed. YMAA Publication Center, 1999, 2010

Tài Chí Qìgōng: The Internal Foundation of Tài Chí Chuán, 2nd ed. rev. YMAA Publication Center, 1997, 1990, 2013

Tài Chí Secrets of the Ancient Masters: Selected Readings with Commentary. YMAA Publication Center, 1999

Tài Chí Secrets of the Wǔ and Lǐ Styles: Chinese Classics, Translation, Commentary. YMAA Publication Center, 2001

Tài Chí Secrets of the Wú Style: Chinese Classics, Translation, Commentary. YMAA Publication Center, 2002

Tài Chí Secrets of the Yáng Style: Chinese Classics, Translation, Commentary. YMAA Publication Center, 2001

Tài Chí Sword Classical Yáng Style: The Complete Long Form, Qìgōng, and Applications, 2nd ed. YMAA Publication Center, 1999, 2014

Tàijí Chín Ná: The Seizing Art of Tàijíquan, 2nd ed. YMAA Publication Center, 1995, 2014

Tàijíquan Theory of Dr. Yáng, Jwìng-Mǐng: The Root of Tàijíquan. YMAA Publication Center, 2003

Xíngyìquán: Theory and Applications, 2nd ed. YMAA Publication Center, 1990, 2003 Yáng Style Tài Chí Chuán. Unique Publications, Inc., 1981

Videos by Dr. Yáng, Jwìng-Mǐng

Advanced Practical Chín Ná in Depth, YMAA Publication Center, 2010

Analysis of Shàolín Chín Ná. YMAA Publication Center, 2004

Bāguàzhǎng (Eight Trigrams Palm Kūng Fū). YMAA Publication Center, 2005

Chín Ná in Depth: Courses 1–4. YMAA Publication Center, 2003

Chín Ná in Depth: Courses 5–8. YMAA Publication Center, 2003

Chín Ná in Depth: Courses 9–12. YMAA Publication Center, 2003

Five Animal Sports Qìgōng. YMAA Publication Center, 2008

Knife Defense: Traditional Techniques. YMAA Publication Center, 2011

Meridian Qìgōng. YMAA Publication Center, 2015

Neigong. YMAA Publication Center, 2015

Northern Shàolín Sword. YMAA Publication Center, 2009

Qìgōng Massage. YMAA Publication Center, 2005

Saber Fundamental Training. YMAA Publication Center, 2008

Shàolín Kūng Fū Fundamental Training. YMAA Publication Center, 2004

Shàolín Long Fist Kūng Fū: Basic Sequences. YMAA Publication Center, 2005

Shàolín Saber Basic Sequences. YMAA Publication Center, 2007

Shàolín Staff Basic Sequences. YMAA Publication Center, 2007

Shàolín White Crane Gōng Fū Basic Training: Courses 1 & 2. YMAA Publication Center, 2003

Shàolín White Crane Gōng Fū Basic Training: Courses 3 & 4. YMAA Publication Center, 2008

Shàolín White Crane Hard and Soft Qìgōng. YMAA Publication Center, 2003

Shuāi Jiāo: Kūng Fū Wrestling. YMAA Publication Center, 2010

Simple Qìgōng Exercises for Arthritis Relief. YMAA Publication Center, 2007

Simple Qìgōng Exercises for Back Pain Relief. YMAA Publication Center, 2007

Simple Qìgōng Exercises for Health: The Eight Pieces of Brocade. YMAA Publication Center, 2003

Staff Fundamental Training: Solo Drills and Matching Practice. YMAA Publication Center, 2007

Sword Fundamental Training. YMAA Publication Center, 2009

Tài Chí Ball Qìgōng: Courses 1 & 2. YMAA Publication Center, 2006

Tài Chí Ball Qìgōng: Courses 3 & 4. YMAA Publication Center, 2007

Tài Chí Chuán: Classical Yáng Style. YMAA Publication Center, 2003

Tài Chí Fighting Set: 2-Person Matching Set. YMAA Publication Center, 2006

Tài Chí Pushing Hands: Courses 1 & 2. YMAA Publication Center, 2005

Tài Chí Pushing Hands: Courses 3 & 4. YMAA Publication Center, 2006

Tài Chí Qìgōng. YMAA Publication Center, 2005

Tài Chí Sword, Classical Yáng Style. YMAA Publication Center, 2005

Tài Chí Symbol: Yīn/Yáng Sticking Hands. YMAA Publication Center, 2008

Tàijí 37 Postures Martial Applications. YMAA Publication Center, 2008

Tàijí Chín Ná in Depth. YMAA Publication Center, 2009

Tàijí Saber: Classical Yáng Style. YMAA Publication Center, 2008

Tàijí Wrestling: Advanced Takedown Techniques. YMAA Publication Center, 2008

Understanding Qìgōng, DVD 1: What is Qìgōng? The Human Qì Circulatory System. YMAA Publication Center, 2006

Understanding Qìgōng, DVD 2: Key Points of Qìgōng & Qìgōng Breathing. YMAA Publication Center, 2006

Understanding Qìgōng, DVD 3: Embryonic Breathing. YMAA Publication Center, 2007

Understanding Qìgōng, DVD 4: Four Seasons Qìgōng. YMAA Publication Center, 2007

Understanding Qìgōng, DVD 5: Small Circulation. YMAA Publication Center, 2007

Understanding Qìgōng, DVD 6: Martial Arts Qìgōng Breathing. YMAA Publication Center, 2007

Xíngyìquán: Twelve Animals Kūng Fū and Applications. YMAA Publication Center, 2008

Yáng Tài Chí for Beginners. YMAA Publication Center, 2012

YMAA 25-Year Anniversary. YMAA Publication Center, 2009

BOOKS FROM YMAA

101 REFLECTIONS ON TAI CHI CHUAN
108 INSIGHTS INTO TAI CHI CHUAN
A WOMAN'S QIGONG GUIDE
ADVANCING IN TAE KWON DO
ANALYSIS OF SHAOLIN CHIN NA 2ND ED
ANCIENT CHINESE WEAPONS
ART AND SCIENCE OF STAFF FIGHTING
THE ART AND SCIENCE OF SELF-DEFENSE
ART AND SCIENCE OF STICK FIGHTING
ART OF HOJO UNDO
ARTHRITIS RELIEF, 3D ED.
BACK PAIN RELIEF, 2ND ED.
BAGUAZHANG, 2ND ED.
BRAIN FITNESS
CHIN NA IN GROUND FIGHTING
CHINESE FAST WRESTLING
CHINESE FITNESS
CHINESE TUI NA MASSAGE
COMPLETE MARTIAL ARTIST
COMPREHENSIVE APPLICATIONS OF SHAOLIN CHIN NA
CONFLICT COMMUNICATION
DAO DE JING: A QIGONG INTERPRETATION
DAO IN ACTION
DEFENSIVE TACTICS
DIRTY GROUND
DR. WU'S HEAD MASSAGE
ESSENCE OF SHAOLIN WHITE CRANE
EXPLORING TAI CHI
FACING VIOLENCE
FIGHT LIKE A PHYSICIST
THE FIGHTER'S BODY
FIGHTER'S FACT BOOK 1&2
FIGHTING ARTS
FIGHTING THE PAIN RESISTANT ATTACKER
FIRST DEFENSE
FORCE DECISIONS: A CITIZENS GUIDE
INSIDE TAI CHI
JUDO ADVANTAGE
JUJI GATAME ENCYCLOPEDIA
KARATE SCIENCE
KATA AND THE TRANSMISSION OF KNOWLEDGE
KRAV MAGA COMBATIVES
KRAV MAGA FUNDAMENTAL STRATEGIES
KRAV MAGA PROFESSIONAL TACTICS
KRAV MAGA WEAPON DEFENSES
LITTLE BLACK BOOK OF VIOLENCE
LIUHEBAFA FIVE CHARACTER SECRETS
MARTIAL ARTS OF VIETNAM
MARTIAL ARTS INSTRUCTION
MARTIAL WAY AND ITS VIRTUES
MEDITATIONS ON VIOLENCE
MERIDIAN QIGONG EXERCISES
MINDFUL EXERCISE
MIND INSIDE TAI CHI
MIND INSIDE YANG STYLE TAI CHI CHUAN
NATURAL HEALING WITH QIGONG
NORTHERN SHAOLIN SWORD, 2ND ED.
OKINAWA'S COMPLETE KARATE SYSTEM: ISSHIN RYU
PRINCIPLES OF TRADITIONAL CHINESE MEDICINE
PROTECTOR ETHIC
QIGONG FOR HEALTH & MARTIAL ARTS 2ND ED.
QIGONG FOR TREATING COMMON AILMENTS
QIGONG MASSAGE
QIGONG MEDITATION: EMBRYONIC BREATHING
QIGONG GRAND CIRCULATION
QIGONG MEDITATION: SMALL CIRCULATION
QIGONG, THE SECRET OF YOUTH: DA MO'S CLASSICS
REDEMPTION
ROOT OF CHINESE QIGONG, 2ND ED.
SAMBO ENCYCLOPEDIA
SCALING FORCE
SELF-DEFENSE FOR WOMEN
SHIN GI TAI: KARATE TRAINING
SIMPLE CHINESE MEDICINE
SIMPLE QIGONG EXERCISES FOR HEALTH, 3RD ED.
SIMPLIFIED TAI CHI CHUAN, 2ND ED.
SOLO TRAINING 1&2
SPOTTING DANGER BEFORE IT SPOTS YOU
SPOTTING DANGER BEFORE IT SPOTS YOUR KIDS
SPOTTING DANGER BEFORE IT SPOTS YOUR TEENS
SUMO FOR MIXED MARTIAL ARTS
SUNRISE TAI CHI
SURVIVING ARMED ASSAULTS
TAE KWON DO: THE KOREAN MARTIAL ART
TAEKWONDO BLACK BELT POOMSAE
TAEKWONDO: A PATH TO EXCELLENCE
TAEKWONDO: ANCIENT WISDOM
TAEKWONDO: DEFENSE AGAINST WEAPONS
TAEKWONDO: SPIRIT AND PRACTICE
TAI CHI BALL QIGONG: FOR HEALTH AND MARTIAL ARTS
THE TAI CHI BOOK
TAI CHI CHIN NA, 2ND ED.
TAI CHI CHUAN CLASSICAL YANG STYLE, 2ND ED.
TAI CHI CHUAN MARTIAL POWER, 3RD ED.
TAI CHI CONCEPTS AND EXPERIMENTS
TAI CHI CONNECTIONS
TAI CHI DYNAMICS
TAI CHI FOR DEPRESSION
TAI CHI IN 10 WEEKS
TAI CHI PUSH HANDS
TAI CHI QIGONG, 3RD ED.
TAI CHI SECRETS OF THE ANCIENT MASTERS
TAI CHI SECRETS OF THE WU & LI STYLES
TAI CHI SECRETS OF THE WU STYLE
TAI CHI SECRETS OF THE YANG STYLE
TAI CHI SWORD: CLASSICAL YANG STYLE, 2ND ED.
TAI CHI SWORD FOR BEGINNERS
TAI CHI WALKING
TAIJIQUAN THEORY OF DR. YANG, JWING-MING
FIGHTING ARTS
TRADITIONAL CHINESE HEALTH SECRETS
TRADITIONAL TAEKWONDO
TRAINING FOR SUDDEN VIOLENCE
TRIANGLE HOLD ENCYCLOPEDIA
TRUE WELLNESS SERIES (MIND, HEART, GUT)
WARRIOR'S MANIFESTO
WAY OF KATA
WAY OF SANCHIN KATA
WAY TO BLACK BELT
WESTERN HERBS FOR MARTIAL ARTISTS
WILD GOOSE QIGONG
WINNING FIGHTS
XINGYIQUAN

AND MANY MORE . . .

VIDEOS FROM YMAA

ANALYSIS OF SHAOLIN CHIN NA
BAGUA FOR BEGINNERS 1 & 2
BAGUAZHANG: EMEI BAGUAZHANG
BEGINNER QIGONG FOR WOMEN 1 & 2
BEGINNER TAI CHI FOR HEALTH
CHEN TAI CHI CANNON FIST
CHEN TAI CHI FIRST FORM
CHEN TAI CHI FOR BEGINNERS
CHIN NA IN-DEPTH SERIES
FACING VIOLENCE: 7 THINGS A MARTIAL ARTIST MUST KNOW
FIVE ANIMAL SPORTS
FIVE ELEMENTS ENERGY BALANCE
INFIGHTING
INTRODUCTION TO QI GONG FOR BEGINNERS
JOINT LOCKS
KNIFE DEFENSE
KUNG FU BODY CONDITIONING 1 & 2
KUNG FU FOR KIDS AND TEENS SERIES
LOGIC OF VIOLENCE
MERIDIAN QIGONG
NEIGONG FOR MARTIAL ARTS
NORTHERN SHAOLIN SWORD
QI GONG 30-DAY CHALLENGE
QI GONG FOR ANXIETY
QI GONG FOR ARMS, WRISTS, AND HANDS
QIGONG FOR BEGINNERS: FRAGRANCE
QI GONG FOR BETTER BALANCE
QI GONG FOR BETTER BREATHING
QI GONG FOR CANCER
QI GONG FOR DEPRESSION
QI GONG FOR ENERGY AND VITALITY
QI GONG FOR HEADACHES
QI GONG FOR THE HEALTHY HEART
QI GONG FOR HEALTHY JOINTS
QI GONG FOR HIGH BLOOD PRESSURE
QIGONG FOR LONGEVITY
QI GONG FOR STRONG BONES
QI GONG FOR THE UPPER BACK AND NECK
QIGONG FOR WOMEN WITH DAISY LEE
QIGONG FLOW FOR STRESS & ANXIETY RELIEF
QIGONG MASSAGE
QIGONG MINDFULNESS IN MOTION
QI GONG—THE SEATED WORKOUT
QIGONG: 15 MINUTES TO HEALTH
SABER FUNDAMENTAL TRAINING
SAI TRAINING AND SEQUENCES
SANCHIN KATA: TRADITIONAL TRAINING FOR KARATE POWER
SCALING FORCE
SEARCHING FOR SUPERHUMANS
SHAOLIN KUNG FU FUNDAMENTAL TRAINING 1 & 2
SHAOLIN LONG FIST KUNG FU BEGINNER—INTERMEDIATE—ADVANCED SERIES
SHAOLIN SABER: BASIC SEQUENCES
SHAOLIN STAFF: BASIC SEQUENCES
SHAOLIN WHITE CRANE GONG FU BASIC TRAINING SERIES
SHUAI JIAO: KUNG FU WRESTLING
SIMPLE QIGONG EXERCISES FOR HEALTH
SIMPLE QIGONG EXERCISES FOR ARTHRITIS RELIEF
SIMPLE QIGONG EXERCISES FOR BACK PAIN RELIEF
SIMPLIFIED TAI CHI CHUAN: 24 & 48 POSTURES
SIMPLIFIED TAI CHI FOR BEGINNERS 48
SIX HEALING SOUNDS
SUN TAI CHI
SWORD: FUNDAMENTAL TRAINING
TAEKWONDO KORYO POOMSAE
TAI CHI BALL QIGONG SERIES
TAI CHI BALL WORKOUT FOR BEGINNERS
TAI CHI CHUAN CLASSICAL YANG STYLE
TAI CHI FIGHTING SET
TAI CHI FIT: 24 FORM
TAI CHI FIT: ALZHEIMER'S PREVENTION
TAI CHI FIT: CANCER PREVENTION
TAI CHI FIT FOR VETERANS
TAI CHI FIT: FOR WOMEN
TAI CHI FIT: FLOW
TAI CHI FIT: FUSION BAMBOO
TAI CHI FIT: FUSION FIRE
TAI CHI FIT: FUSION IRON
TAI CHI FIT: HEALTHY BACK SEATED WORKOUT
TAI CHI FIT: HEALTHY HEART WORKOUT
TAI CHI FIT IN PARADISE
TAI CHI FIT: OVER 50
TAI CHI FIT OVER 50: BALANCE EXERCISES
TAI CHI FIT OVER 50: SEATED WORKOUT
TAI CHI FIT OVER 60: GENTLE EXERCISES
TAI CHI FIT OVER 60: HEALTHY JOINTS
TAI CHI FIT OVER 60: LIVE LONGER
TAI CHI FIT: STRENGTH
TAI CHI FIT: TO GO
TAI CHI FOR WOMEN
TAI CHI FUSION: FIRE
TAI CHI QIGONG
TAI CHI PUSHING HANDS SERIES
TAI CHI SWORD: CLASSICAL YANG STYLE
TAI CHI SWORD FOR BEGINNERS
TAI CHI SYMBOL: YIN YANG STICKING HANDS
TAIJI & SHAOLIN STAFF: FUNDAMENTAL TRAINING
TAIJI CHIN NA IN-DEPTH
TAIJI 37 POSTURES MARTIAL APPLICATIONS
TAIJI SABER CLASSICAL YANG STYLE
TAIJI WRESTLING
TRAINING FOR SUDDEN VIOLENCE
UNDERSTANDING QIGONG SERIES
WATER STYLE FOR BEGINNERS
WHITE CRANE HARD & SOFT QIGONG
YANG TAI CHI FOR BEGINNERS
YOQI: MICROCOSMIC ORBIT QIGONG
YOQI QIGONG FOR A HAPPY HEART
YOQI:QIGONG FLOW FOR HAPPY MIND
YOQI:QIGONG FLOW FOR INTERNAL ALCHEMY
YOQI QIGONG FOR HAPPY SPLEEN & STOMACH
YOQI QIGONG FOR HAPPY KIDNEYS
YOQI QIGONG FLOW FOR HAPPY LUNGS
YOQI QIGONG FLOW FOR STRESS RELIEF
YOQI: QIGONG FLOW TO BOOST IMMUNE SYSTEM
YOQI SIX HEALING SOUNDS
YOQI: YIN YOGA 1
WU TAI CHI FOR BEGINNERS
WUDANG KUNG FU: FUNDAMENTAL TRAINING
WUDANG SWORD
WUDANG TAIJIQUAN
XINGYIQUAN
YANG TAI CHI FOR BEGINNERS

AND MANY MORE . . .